CHROMATIN REMODELLING

Edited by **Danuta Radzioch**

Chromatin Remodelling
http://dx.doi.org/10.5772/50815
Edited by Danuta Radzioch

Contributors

Shiaw-Yih Lin, Lili Gong, Edward Wang, Luigi Bagella, Irene Marchesi, Elena R. Garcia-Trevijano, Luis Torres, Rosa Zaragoza, Juan R. Viña, Nadezhda Vorobyeva, Danuta Radzioch, Gernot Längst, Laura Manelyte, Mario Garcia-Dominguez, Laurence Wilson, Aude Fahrer, Daniela Zahorakova

Published by InTech

Janeza Trdine 9, 51000 Rijeka, Croatia

Publishing Process Manager Viktorija Zgela
Technical Editor InTech DTP team
Cover InTech Design team

Additional hard copies can be obtained from orders@intechopen.com

Chromatin Remodelling, Edited by Danuta Radzioch
p. cm.
ISBN 978-953-51-1087-3

For EU product safety concerns:
IN TECH d.o.o., Prolaz Marije Krucifikse Kozulić 3, 51000 Rijeka, Croatia,
info@intechopen.com or visit our website at intechopen.com.

Meet the editor

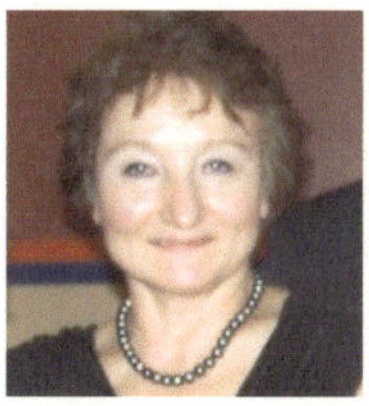

Dr. Danuta Radzioch, Ph.D., is a Full Professor at the Faculty of Medicine of McGill University, Department of Medicine and Department of Human Genetics, Montreal, Canada. She defended her Ph.D. dissertation in the field of molecular biology of cancer at the Jagiellonian University (1982), Cracow, Poland and completed post-doctoral training (1984-1987) at the National Institute of Health, National Cancer Institute (Frederick Cancer Research Facility, USA) in the field of molecular immunoregulation. Dr. Radzioch worked at the Frederick Cancer Research Facility until 1989. In 1989 she had become appointed as an Assistant Professor of Medicine at McGill University. She became an Associate Professor with Tenure in 1996 and full Professor in 2003 at the Department of Experimental Medicine and at the Department of Human Genetics. Dr. Radzioch published 145 scientific papers and 6 books and book chapters. She has co-authored five patents and two Orphan Drug designation applications: one already approved by U.S. Food and Drug Administration (FDA) and the other submitted to European Medicines Evaluation Agency (EMEA) for a new promising drug called fenretinide, a derivative of Vitamin A, for the treatment of CF patients suffering from chronic bacterial lung infections with P. aeruginosa. Her current fields of research are focused on regulation of inflammatory response in Cystic fibrosis, genetic regulation of airway hyperresponsiveness and allergic asthma, safety of novel methods of delivery of anticancer drugs and on the molecular mechanisms of gene expression regulation during the course of infection and inflammation. Her current research explores transcriptional regulation which involves chromatin remodelling and posttranscriptional processes of gene expression regulation by the RNA-binding proteins.

Contents

Preface

In the eukaryotic cells, DNA, histone proteins and associated macromolecules are tightly packaged into chromatin. The basic unit of chromatin is the nucleosome – a DNA fragment wrapped around an octamer core of histone proteins. During the past two decades the field of chromatin research has advanced at an incredible pace due to the development of novel techniques. It has become increasingly clear that, rather than simply representing packaged DNA, chromatin organization undergoes dynamic changes and plays a key role in controlling genome activities throughout life, from the onset of embryonic development to cell, tissue and organ differentiation. The term "chromatin remodelling" is widely used to describe changes in chromatin structure which is controlled by histone-modifying enzymes, chromatin remodelling complexes, non-histone DNA-binding proteins and noncoding RNAs. Many human diseases such as cancer, various genetic syndromes, autism and infectious disease have been linked to the disruption of these control processes by genetic, environmental or microbial factors. Therefore, to unravel the mechanisms by which they operate is one of the most exciting and rapid developing fields of modern biology and will contribute to new ways in treatment of these diseases.

The chapters in this book will focus on recent advances in our understanding of the mechanisms that govern the dynamic structural of chromatin, thereby providing important insights into gene regulation, DNA repair, and human diseases.

The book begins with the section "Molecular basis for chromatin structure and regulation" dealing with the molecular mechanisms underlying chromatin dynamics. In the first chapter "Chromatin Remodelers and Their Way of Action" written by Laura Manelyte and Gernot Langst, the authors give an overview of four major families of chromatin remodelers including SWI/SNF, ISWI, CHD and INO80 family. The domain compositions, components and basic functions of these remodelers have been described and the following three aspects related to the functions of chromatin remodelers have been highlighted: 1) Mechanisms of nucleosome positioning in vitro and in vivo; 2) Targeting of remodelling machines to genomic loci and their specific interaction with the modified substrate and histone variants; 3) Regulation of remodeler activity. This chapter provides an excellent knowledge in understanding the mechanisms of chromatin remodelling by ATP-dependent chromatin remodelers.

Sumoylation is a post-translational modification of proteins by attachment of the small polypeptide SUMO (small ubiquitin-like modifier), which plays an important role in various cellular processes, such as nuclear-cytosolic transport, transcriptional regulation, apoptosis, protein stability, signal transduction, cell cycle progression and differentiation. In the second chapter "SUMO Tasks in Chromatin Remodeling" written by Mario Garcia-Dominguez, the prominent function of SUMO in transcriptional regulation, in the context of chromatin structure and dynamic, has been discussed. The author describes in detail the different ways by which SUMO is involved in chromatin remodeling: 1) histone modification; 2) modulation of transcription factors activity, and 3) architecture of protein complexes associated to the chromatin, especially those associated to the heterochromatin. This chapter provides a versatile view on molecular mechanisms of chromatin remodeling regulated by sumoylation.

Chapters 3 to 5 are classified into section 2 "Chromatin remodeling in regulating gene expression". It is clear that SW/SNF chromatin remodeling complex plays an important role in the process of RNA polymerase II-mediated transcription. SWI/SNF complex not only assists transcription events by remodeling nucleosomes but also participates in early event in transcription through interaction with transcription factors and the recruitment of RNA polymerase II. Recent studies have suggested that this complex has an activity beyond transcription initiation as it can regulate the transcription elongation rate with a consequence on alternative splicing. In particular, this complex has been shown to be associated with pre-mRNP. dSWI/SNF complex contains two subcomplexes PBAP and BAP. Which of them is involved in transcription elongation? This question is answered in chapter 3 "SWI/SNF Chromatin Remodeling Complex Involved in RNA Polymerase II Elongation Process in Drosophila Melanogaster" written by authors Nadezhda E. Vorobyeva, Marina U. Mazina and Semen A. Doronin. Chapter 3 is presenting results of an original research. In this article, the authors generated two specific antibodies against OSA and BAP 170, respectively. The OSA is the specific subunit of BAP and the BAP 170 is the specific subunit of PBAP. Using chromatin immunoprecipitation assay, the authors found that both BAP and PBAP subcomplexes bind to the promoter but not to the coding region of ftz-f1 gene before transcription induction. Interestingly, in response to transcription induction, only PBAP but not BAP is found to be accumulated at the coding region of this gene. Similar results are observed when performing the same experiments using another gene (hsp70 gene). Based on these results, the authors suggest that PABP subcomplex is involved in the transcription elongation mediated by RNA polymerase II.

In chapter 4 titled "Condensins, Chromatin Remodeling and Gene Transcription", authors Laurence O.W. Wilson and Aude M. Fahrer discuss the role of condensins in the regulation of gene transcription. Condensins belong to an ancient family of protein complexes capable of manipulating chromatin structure. In eukaryotes, condensin I and condensin II are vital for the proper formation and resolution of sister chromosomes. In recent years, evidence has gradually demonstrated that condensins are much more than architects of chromatin structure; they are also important regulators of gene transcription. However, the vital role of condensins makes the study of these complexes difficult. In this chapter, the authors introduce several different methods to investigate the roles of condensins in chromatin structure change and gene regulation. A special focus is placed on two particular examples of condensin in regulating gene transcription: dosage compensation in C. elegans and thymocyte development in mice.

Id2 (inhibitor of DNA binding 2, dominant-negative helix-loop-helix protein) belongs to a family of helix-loop-helix proteins which plays a central role in the regulation of cell growth and differentiation and cancer. In chapter 5 "The Role of Id2 in the Regulation of Chromatin Structure and Gene Expression" written by Elena R. Garcia-Trevijano, Luis Torres, Rosa Zaragozá and Juan R. Viña, the authors give a broad introduction to the topic. This chapter begins with description of the structure and functions of Id2 protein followed by the molecular mechanisms underlying the role of Id2 as a proliferative factor in normal cell cycle progression, in cancer and in G0-G1 transition in response to mitogenic stimuli are discussed. Id2 is involved in regulation of gene expression as a switch to open or close chromatin structure through modulation of chromatin protein complex at target genes. Finally, the molecular regulation of Id2 activity and expression by phosphorylation and GSH depletion are also discussed.

In section 3 "Chromatin remodeling in DNA damage, development and human disease", four chapters are presented, dealing with the molecular mechanisms underlying the involvement of chromatin remodeling in controlling key physiological or pathological events such as differentiation, development, DNA damage response, tumorigenesis and microbial infection.

Polycomb group (PcG) proteins are highly conserved regulatory factors that were initially discovered in Drosophila. They constitute a global silencing system and play key roles in embryonic development and stem cell maintenance. Deregulation of PcG members contribute to defects in stem cell fates and to tumorigenesis. In mammals, PcG proteins form two main complexes: polycomb-repressive complex 1 and 2 (PRC1, PRC2). They act by modifying chromatin structure and by regulating deposition and recognition of posttranslational histone modifications.

Chapter 6 "Role of Enhancer of Zeste Homolog 2 Polycomb Protein and Its Significance in Tumor Progression and Cell Differentiation" by Irene Marchesi and Luigi Bagella give an overview of molecular biology and function of PCR2 with special emphasis on EZH2, the catalytic subunit of PRC2. The content covers PCR2-mediated silencing mechanism, PCR2 activity regulation, including expression regulation, posttranscriptional modification and recruitment to target genes, as well as the mechanisms underlying the role of EZH2 in neurogenesis, skeletal myogenesis and tumorigenesis.

Cells are inescapably and constantly exposed to a variety of environmental and endogenous agents which can cause DNA damage such as single-strand breaks, double-strand breaks, mismatches and base modifications. To maintain genome stability, cells have developed a global signaling network, known as DNA damage response (DDR) to sense and repair DNA damages. Chromatin remodeling is critical during this process, as chromatin constitutes a natural barrier to associated enzymes and regulatory factors to reach DNA. Aging is a complex process that has long been thought to be a consequence of unprogrammed deleterious events and accumulation of random gene mutation. However, in recent years, DNA damage has been shown to play a central role in premature aging and DNA damage theory of aging has been developed although there are still several unresolved controversies that require further clarification.

In chapter 7 "Chromatin Remodeling in DNA Damage Response and Human Aging" by Lili Gong, Edward Wang and Shiaw-Yih Lin, the authors summarize the current knowledge on DNA damage repair mechanisms, the role of chromatin remodeling in DDR, DDR in heterochromatin and the interplay between DNA damage, chromatin remodeling and human aging. Intracellular pathogens, through a long-standing coexistence with host cells, have evolved mechanisms that provide pathogens with the amazing capacity to adapt and survive in variable and often hostile environments encountered in their hosts. The concept of chromatin modification as a mechanism by which pathogens affect host immune responses to facilitate infection has emerged in recent years.

In chapter 8 "Chromatin Remodeling During Host-Bacterial Pathogen Interaction" written by Yong Zhong Xu, Cynthia Kanagaratham and Danuta Radzioch, the chromatin modifications in host cells induced by bacterial pathogens and their effects on host gene expression and infection are introduced. MAPK, IFN-◎ and transcription factor NF-κB signaling pathways are common targets for bacteria-induced posttranscriptional modifications. These signal pathways selectively affect histone modifications at host target genes therefore affecting the expression of target genes. In this chapter, the potential role of HDAC inhibitors to be used as therapeutic immunomodulators in treatment of infections is also discussed. Defects in epigenetic mechanisms can give rise to several neurological and behavioral phenotypes. Rett syndrome is a pervasive neurodevelopmental disorder that is primarily caused by mutations in MECP2 gene encoding methyl-CpG-binding protein 2 (MeCP2 protein). The functions of this protein are related to DNA methylation process, a key epigenetic mechanism which plays a critical role in gene silencing during chromatin remodeling. Rett syndrome is the first human disorder that shows a link between epigenetic modifications/ chromatin remodeling and neuronal dysfunction.

In chapter 9 "Rett Syndrome", the author Daniela Zahorakova gives a detailed description of the clinical features, diagnosis, as well as the molecular mechanism of Rett syndrome that arises as a consequence of MECP2 gene mutations and disordered chromatin remodeling

I would like to thank Ms. Mirna Cvijic of InTech publisher for helping me on this project, to all the authors of the chapters for their time and effort to contribute to this book. I hope readers will enjoy reading this collection of reviews and research papers, leaving with a sense of anticipation for what lies ahead in the field of chromatin remodeling.

Dr. Danuta Radzioch
Professor, McGill University
Department of Medicine and Department of Human Genetics
Montreal, Canada

Section 1

Molecular Basis for Chromatin Structure and Regulation

Chapter 1

Chromatin Remodelers and Their Way of Action

Laura Manelyte and Gernot Längst

Additional information is available at the end of the chapter

http://dx.doi.org/10.5772/55683

1. Introduction

Chromatin is the packaged form of the eukaryotic genome in the cell nucleus, presenting the substrate for all DNA dependent processes. The basic packaging unit of chromatin is the nucleosome core, a nucleoprotein structure consisting of 8 histone proteins and 147 bp of DNA. Two of each H2A and H2B, H3 and H4, form an octameric, disc like particle on which 1.65 turns of DNA is wrapped [1]. Nucleosomal cores are separated by a linker DNA, with a varying length of 7 bp to 100 bp, with distinct lengths in different organisms and tissues. Even within one cell type the linker length can vary about 40 bp between the actively transcribed and repressed genes [2].

Binding of the DNA to the histone octamer and the bending of the molecule on the protein surface present a strong barrier to sequence specific recognition of the nucleosomal DNA molecule. That's why the packaging of DNA into nucleosomes and higher order structures is generally inhibitory to all kind of DNA dependent processes. To overcome DNA sequence accessibility problems, cells have developed mechanisms to open higher order structures of chromatin and to disrupt nucleosomes allowing the binding of sequence specific regulators. In general, two major mechanisms exist which regulate chromatin accessibility: First, histones can be posttranslationally modified and recruit specific effector proteins to chromatin [3]. Second, specific chromatin remodeling enzymes displace the histone octamers from DNA or translocate them on DNA, thereby exposing or protecting underlying DNA sequences to regulatory factors that control the DNA dependent processes [4].

The presence of 53 different chromatin remodeling enzymes in the human cell suggests specialized functions of these enzymes and the associated complexes. Chromatin remodelers are DNA translocases that apply an ATP-dependent torsional strain to DNA, providing the force to reposition nucleosomes; i.e. moving the histone octamer to a different site on the DNA [4,5]. Diverse remodeling enzymes and complexes have distinct nucleosome positioning activities. In other words, the remodelers interpret the DNA sequence/structure information in different ways, establishing target site-specific nucleosome positioning patterns. The exact nucleosome positions at a given site depends on both, the type of the ATPase motor protein and the composition of the multiprotein complex where it is integrated [6]. The specialized functions of remodeling enzymes may result from their different nucleosome positioning behavior and the distinct targeting to genomic sites.

There is plenty of data available on the remodeling mechanism *in vitro*, however not much is known about the targeting and regulation of the remodelers *in vivo*. It remains unclear whether these complexes form a dynamic chromatin environment or a rather static chromatin structure with defined nucleosome positions in the cell nucleus. Many chromatin remodelers are believed to bind DNA and nucleosomes in a sequence independent manner *in vitro*, however there is mounting evidence for specific chromatin signals that are recognized by chromatin remodelers. This is best demonstrated by the recognition of histone variants, modified histone tails, the preferential binding to nucleosome free regions of DNA and binding to specific DNA and RNA structures and sequences. In addition, interacting proteins and/or accessory domains of the remodeling complexes may serve as an additional layer of signal recognition and recruitment of remodelers to the right place at the right time.

2. Remodeler families

The catalytic subunit of the remodeling enzymes consists of a conserved ATPase domain and unique flanking domains, used for a simplified separation into four distinct families (Fig. 1). The ATPase domain consists of two tandem RecA-like folds (DExx and HELICc), containing seven conserved helicase-related sequence motifs that classify the enzymes as part of the Superfamily 2 grouping of helicase-like proteins [7,8]. Chromatin remodelers are lacking the ability to separate nucleic acid strands, so they are not bona fide helicases. However, they are DNA translocases that use the energy of ATP to create a necessary force to reposition nucleosomes.

In a qualitative and quantitative study, the Snf2 family members were further subdivided into 24 distinct subfamilies based on similarities within the Snf2-specific motifs. Increased genomic complexity is paralleled by an increasing number of subfamilies and members of a given subfamily: the *S.cerevisiae* genome encoding some 6000 genes has 17 Snf2 family members belonging to 13 subfamilies, and the human genome encoding some 21000 genes has 53 Snf2 family genes from 20 subfamilies [8].

2.1. SWI/SNF family

The SWI/SNF complex was first described in *Saccharomyces cerevisiae*. In 1984 genetic screens revealed that the mutations in sucrose non-fermenting (SNF) genes caused defects in expression of the SUC2 gene, which is required for growth on sucrose and raffinose as a carbon sources [9]. Similarly, mutations in SWI genes were identified as defective for expression of the HO gene, which is required for mating type switching (the name Swi is derived from switching defective). Mutations in both SNF and SWI genes cause pleiotropic phenotypes,

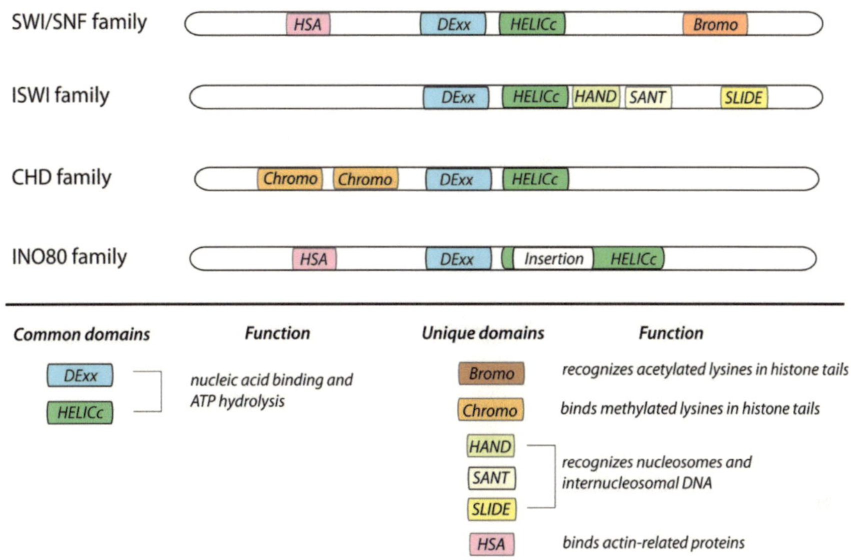

Figure 1. Classical organization of remodeler families defined by their catalytic domain. All remodeling enzymes consist of a shared ATPase domain and unique flanking domains.

suggesting a global role for Swi/Snf in gene expression. However, recent whole-genome expression studies have shown that Swi/Snf controls transcription of a small percentage of all *S. cerevisiae* genes [10]. The SWI/SNF family members are defined by the presence of an N-terminally located HSA (helicase-SANT) domain, which is known to recruit actin and actin-related proteins, and a C-terminally located bromo domain, suggested to bind to the acetylated-lysines of histones. This family of remodeling enzymes was shown to slide and to evict nucleosomes from DNA, but lacking chromatin assembly activities. Remodelers belonging to this family are large, multi-subunit complexes containing 8 or more proteins. Most eukaryotes utilize two related SWI/SNF family remodelers, built around the two related catalytic subunits Swi2/Snf2 or Sth1 in yeast, and BRM or BRG1 in humans (Table 1). Although SWI/SNF is not essential for yeast growth, a genome-wide analysis demonstrated that ~3 to 6% of yeast genes are regulated by SWI/SNF, with functions that contribute to both gene activation and repression [10,11]. On the other hand, RSC complex containing the Sth1 ATPase is essential for growth and about 10-fold more abundant than the SWI/SNF complex. RSC function is required for normal cell cycle progression [12]. Human BAF and PBAF complexes share eight identical subunits and are distinguished by the presence of only several unique subunits: BAF180, BAF200 and BRD7 for PBAF and BAF250a for BAF [13]. Variant subunits are thought to contribute to targeting, assembly and regulation of lineage-specific functions of those complexes. For example only PBAF, but not BAF, is capable of facilitating ligand-dependent transcriptional activation by nuclear receptors *in vitro* and to mediate expression of an interferon-responsive genes [14,15]. Both appear to be associated with lung cancer, as 90% of non-small cell lung carcinomas stained positively for BRG1 and BRM [16]. BRG1 possesses tumor suppressor functions, whereas BRM loss is a contributing factor and potential marker of tumorigenesis in lung, prostate and gastric cancers [17].

Complex	Catalytic subunit	Auxillary subunits	Organism
SWI/SNF	Swi2/Snf2	Swi1/Adr6, Swi3, Swp73, Snf5, Arp7, Arp9, Swp82, Snf11, Taf14, Snf6, Rtt102	*Yeast*
RSC	Sth1	Sth1, Rsc8/Swh3, Rsc6, Sfhl, Arp7, Arp9, Rsc1,2 or 4, Rsc7, Rsc30, Rsc3, Rsc5, Rtt102, Rsc14/Ldb7, Rsc10, Rsc9	
BAF	BRM or BRG1	BAF250, BAF155, BAF170,BAF60(A,B or C), SNF5, BAF57, BAF53(A or B), β-actin, BAF45(A,B,C or D)	*Human*
PBAF	BRG1	BAF180, BAF200, BRD7, BAF155, BAF45(A,B,C or D), BAF170,BAF60(A, B or C), SNF5, BAF57, BAF53(A or B), β-actin	

Table 1. Selected SWI/SNF family remodelers from yeast and human.

2.2. ISWI family

The ISWI (imitation switch) family ATPases harbour a C-terminal SANT domain adjacent to a SLIDE domain (SANT-like ISWI), which together form a nucleosome recognition module that binds to DNA and unmodified H4 tails [4]. The ISWI remodeling enzyme in *Drosophila,* is known to be present in several chromatin remodeling complexes such as NURF, CHRAC and ACF. Snf2H and Snf2L are the mammalian homologues of ISWI, which can act on their own or in the presence of one or more auxilary subunits forming different remodeling complexes with different properties. For example, Snf2H is known to interact with Tip5, RSF1 and WSTF proteins to form NoRC, RSF and WICH complexes. Specialized accessory proteins contain many chromatin binding domains, including histone fold motifs (in CHRAC), plant homeodomain (in Tip5), bromodomains (in BPTF, ACF1, Tip5) and additional DNA-binding motifs (HMGI(Y) in NURF301; AT hooks in Tip5). Many ISWI family complexes (ACF, CHRAC, NoRC) catalyze nucleosome spacing, promote chromatin assembly and confer transcriptional repression. However, NURF escapes theses general rules by disturbing nucleosome spacing and assisting ecdysone dependent transcriptional activation, showing that functional diversity is determined by the additional subunits [4]. The steroid hormone ecdysone directly modulates germline stem cells maintenance, activates transcription and proliferation in a cooperation with the NURF remodeler [18]. In *Drosophila,* loss of ISWI causes global transcriptional defects and results in dramatic alterations of the higher-order structure of chromatin, especially on the male X chromosome [19]. NoRC action correlates with specific changes in nucleosome positioning at the rDNA promoter region, causing heterochromatin formation and gene silencing [20].

Complex	Catalytic subunit	Auxillary subunits	Organism
NURF	ISWI	NURF301, NURF55/p55, NURF38	*Fly*
ACF		ACF1	
CHRAC		ACF1, CHRAC 14, CHRAC 16	
ISWI1a	ISWI1	loc3	*Yeast*
ISWI1b		loc2, loc4	
ISWI2	ISWI2	Itc1	
NURF	Snf2L	BPTF, RbAp46 or RbAP48	*Human*
ACF	Snf2H	ACF1	
CHRAC		ACF1, CHRAC17, CHRAC15	
NoRC		Tip5	
RSF		Rsf1	
WICH		Wstf	

Table 2. Selected SWI/SNF family remodelers.

2.3. CHD family

The CHD (Chromodomain-Helicase-DNA binding) family is defined by the presence of two chromodomains, arranged as a tandem, N-terminal of the ATPase domain. Additional structural motifs are used to further divide the CHD family into the subfamilies CHD1, Mi-2 and CHD7 [8,21].

Members of the CHD1 subfamily contain a C-terminal DNA-binding domain that preferentially binds to AT-rich DNA *in vitro* (members are Chd1 and Chd2 proteins in higher eukaryotes) [22,23]. Recently, the crystal structure of the DNA binding domain of Chd1, revealed a SANT-SLIDE like fold. This domain was shown to be required for the remodeling activity of Chd1 *in vitro* and *in vivo* [24].

The Mi-2 subfamily members contain a pair of PHD domains (plant homeodomain) in their N-terminal part (human Chd3 and Chd4, also known as Mi-2α and Mi-2β in *Drosophila,* respectively), implicated in nucleosome binding [25].

The CHD7 subfamily members have additional C-terminal domains, like the SANT or BRK domains (Chd5 to Chd9 proteins).

The biological properties of CHD family members are highly heterogenous. Some exist as monomers *in vivo*; others are subunits of multiprotein complexes, many of which have not yet been fully characterized [26]. The best studied is the NURD (nucleosome remodeling and deacetalase) complex, containing Chd3/Chd4, histone deacetylases (HDAC1/2) and methyl CpG-binding domain (MBD) proteins. It was shown to be involved in transcriptional repression of a specific set of genes during *C.elegans*, *D.melanogaster* and mammalian development [26]. Chd1 together with Isw1 are also termed nucleosome-spacing enzymes that are required to maintain nucleosomal organization in yeast [27]. To date, Chd3, Chd4, Chd5 and Chd7 have been implicated in human disease processes. Chd3 and Chd4 have been identified as autoantigens in patients with dermatomyositis, a connective-tissue disease characterized by inflammation of both muscles and skin. Chd3 is associated with Hodgkin's lymphoma and Chd5 is associated with neuroblastoma, a malignant neoplasm of the peripheral sympathetic nervous system frequently affecting infants and children [28]. Haploinsufficiency of Chd7 in humans results in the CHARGE syndrome. Chd7 is essential for the develompment of multipotent migratory neural crest cells, which contribute to the formation of many tissues affected in CHARGE syndrome [29].

Complex	Catalytic subunit	Auxillary subunits	Organism
Chd1	Chd1		*Fly*
Chd2	Chd2		
NuRD	Mi-2	MBD2/3, MTA, RPD3, p55, p66/68	
Chd1	Chd1		*Human*
Chd2	Chd2		
NuRD	Chd3/Chd4	MBD3, MTA1/2/3, HDAC1/2, RbAp46/48, p66α/β, DOC-1?	
	Chd5	Unknown	
	Chd7	PARP1, PBAF complex	

Table 3. Selected CHD family remodelers.

2.4. INO80 family

The specific feature of the remodeling enzymes belonging to the INO80 (inositol requiring 80) family is the split ATPase domain. This unique module retains ATPase activity, and acts as a scaffold for the association with the RuvB-like proteins, Rvb1 and Rvb2. RuvB is a bacterial ATP-dependent helicase that forms a double hexamer around Holliday junctions to promote their migration during homologous recombination [30]. Unlike remodelers of other families, the INO80 complex exhibits DNA helicase activity and binds to specialized DNA structures *in vitro*. These DNA structures resemble Holliday junctions and replication forks consistent with the function of the complex in homologous recombination and DNA replication [31,32]. Yeast INO80 was shown to control the genome-wide distribution and dynamics of the histone variant H2A.Z. INO80 and SWR1 were shown to exhibit histone-exchange activity, being capable to replace nucleosomal H2A.Z/H2B with free H2A/H2B dimers [33,34]. Both remodeling complexes can slide nucleosomes *in vitro* on a reconstituted chromatin template and evict histones from DNA [35-37]. In addition to the role of INO80 in recombination and DNA replication, it is suggested to regulate the transcription level of about 20% of the yeast genes and to participate in DNA double-strand break repair via the interaction with γ–H2AX and recruit the MRX and Mec1 complexes to the DNA damage site [33].

http://dx.doi.org/10.5772/55683

Complex	Catalytic subunit	Auxillary subunits	Organism
INO80	Ino80	Rvb1, Rvb2, Arp5, Arp8, Arp4, Act1, Taf14, Ies1, Ies2, Ies3, Ies4, Ies5, Ies6, Nhp10	*Yeast*
SWR1	Swr1	Rvb1, Rvb2, Arp6, Arp4, Act1, Yaf9, Swc4/Eaf2, Swc2, Swc3, Swc4, Swc5, Swc6, Yaf9, Bdf1, Swc7, H2AZ, H2B	

Table 4. Selected INO80 family remodelers.

3. Translocation mechanism of chromatin remodelers

Chromatin remodelers use the energy of ATP hydrolysis to assemble, reposition or evict histones from DNA. Nucleosome repositioning by remodelers can be described as a 3-step mechanism: 1) initiation step that requires the recognition and specific binding to the substrate, 2) several translocation steps with varying step-lengths and kinetics depending on the particular remodeling enzyme and on the properties of the underlying DNA sequence, 3) release step, which occurs at energetically favourable positions depending on the combination of remodeler and DNA sequence/structure at this site [6,38]. This chapter will focus on the mechanisms of the translocation step.

Proposed models for nucleosome remodeling suggest that only a minor fraction of the 358 direct and indirect histone-DNA interactions are disrupted at a given time of the reaction, as the energy of ATP hydrolysis would not be sufficient to fully disrupt the nucleoprotein structure [39,40]. One of the first mechanisms proposed, is the "twist diffusion model" describing moving of the DNA over the histone octamer surface in 1 bp intervals. Thus, a single base pair distortion is continuously propagated through the nucleosome, transiently storing one additional basepair in the realm of the nucleoprotein structure. This model is supported by nucleosomal crystal structures exhibiting such a single-basepair "twist defect" [39,41]. However, several studies could not confirm such a translocation model. Experiments using nicked or gapped DNA substrates that uncouple DNA rotation mediated processes still allowed SWI/SNF and ISWI dependent nucleosome remodeling, arguing against a sole twist-diffusion mechanism [42-44].

Alternatively, it was suggested that nucleosomes are repositioned according to the "loop recapture model", proposing a detachment of a DNA segment from the histone octamer surface at the entry site of the nucleosome. The exposed octamer surface would interact with more distant regions of the DNA molecule, resulting in the formation of a DNA loop on the histone octamer surface. This DNA loop would translocate over the octamer surface in an energy-neutral process, by releasing and rebinding adjacent sequences on the protein surface. DNA loop propagation would change the translational position of the nucleosome, according to the size of the DNA loop [45]. This model is strengthened by biochemical and recent single molecule studies. ACF remodeling complex was shown to cause the unwrapping of DNA, roughly 20 and 40 bp, from the nucleosomal border [46]. ATP dependent translocation of SWI/SNF and RSC on DNA and nucleosomal templates produces DNA loops and nucleosome remodeling by RSC was shown to produce a remodeled intermediate containing internal DNA loops [47].

Nucleosomal translocation and its step-size depend on the size of the DNA loop, a parameter that depends on the nature of the remodeling enzyme. Single molecule studies with the remodeling complex ACF suggested an initial step size of 7 bp and subsequent steps of 3-4 bp [48], whereas RSC was shown to exhibit a step size of 2 bp [49]. Within a strong nucleosomal positioning sequence both recombinant *Drosophila* Mi-2 and native RSC from yeast repositioned the nucleosome at 10 bp intervals, which are intrinsic to the positioning sequence. Furthermore, RSC-catalysed nucleosome translocation was noticeably more efficient when beyond the influence of this sequence. Interestingly, under limiting ATP conditions RSC preferred to position the nucleosome with 20 bp intervals within the positioning sequence, suggesting that native RSC preferentially translocates nucleosomes with 15 to 25 bp DNA steps [38]. Lately, it was proposed that loops do not freely diffuse about the exterior of the nucleosome but rather feed through specific restriction points by threading past fixed constrictions [47].

4. Targeting remodelers: Signals

One of the enigmas is the cellular requirement for 53 types of remodeling enzymes in humans that are capable to form hundreds to thousands of different remodeling complexes [6]. Such high numbers already suggest specialized functions for individual complexes and that remodeling enzymes mobilize nucleosomes in a specific manner. Many chromatin remodelers bind to DNA and nucleosomes in a sequence independent manner *in vitro*, albeit they exhibit complex specific features in nucleosome positioning and many of the complex subunits recognize specific chromatin features, targeting the complexes to defined genomic regions *in vivo*. The redundancy of enzymes and remodeling complexes suggest that they establish local and context specific chromatin structures and thereby regulate the DNA dependent processes. This chapter addresses the known and potential targeting mechanisms via DNA binding factors, the recognition of local chromatin features via functional RNA molecules and the impact of sequence context on the local chromatin structures (Fig. 2).

4.1. Direct chromatin targets

4.1.1. DNA and RNA sequence/structure

Mechanistical analysis of the nucleosome remodeling process revealed that binding of a remodeling complex to a mononucleosomal substrate results in a specific and ATP-dependent repositioning of the nucleosome on the DNA [50,51]. An *in vitro* study compared 7 different remodelers on different nucleosomal templates [6]. It appeared that each enzyme placed the nucleosomes at distinct positions and that even the same remodeling enzyme present in a

http://dx.doi.org/10.5772/55683

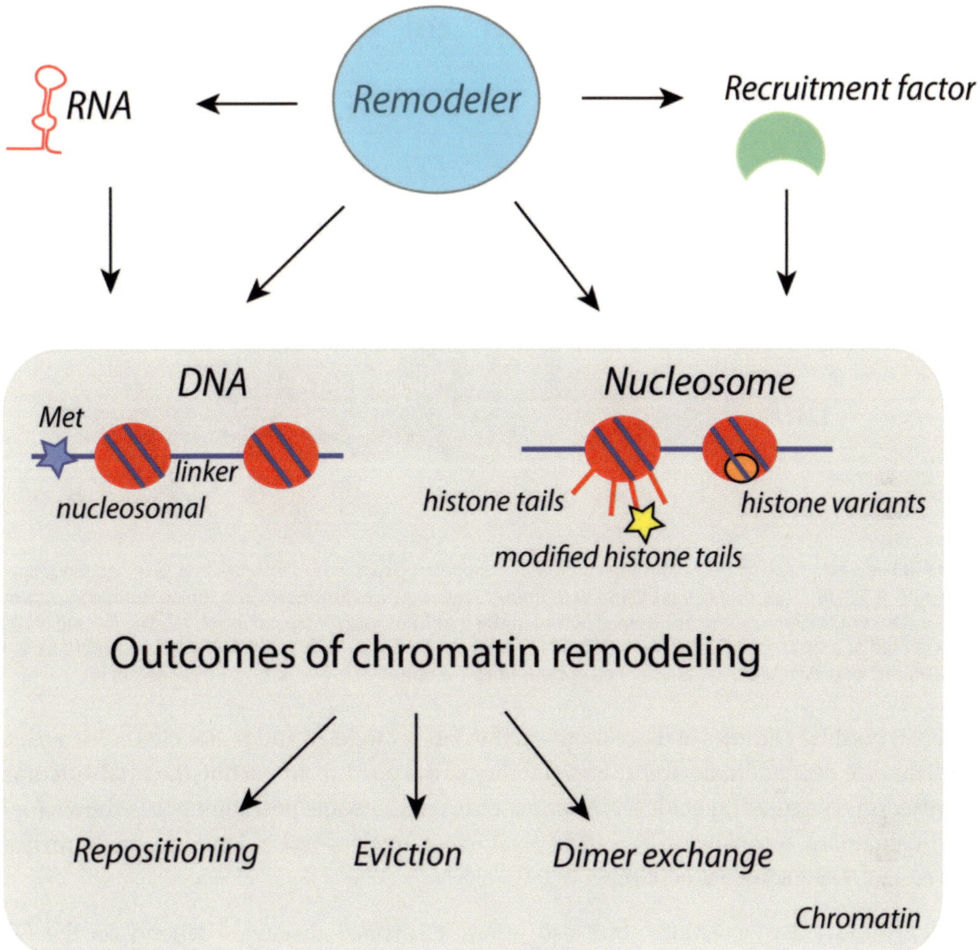

Figure 2. Targeting signals for chromatin remodeling complexes.

different complexes with various non-catalytic subunits, changed the outcome of the remodeling reaction (Fig. 3). Additionally, recent genome-wide studies compared 4 different remodeling complexes and similarly, it was observed that each remodeler exhibits a unique set of genomic targets correlating with distinct chromatin signatures [52]. Thus, these data suggest that the remodelers are capable to recognize the underlying DNA sequence/structure and accordingly establish specific chromatin structures.

The remodeling complexes contain DNA-binding motifs that are present in the catalytic or/and in accessory subunits (Fig. 1). For example, catalytic subunit Snf2H contains a SANT-SLIDE domain and in addition the WAC and AT hook motifs in the Acf1 and Tip5 proteins [4, 53-57]. These modules allow the specific recognition of DNA sequences and determine the outcome of a remodeling reaction, as it was shown by exchanging such domains between remodeling enzymes [38,58-60]. Nucleosome positioning is most probably affected by the

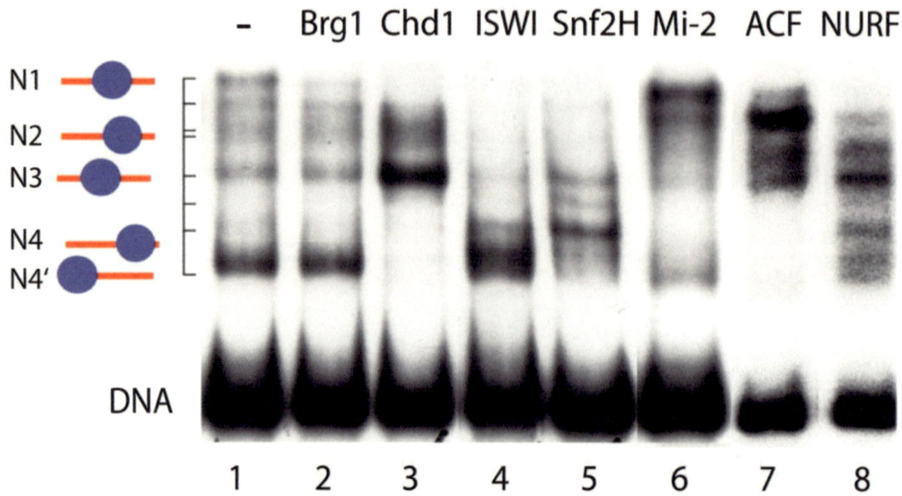

Figure 3. Bandshift assay showing that the chromatin remodelers position nucleosomes in a DNA sequence-specific manner. The 350 bp DNA, containing the hsp70 promoter sequence, was assembled into the nucleomes via salt dialysis. Five different single-nucleosomes were observed in the bandshift assay (mapped as N1, N2, N3, N4 and N4') and this was used as a substrate for seven recombinant chromatin remodelers (lane 1). Brg1, Chd1, ISWI, Snf2H, Mi-2, ACF and NURF in the presence of ATP repositioned nucleosomes in a remodeler-specific manner (lanes 2-8) [6].

different binding affinities of those motifs to the non-remodeled and remodeled substrates and the sequence dependent flexibility and stability of the particle, impacting the final outcome of the reaction. The role of specific DNA sequences in nucleosome positioning was shown for the ISWI-containing complex ACF, which positions a nucleosome relative to an intrinsically curved DNA sequence element [6].

Not only individual positions, but also internucleosomal distances depend on the DNA binding domains of the enzymes. ACF interacts with linker DNA and is capable to sense its length [61]. This structural element appears to play a key role in the positioning of nucleosomes in regular arrays, as the remodeler-induced mobility of the nucleosome is biased towards the longer flanking DNA [62]. Similarly, the Chd1 remodeler was described to sense the length of linker DNA [63].

Moreover, unusual DNA structures like quadruplexes could represent specific targeting signals. ATRX recognises G-rich repeat sequences, which are prevalent in telomeres [64]. These repeat sequences likely to form G-quadruplex (G4) structures, and ATRX preferentially binds to such a G4 structure *in vitro*. Such alternative DNA structures are believed to destabilize the genome and it is enticing to think that ATRX is responsible for stabilizing G-rich regions of the genome by remodeling G4 DNA and incorporating H3.3-containing nucleosomes [64].

Methylated CpG islands in the DNA were shown to be recognized by MBD (methyl-binding domain) domains, so it can serve as a targeting signal for particular remodelers. For example, MBD2 recruits the NuRD complex to methylated promoters [65]. The related TAM domain (MBD-like) in Tip5, the noncatalytic subunit of the NoRC complex, does not recognise methylated DNA, but binds to the pRNA (promoter RNA). The pRNA is folded into the hairpin-like structure which is bound by NoRC and participates in the recruitment NoRC to the rRNA gene promoter region [56,66-68].

4.1.2. Histone modifications

The histone code hypothesis suggests that individual covalent modifications of histones or combinations of these modifications are recognized by specific readers which determine downstream events [3]. Chromatin remodeling complexes contain histone code reader domains, allowing the targeting to specifically modified chromatin domains and thereby enabling the establishment of a remodeler dependent nucleosomal positioning landscape.

The SWI/SNF type of remodelers contain bromodomains, interacting specifically with acetylated lysines on the histone tails [69]. Acetylation of the histone H3 N-terminal tail facilitated the recruitment and nucleosome mobilization by SWI/SNF and RSC. Tetra-acetylated H3 tails, but not tetra-acetylated H4 tails, increased the affinity of RSC and SWI/SNF for nucleosomes, which is dependent on the SWI/SNF bromodomain, but is not further enhanced by additional bromodomains present in RSC [70]. By contrast, the SANT domain of the ISWI type of remodelers is known to interact with unmodified histone tails. The H4 tail has been shown to play a decisive role in ISWI remodeling, in that both, the complete removal of the H4 tail [71,72] and its site-specific acetylation suppress the remodeling action of ISWI [73]. Human Chd1 protein interacts with H3K4me2/3 via its double chromodomains, which fold into a functional unit. On the other hand, nucleosomal H3K4 methylation reduces the affinity of the NuRD complex for H3 tail binding. It was shown that the second PHD finger of Chd4 preferentially interacts with unmodified H3K4 and H3K9me3 [74,75]. Full-length NURF301 the large subunit of the ISWI containing NURF complex contains a C-terminal bromodomain and a juxtaposed PHD finger that bind H3K4me3 and H4K16Ac, respectively. However, a NURF301 isoform lacking these C-terminal domains is also detected in cells, suggesting that alternative splicing can change targeting signals and localisation of the complexes within the genome. It was concluded, that the specific recognition of the posttranslational marks by NURF is important for the regulation of primary spermatocyte differentiation in *Drosophila* [76].

4.1.3. Histone variants

Non-canonical histone variants differ from the canonical histones at the level of their primary sequence, which can range from a few amino acid changes to large domains. These variants show distinct regulatory mechanisms for their expression and deposition, resulting in the establishment of chromatin domains with specific properties. The exchange of canonical histones for the variant ones is an active process, requiring the activity of remodeling enzymes and the action of RNA and DNA polymerases that actively displace the histones from DNA [77].

Analyzing the dynamic changes in the composition of histone variants in nuclear-transferred embryos revealed that the donor cell-derived histone H3 variants H3.1, H3.2, and H3.3, as well as H2A and H2A.Z, were rapidly eliminated from the chromatin of nuclei transplanted into enucleated oocytes. In parallel to this removal, oocyte-stored histone H3 variants and H2A.X were incorporated into the transplanted nuclei, while the incorporation of H2A and H2A.Z was minimal or not detected. The incorporation of these variant histones was independent of DNA replication suggesting an active process depending on the remodeling complexes [78].

An ATRX (α-thalassemia X-linked mental retardation protein) – Daxx (death domain associated protein) complex can effectively assemble H3.3-containing nucleosomes in murine embryonic stem cells. It was shown that ATRX recruits Daxx to telomeres, and both complex subunits are required for H3.3 deposition at telomeric chromatin [79]. Chd1 in *Drosophila* embryos is required for the incorporation of the H3.3 variant into the male pronucleus, enabling the paternal genome to participate in zygotic mitosis [80]. The exchange of H2A.Z for H2A by the yeast SWR1 complex is in mechanistical terms the best described model system. H2A.Z replacement studied *in vitro* occurs in a stepwise and unidirectional fashion, exchanging one H2A.Z-H2B dimer at a time. Thereby heterotypic nucleosomes, containing one H2A.Z and one H2A molecule are established as intermediates and the homotypic H2A.Z nucleosomes as end products are generated in a second exchange step. The ATPase activity of SWR1 is specifically stimulated by H2A-containing nucleosomes without active displacement of histone H2A. Remarkably, the addition of free H2A.Z-H2B dimers results in a further stimulation of its ATPase activity and the combined eviction of nucleosomal H2A-H2B and deposition of H2A.Z-H2B. These results suggest that the combination of H2A-containing nucleosome and the presence of free H2A.Z-H2B dimer act as effector and substrate for SWR1 to govern the specificity and outcome of the replacement reaction [81]. Chromatin remodeling enzymes are also involved in the modification and dynamics of the histone variant H2A.X, which is phosphorylated upon DNA damage and repair. The WICH (WSTF-Snf2H) chromatin remodeling complex exhibits a novel kinase domain capable to phosphorylate Y142 on H2A.X. Both proteins, WSTF and Snf2H were also shown to bind to H2A.X in co-immunoprecipitation experiments [82]. In addition, it was recently shown that the activity of the Lsh remodeling enzyme is necessary for the efficient phosphorylation of H2A.X at DNA double-strand breaks and the successful repair of DNA damage [83].

4.2. Indirect chromatin targets

4.2.1. Sequence specific DNA binding proteins

The DNA-sequence dependent recruitment of remodelers is not necessarily mediated by the remodeling complex subunits themselves but can also occur via transient interactions with other sequence specific DNA binding proteins. For example, the NuRD complex is recruited to the various promoters of the target genes via interaction with several transcription factors and co-regulators such as NAB2, Ikaros, FOG1, BCL11B and several other factors described by Brehm and colleagues [26]. Genome wide expression, genetic and biochemical analysis established that TramTrack69, MEP1, and the *Drosophila* remodeling enzyme Mi-2 cooperate to control transcription levels of target genes [84]. It was also shown that Mi-2 binds to SUMO and to SUMO-ylated proteins giving rise to the hypothesis that this is a common signal for the Mi-2 recruitment. Similarly, Brg1 containing complexes are targeted via Sox10 to two key target genes in the Schwann cells [85]. Recruitment of SWI/SNF to the target genes of ERα requires the nuclear receptor co-activator protein Flightless-I, which then directly binds to both, the ER and the BAF53 subunit of the SWI/SNF complex [86]. The ISWI subfamily containing remodeling complex NoRC is directly recruited to the rRNA gene by the transcription factor TTF-I, inducing gene silencing and heterochromatin formation [56].

4.2.2. Poly(ADP-ribose) polymer

Several studies demonstrated the targeting of Chd4 to sites of DNA double strand breaks in a PARP dependent manner [87]. The enzyme was shown to bind to the poly(ADP-ribose) polymer *in vitro*. Also ALC1 binds to PAR via its macrodomain and is recruited to sites of DNA damage [88].

5. Targeting remodelers: Search mechanism

The human genome is packaged into some 30 millions of nuclesosomes that have to be organized into functional chromatin domains with specific local structures. In order to identify target sites or to detect nucleosomes that have to be repositioned, the remodeling complexes have to detect such sites in chromatin very quickly. Potential genome screening mechanisms by the remodelers are discussed in this chapter.

5.1. Release/termination model

In the seventies, JJ Hopfield introduced the kinetic proofreading mechanism for reducing errors in biological systems. He used Michaelis Menten kinetics to explain how enzymes discriminate between different substrates [89]. A similar kinetic proofreading mechanism can be used to describe the action of remodelers, where "good" substrates are characterized by a high affinity of the remodeler for the nucleosome substrate (low value of Michaelis-Menten constant K_M) and a high catalytic conversion rate k_{cat}, efficiently moving the nucleosome to the end position of the translocation reaction. Thus, the k_{cat}/K_M ratio is high as expected for an efficient catalytic process. The opposite would be true for "bad" nucleosomal substrates, i. e. having a low k_{cat}/K_M ratio. According to this model, remodeler bind to "good" substrates and move them as long, as they are converted to "bad" substrates, exhibiting a lower affinity for the remodeler. The remodelers are released from the low affinity substrates, a mechanism termed "release model" (Fig. 4). In an alternative "arrest model", all nucleosomal substrates are recognized with similar affinities, but remodeler has a slow translocation rate on a "bad" substrate. *In vitro* binding assays showed that the Chd1 and ACF complexes were bound with lower afiinity to the nucleosomes at positions that reflected the end points of the remodeling reaction, suggesting that those enzymes function according to the release model (Fig. 4) [6].

5.2. The continuous sampling mechanism

Many proteins in the nucleus, including several remodelers are highly mobile as revealed by fluorescence recovery after photobleaching (FRAP) experiments. For proteins that do not

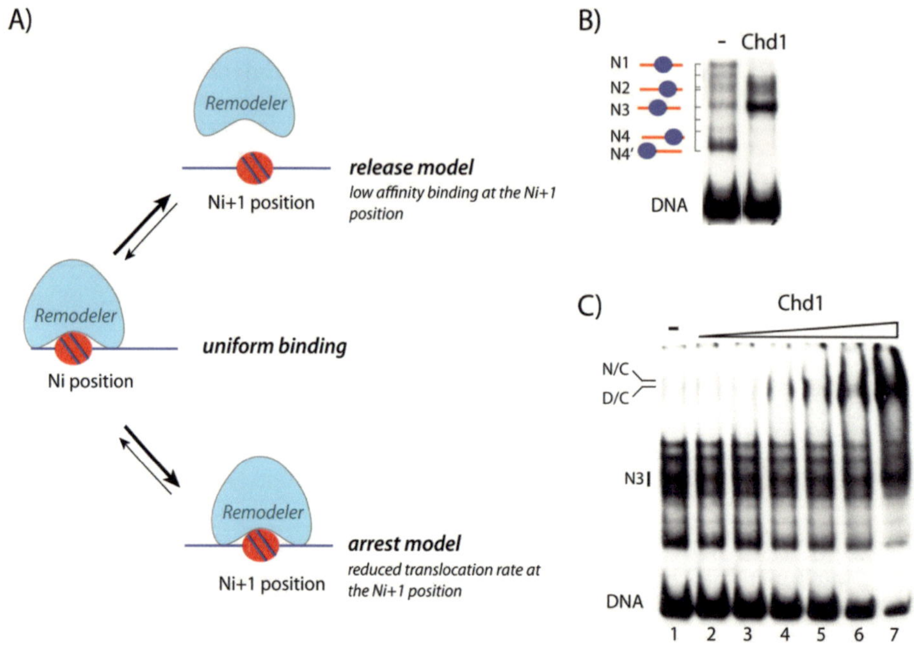

Figure 4. Model describing the affinity of remodelers to nucleosomes at different positions on the DNA. A) In the release model, the remodeling complex has a weaker binding affinity to the end-positioned nucleosome in comparison to any other nucleosome. In the arrest model, the remodeler binds all nucleosomes with similar affinity, but the translocation rate constant is much slower on a nucleosome present in the final position. B) Chd1 positions nucleosomes according to the release mechanism. Nucleosome position-dependent differences in the affinity of the remodeling complexes to the nucleosomal substrate were analyzed by bandshift assays. Remodeling reaction of Chd1 on mononucleosomal substrates reconstituted on a 350 bp DNA fragment containing hsp70 promoter region. Chd1 positions nulceosomes to the N3 and N2 positions. C) Binding reaction of Chd1 to the nucleosomes. The position of the DNA–Chd1 (D/C) and the nucleosome–Chd1 (N/C) complexes are indicated. The position of the N3 nucleosome is shown by a black box. Nucleosomes positioned at this site are bound by Chd1 with the lowest affinity. This position is at the same time the preferred endpoint of the remodeling reaction [6].

interact with any cellular structures, FRAP kinetics are a direct reflection of their translational motion properties. In contrast, proteins that bind to immobile structures such as chromatin, exhibit a slower overall mobility. The mobility of ISWI family remodelers Snf2H, Snf2L and Snf2L+13 (an ATPase inactive variant of the Snf2L) was studied in living U2OS cells. During G1/2 phase only 1-4% of the enzymes were immobilized [90], whereas the rest could be fitted by the free-diffusion model, suggesting only transient binding events. Additionally, chip-seq experiments with remodeling enzymes support the transient binding events. These experiments revealed that the localization pattern of wild-type Isw2p did not correlate with known sites of Isw2 function *in vivo*. In contrast, the catalytically inactive Isw2p–K215R was preferentially enriched at the known Isw2 target sites. This suggests, that in the absence of ATP hydrolysis the target sites remain high affinity binding sites, whereas the ATPase active enzyme does not bind to the remodeled nucleosomes [91]. These results indicate a continuous sampling mechanism (Fig. 5), by which the remodeler continuously screens the genomic nucleosomes for "good" substrates, converting them into the "bad" ones. Most of the binding

http://dx.doi.org/10.5772/55683

events seem to be unproductive, meaning that the remodeling reaction does not occur. From the experimentally determined relatively high remodeling enzyme concentrations (in the range of μM) and short chromatin bound residence times around 100 ms, average sampling times of tens of seconds to minutes were calculated for Snf2H containing remodelers to probe 99% of all genomic nucleosomes. Thus, a combination of high remodeler concentrations, short residence times in the chromatin bound state and fast 3D diffusive translocations in the intervening periods appears to be an efficient mechanism to keep nucleosomes in place [90,92].

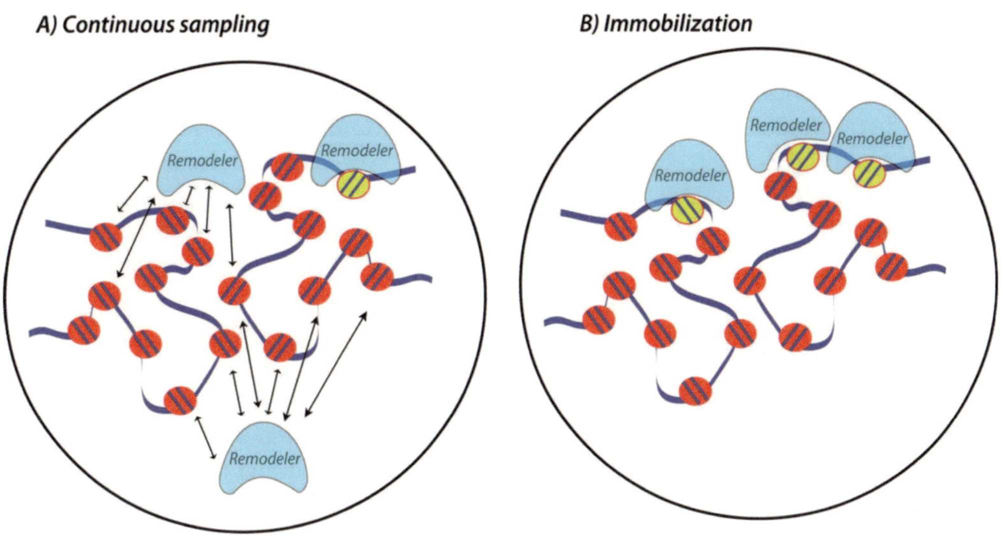

Figure 5. Genome-wide search for nucleosomal targets by remodeling enzymes. A) Continuous sampling mechanism. It is a diffusion-driven, rapid sampling of nonspecific sites with the remodeling enzymes binding only transiently to the nucleosomes. Most binding events are non-productive, as the nucleosomes are well positioned. B) Immobilization mechanism. Remodelers are recruited to the particular sites where they change nucleosomal positions. Targeting is achieved upon recognition of specific signals like histone modifications, chromatin-associated proteins, structural features of the chromatin environment or even by small molecules such as hormones.

5.3. Immobilization

In parallel with the continuous sampling mechanism, remodeling complexes are engaged by specific recruitment or immobilization at specific target sites. The respective mechanisms are described in chapter 4. For example, when cells were treated with dexamethasone, BRG1 and BRM were concentrated in a single spot in the nucleus, as revealed by immunofluorescence. The site coincided with the multimerized MMTV DNA and RNA FISH signals, showing that the enzymes are recruited to the MMTV array in a hormone-dependent manner. In this case the recruitment of the SWI/SNF machine results in the maintenance of an active chromatin structure that is compatible with transcription [93]. In other cases, like the nucleolar remodeling complex NoRC recruitment to the rRNA genes, continuous targeting results in gene repression via changes of the promoter nucleosome positioning that are incompatible with transcription initiation factor binding and further leads to the heterochromatin formation [20,94].

5.4. Nuclear dynamics of chromatin remodeling enzymes

Cells express a plethora of different remodeling complexes that act simultaneously on the cellular chromatin. The remodeler complexes diffuse freely through the nucleus, searching for "good" nucleosomes. "Good" nucleosomal substrates for the one machine may represent "bad" substrates for the other machine, suggesting that an active, free diffusing pool of remodeling complexes continuously changes the local chromatin structure. Upon specific signals individual machines are recruited to the specific sites to establish local chromatin structures correlating with a persistent activation or repression of certain DNA dependent processes. We hypothesize that the mixture of remodeling complexes in the cell, with their complex-specific remodeling patterns would continuously changes local chromatin structures, depending on complex that is currently recruited to such sites. Overall the action of the diverse remodeling complexes suggests that chromatin is continuously switching local nucleosome positions according to the levels, activity and set of remodeling complexes in a given cell [95].

6. Regulation of remodeler activity

As mentioned above, the individual accessory proteins of the remodeling complexes contain a diverse set of histones, DNA and nucleosome recognition motifs and these proteins change the outcome of nucleosome remodeling reactions. Accordingly, these proteins significantly determine the targeting to genomic regions and the qualitative outcome of a remodeling reaction. In this chapter, we want to focus on the regulation of the overall activity of remodeling enzymes by metabolites and modifications. Subunits of chromatin remodeling complexes often contain domains capable of recognizing specific posttranslational modifications on histone tails. However, significantly less is known about the functions of posttranslational modifications on remodeling complexes themselves and our understanding of its role is only beginning to emerge.

Phosphorylation. The first example of phosphoregulation of a remodeler was the mitotic phosphorylation of human SWI/SNF, which inhibits remodeling activity, with subsequent dephosphorylation by hPP2A restoring remodeling activity. It was suggested that the phosphorylated form would promote global repression of chromatin remodeling during mitosis [96]. In *Drosophila,* Mi-2 undergoes constitutive phosphorylation at N-terminus and CK2 was identified as a major kinase. Dephosphorylated Mi-2 displays increased affinity for the nucleosomal substrate, which in turn leads to an increased nucleosome-stimulated ATPase and remodeling activity. It was even postulated that it might be a common regulatory mechanism for CHD family remodelers [97]. Whether and how the phosphorylation alters the biochemical activity of INO80 is not known, but upon exposure to DNA damage, it was found that yeast INO80 complex is phosphorylated on the Les4 subunit in a Mec1/Tel1-dependent manner [98].

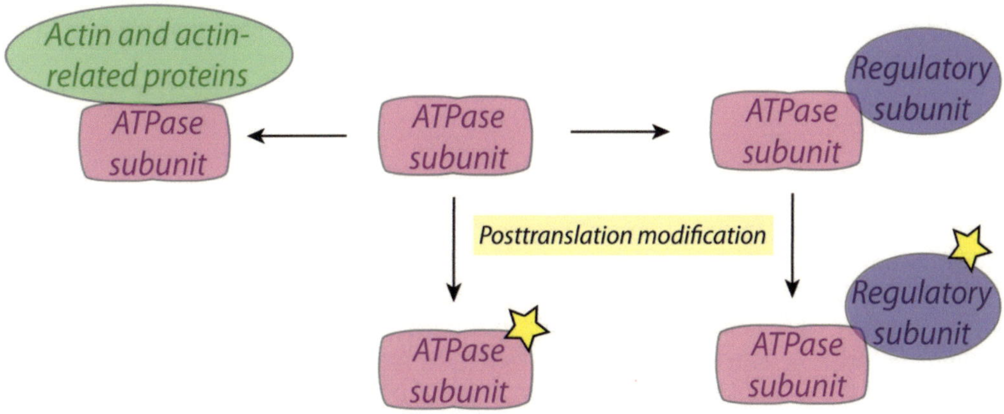

Figure 6. Different regulation possibilities of remodeler activity.

Acetylation. The acetyltransferase MOF acetylates TIP5, the largest subunit of NoRC, at position K633, adjacent to the TIP5 RNA-binding domain, and that the NAD(+)-dependent deacetylase SIRT1 removes the acetyl group. Acetylation regulates the interaction of NoRC with pRNA, which in turn affects heterochromatin formation, nucleosome positioning and rDNA silencing. Significantly, NoRC acetylation is responsive to the intracellular energy status and fluctuates during S-phase. Activation of SIRT1 on glucose deprivation leads to deacetylation of K633, enhanced pRNA binding and an increase in heterochromatic histone marks [99]. The acetylation of yeast Rsc4 does not significantly affect RSC catalytic activity or its ability to recognize acetylated nucleosomes, but K25 acetylation mark plays a key role in resistance to DNA damage, in a manner that appears to be regulated by its interaction with bromodomain 1. Moreover, Rsc4 acetylation acts in parallel with the INO80-remodeling complex to promote S-phase progression in cells subject to replication stress [100]. *Drosophila* ISWI is acetylated at position K753 *in vivo* and *in vitro* by the histone acetyltransferase GCN5. The acetylated form of ISWI represents a minor species presumably associated with the nucleosome remodeling factor NURF and may contribute during metaphase chromosome condensation [101]. Human Brm was shown to be acetylated at multiple locations, but two sites, clustered in the C-terminal region, appear to play a central role in the regulation. Mutation of these sites into non-acetylatable versions creates a Brm protein with increased activity in terms of inhibition of colony formation and transcriptional activation [102].

PARylation. In *Drosophila*, ISWI is poly-ADP-ribosylated (PARylated) by the enzyme PARP. PARylated ISWI binds weaker to the nucleosomes and DNA and displays weak nucleosome-stimulated ATPase activity. Moreover, the amount of ISWI bound to chromatin is affected by PARP activity, suggesting that PARP and ISWI might compete for common chromatin target sites and antagonize on chromosome condensation [103]. A different scenario is reported in the nucleolus of human embryonic kidney cell line, where PARP1/ARTD1-mediated parylation of TIP5, a noncatalytic subunit of NoRC complex, promotes the silencing of rDNA chromatin during replication. It is reported that upon of pRNA binding TIP5 undergoes conformational change [67] which might favour the association of PARP1 and subsequently Tip5 is parylated. It was postulated that PARP1 enzymatic activity facilitates formation of silent rDNA chromatin and transcriptional silencing [104].

7. Conclusion

Global chromatin structure is a result of the combination of chromatin remodelers present in the cell. The ability to form various complexes with different activities and the concentration of the remodelers influences the nucleosomal positions genome-wide. Much data have been accumulated from *in vitro* experiments addressing the mechanistical questions of chromatin remodelers, but the recent studies have begun to reveal how these proteins find their place of action in the cell. From our current knowledge it seems that the local chromatin structures undergo a continuous change due to a continuous and random binding of different remodeling complexes. A large fraction of the remodeling complexes diffuse freely through the nucleus and act on nucleosomal substrates. In addition, the specific cellular signals are responsible for the fast recruitment of the individual machines to the specialized DNA sites correlating with a persistent activation or repression of particular DNA dependent processes, establishing persistent changes in chromatin structure.

Acknowledgements

We apologize to all colleagues whose work could not be cited due to space limitations. Work in the G.L. laboratory is funded by the DFG, EraSysBio+ and Baygene. Funding for open access charge: Regensburg University Library.

Author details

Laura Manelyte and Gernot Längst

University of Regensburg, Regensburg, Germany

References

[1] van Holde KE, Johnson C, Ho PS. Principles of Physical Biochemistry. 1st ed. Prentice Hall; 1998. p. 657.

[2] Grigoryev S. Nucleosome spacing and chromatin higher-order folding. Nucleus. 2012 Sep. 18;3(6).

[3] Strahl BD, Allis CD. The language of covalent histone modifications. Nature. 2000 Jan. 6;403(6765):41–45.

[4] Clapier CR, Cairns BR. The Biology of Chromatin Remodeling Complexes. Annu. Rev. Biochem. 2009 Jun.;78(1):273–304.

[5] Bowman GD. Mechanisms of ATP-dependent nucleosome sliding. Current Opinion in Structural Biology. 2010 Feb.;20(1):73–81.

[6] Rippe K, Schrader A, Riede P, Strohner R, Lehmann E, Längst G. DNA sequence- and conformation-directed positioning of nucleosomes by chromatin-remodeling complexes. Proc. Natl. Acad. Sci. U.S.A. 2007 Oct. 2;104(40):15635–15640.

[7] Eisen JA, Sweder KS, Hanawalt PC. Evolution of the SNF2 family of proteins: subfamilies with distinct sequences and functions. Nucleic Acids Res. 1995 Jul. 25;23(14): 2715–2723.

[8] Flaus A, Martin DMA, Barton GJ, Owen-Hughes T. Identification of multiple distinct Snf2 subfamilies with conserved structural motifs. Nucleic Acids Res. 2006;34(10): 2887–2905.

[9] Neigeborn L, Carlson M. Genes affecting the regulation of SUC2 gene expression by glucose repression in Saccharomyces cerevisiae. Genetics. 1984 Dec.;108(4):845–858.

[10] Sudarsanam P, Iyer VR, Brown PO, Winston F. Whole-genome expression analysis of snf/swi mutants of Saccharomyces cerevisiae. Proc. Natl. Acad. Sci. U.S.A. 2000 Mar. 28;97(7):3364–3369.

[11] Holstege FC, Jennings EG, Wyrick JJ, Lee TI, Hengartner CJ, Green MR, et al. Dissecting the regulatory circuitry of a eukaryotic genome. Cell. 1998 Nov. 25;95(5):717–728.

[12] Muchardt C, Yaniv M. When the SWI/SNF complex remodels 1/4 the cell cycle. Oncogene. 2001 May 28;20(24):3067–3075.

[13] Wilson BG, Roberts CWM. SWI/SNF nucleosome remodellers and cancer. Nat Rev Cancer. 2011 Jul.;11(7):481–492.

[14] Lemon B, Inouye C, King DS, Tjian R. Selectivity of chromatin-remodelling cofactors for ligand-activated transcription. Nature. 2001 Nov.;414(6866):924–928.

[15] Yan Z. PBAF chromatin-remodeling complex requires a novel specificity subunit, BAF200, to regulate expression of selective interferon-responsive genes. Genes & Development. 2005 Jul. 15;19(14):1662–1667.

[16] Reisman DN, Sciarrotta J, Wang W, Funkhouser WK, Weissman BE. Loss of BRG1/BRM in human lung cancer cell lines and primary lung cancers: correlation with poor prognosis. Cancer Research. 2003 Feb. 1;63(3):560–566.

[17] Weissman B, Knudsen KE. Hijacking the chromatin remodeling machinery: impact of SWI/SNF perturbations in cancer. Cancer Research. 2009 Nov. 1;69(21):8223–8230.

[18] Ables ET, Drummond-Barbosa D. The steroid hormone ecdysone functions with intrinsic chromatin remodeling factors to control female germline stem cells in Drosophila. Cell Stem Cell. 2010 Nov. 5;7(5):581–592.

[19] Sala A, Toto M, Pinello L, Gabriele A, Di Benedetto V, Ingrassia AMR, et al. Genome-wide characterization of chromatin binding and nucleosome spacing activity of the nucleosome remodelling ATPase ISWI. The EMBO Journal. 2011 May 4;30(9):1766–1777.

[20] Grummt I, Längst G. Epigenetic control of RNA polymerase I transcription in mammalian cells. Biochim. Biophys. Acta. 2012 Oct. 12.

[21] Sims JK, Wade PA. SnapShot: Chromatin remodeling: CHD. Cell. 2011 Feb. 18;144(4): 626–626.e1.

[22] Delmas V, Stokes DG, Perry RP. A mammalian DNA-binding protein that contains a chromodomain and an SNF2/SWI2-like helicase domain. Proc. Natl. Acad. Sci. U.S.A. 1993 Mar. 15;90(6):2414–2418.

[23] Stokes DG, Perry RP. DNA-binding and chromatin localization properties of CHD1. Molecular and Cellular Biology. 1995 May;15(5):2745–2753.

[24] Ryan DP, Sundaramoorthy R, Martin D, Singh V, Owen-Hughes T. The DNA-binding domain of the Chd1 chromatin-remodelling enzyme contains SANT and SLIDE domains. The EMBO Journal. 2011 Jul. 6;30(13):2596–2609.

[25] Watson AA, Mahajan P, Mertens HDT, Deery MJ, Zhang W, Pham P, et al. The PHD and chromo domains regulate the ATPase activity of the human chromatin remodeler CHD4. Journal of Molecular Biology. 2012 Sep. 7;422(1):3–17.

[26] Murawska M, Brehm A. CHD chromatin remodelers and the transcription cycle. Transcription. 2011 Oct.;2(6):244–253.

[27] Gkikopoulos T, Schofield P, Singh V, Pinskaya M, Mellor J, Smolle M, et al. A role for Snf2-related nucleosome-spacing enzymes in genome-wide nucleosome organization. Science. 2011 Sep. 23;333(6050):1758–1760.

[28] Marfella CGA, Imbalzano AN. The Chd family of chromatin remodelers. Mutat. Res. 2007 May 1;618(1-2):30–40.

[29] Bajpai R, Chen DA, Rada-Iglesias A, Zhang J, Xiong Y, Helms J, et al. CHD7 cooperates with PBAF to control multipotent neural crest formation. Nature. 2010 Feb. 18;463(7283):958–962.

[30] West SC. Processing of recombination intermediates by the RuvABC proteins. Annu. Rev. Genet. 1997;31:213–244.

[31] Shen X, Mizuguchi G, Hamiche A, Wu C. A chromatin remodelling complex involved in transcription and DNA processing. Nature. 2000 Aug. 3;406(6795):541–544.

[32] Wu S, Shi Y, Mulligan P, Gay F, Landry J, Liu H, et al. A YY1-INO80 complex regulates genomic stability through homologous recombination-based repair. Nature Publishing Group. 2007 Dec.;14(12):1165–1172.

[33] Bao Y, Shen X. SnapShot: Chromatin remodeling: INO80 and SWR1. Cell. 2011 Jan. 7;144(1):158–158.e2.

[34] Papamichos-Chronakis M, Watanabe S, Rando OJ, Peterson CL. Global regulation of H2A.Z localization by the INO80 chromatin-remodeling enzyme is essential for genome integrity. Cell. 2011 Jan. 21;144(2):200–213.

[35] Shen X, Ranallo R, Choi E, Wu C. Involvement of actin-related proteins in ATP-dependent chromatin remodeling. Mol. Cell. 2003 Jul.;12(1):147–155.

[36] Tsukuda T, Fleming AB, Nickoloff JA, Osley MA. Chromatin remodelling at a DNA double-strand break site in Saccharomyces cerevisiae. Nature. 2005 Nov. 17;438(7066):379–383.

[37] van Attikum H, Fritsch O, Gasser SM. Distinct roles for SWR1 and INO80 chromatin remodeling complexes at chromosomal double-strand breaks. The EMBO Journal. 2007 Sep. 19;26(18):4113–4125.

[38] van Vugt JJFA, de Jager M, Murawska M, Brehm A, van Noort J, Logie C. Multiple Aspects of ATP-Dependent Nucleosome Translocation by RSC and Mi-2 Are Directed by the Underlying DNA Sequence. Freitag M, editor. PLoS ONE. 2009 Jul. 23;4(7):e6345.

[39] Davey CA, Sargent DF, Luger K, Maeder AW, Richmond TJ. Solvent mediated interactions in the structure of the nucleosome core particle at 1.9 a resolution. Journal of Molecular Biology. 2002 Jun. 21;319(5):1097–1113.

[40] Längst G, Becker PB. Nucleosome remodeling: one mechanism, many phenomena? Biochimica et Biophysica Acta (BBA) - Gene Structure and Expression. 2004 Mar.; 1677(1-3):58–63.

[41] Luger K, Mäder AW, Richmond RK, Sargent DF, Richmond TJ. Crystal structure of the nucleosome core particle at 2.8 A resolution. Nature. 1997 Sep. 18;389(6648):251–260.

[42] Aoyagi S, Wade PA, Hayes JJ. Nucleosome sliding induced by the xMi-2 complex does not occur exclusively via a simple twist-diffusion mechanism. J. Biol. Chem. 2003 Aug. 15;278(33):30562–30568.

[43] Aoyagi S, Hayes JJ. hSWI/SNF-catalyzed nucleosome sliding does not occur solely via a twist-diffusion mechanism. Molecular and Cellular Biology. 2002 Nov.;22(21): 7484–7490.

[44] Langst G, Becker PB. ISWI induces nucleosome sliding on nicked DNA. Mol. Cell. 2001 Nov.;8(5):1085–1092.

[45] Schiessel H, Widom J, Bruinsma RF, Gelbart WM. Polymer reptation and nucleosome repositioning. Phys. Rev. Lett. 2001 May 7;86(19):4414–4417.

[46] Strohner R, Wachsmuth M, Dachauer K, Mazurkiewicz J, Hochstatter J, Rippe K, et al. A "loop recapture" mechanism for ACF-dependent nucleosome remodeling. Nature Publishing Group. 2005 Jul. 17;12(8):683–690.

[47] Liu N, Peterson CL, Hayes JJ. SWI/SNF- and RSC-catalyzed nucleosome mobilization requires internal DNA loop translocation within nucleosomes. Molecular and Cellular Biology. 2011 Oct.;31(20):4165–4175.

[48] Blosser TR, Yang JG, Stone MD, Narlikar GJ, Zhuang X. Dynamics of nucleosome remodelling by individual ACF complexes. Nature. Nature Publishing Group; 2009 Dec. 14;462(7276):1022–1027.

[49] Sirinakis G, Clapier CR, Gao Y, Viswanathan R, Cairns BR, Zhang Y. The RSC chromatin remodelling ATPase translocates DNA with high force and small step size. The EMBO Journal. 2011 Jun. 15;30(12):2364–2372.

[50] Langst G, Bonte EJ, Corona DF, Becker PB. Nucleosome movement by CHRAC and ISWI without disruption or trans-displacement of the histone octamer. Cell. 1999 Jun. 25;97(7):843–852.

[51] Hamiche A, Sandaltzopoulos R, Gdula DA, Wu C. ATP-dependent histone octamer sliding mediated by the chromatin remodeling complex NURF. Cell. 1999 Jun. 25;97(7):833–842.

[52] Moshkin YM, Chalkley GE, Kan TW, Reddy BA, Ozgur Z, van Ijcken WFJ, et al. Remodelers organize cellular chromatin by counteracting intrinsic histone-DNA sequence preferences in a class-specific manner. Molecular and Cellular Biology. 2012 Feb.;32(3):675–688.

[53] Grüne T, Brzeski J, Eberharter A, Clapier CR, Corona DFV, Becker PB, et al. Crystal Structure and Functional Analysis of a Nucleosome Recognition Module of the Remodeling Factor ISWI. Mol. Cell. 2003 Aug.;12(2):449–460.

[54] Fyodorov DV, Kadonaga JT. Binding of Acf1 to DNA involves a WAC motif and is important for ACF-mediated chromatin assembly. Molecular and Cellular Biology. 2002 Sep.;22(18):6344–6353.

[55] Poot RA, Dellaire G, Hülsmann BB, Grimaldi MA, Corona DF, Becker PB, et al. HuCHRAC, a human ISWI chromatin remodelling complex contains hACF1 and two novel histone-fold proteins. The EMBO Journal. 2000 Jul. 3;19(13):3377–3387.

[56] Strohner R, Nemeth A, Jansa P, Hofmann-Rohrer U, Santoro R, Langst G, et al. NoRC--a novel member of mammalian ISWI-containing chromatin remodeling machines. The EMBO Journal. 2001 Sep. 3;20(17):4892–4900.

[57] Jordan-Sciutto KL, Dragich JM, Rhodes JL, Bowser R. Fetal Alz-50 clone 1, a novel zinc finger protein, binds a specific DNA sequence and acts as a transcriptional regulator. J. Biol. Chem. 1999 Dec. 3;274(49):35262–35268.

[58] Stockdale C, Flaus A, Ferreira H, Owen-Hughes T. Analysis of nucleosome repositioning by yeast ISWI and Chd1 chromatin remodeling complexes. J. Biol. Chem. 2006 Jun. 16;281(24):16279–16288.

[59] Sims HI, Lane JM, Ulyanova NP, Schnitzler GR. Human SWI/SNF drives sequence-directed repositioning of nucleosomes on C-myc promoter DNA minicircles. Biochemistry. 2007 Oct. 9;46(40):11377–11388.

[60] Partensky PD, Narlikar GJ. Chromatin Remodelers Act Globally, Sequence Positions Nucleosomes Locally. Journal of Molecular Biology. Elsevier Ltd; 2009 Aug. 7;391(1): 12–25.

[61] Racki LR, Yang JG, Naber N, Partensky PD, Acevedo A, Purcell TJ, et al. The chromatin remodeller ACF acts as a dimeric motor to space nucleosomes. Nature. Nature Publishing Group; 2009 Dec. 14;462(7276):1016–1021.

[62] Yang JG, Madrid TS, Sevastopoulos E, Narlikar GJ. The chromatin-remodeling enzyme ACF is an ATP-dependent DNA length sensor that regulates nucleosome spacing. Nature Publishing Group. 2006 Nov. 12;13(12):1078–1083.

[63] McKnight JN, Jenkins KR, Nodelman IM, Escobar T, Bowman GD. Extranucleosomal DNA binding directs nucleosome sliding by Chd1. Molecular and Cellular Biology. 2011 Dec.;31(23):4746–4759.

[64] Law MJ, Lower KM, Voon HPJ, Hughes JR, Garrick D, Viprakasit V, et al. ATR-X syndrome protein targets tandem repeats and influences allele-specific expression in a size-dependent manner. Cell. 2010 Oct. 29;143(3):367–378.

[65] Zhang Y, Ng HH, Erdjument-Bromage H, Tempst P, Bird A, Reinberg D. Analysis of the NuRD subunits reveals a histone deacetylase core complex and a connection with DNA methylation. Genes & Development. 1999 Aug. 1;13(15):1924–1935.

[66] Mayer C, Schmitz K-M, Li J, Grummt I, Santoro R. Intergenic Transcripts Regulate the Epigenetic State of rRNA Genes. Mol. Cell. 2006 May;22(3):351–361.

[67] Mayer C, Neubert M, Grummt I. The structure of NoRC-associated RNA is crucial for targeting the chromatin remodelling complex NoRC to the nucleolus. EMBO reports. 2008 Jul. 4;9(8):774–780.

[68] Schmitz KM, Mayer C, Postepska A, Grummt I. Interaction of noncoding RNA with the rDNA promoter mediates recruitment of DNMT3b and silencing of rRNA genes. Genes & Development. 2010 Oct. 15;24(20):2264–2269.

[69] Kassabov SR, Zhang B, Persinger J, Bartholomew B. SWI/SNF unwraps, slides, and rewraps the nucleosome. Mol. Cell. 2003 Feb.;11(2):391–403.

[70] Chatterjee N, Sinha D, Lemma-Dechassa M, Tan S, Shogren-Knaak MA, Bartholomew B. Histone H3 tail acetylation modulates ATP-dependent remodeling through multiple mechanisms. Nucleic Acids Res. 2011 Oct.;39(19):8378–8391.

[71] Dang W, Kagalwala MN, Bartholomew B. Regulation of ISW2 by Concerted Action of Histone H4 Tail and Extranucleosomal DNA. Molecular and Cellular Biology. 2006 Oct. 2;26(20):7388–7396.

[72] Clapier CR, Langst G, Corona DF, Becker PB, Nightingale KP. Critical role for the histone H4 N terminus in nucleosome remodeling by ISWI. Molecular and Cellular Biology. 2001 Feb.;21(3):875–883.

[73] Corona DFV, Clapier CR, Becker PB, Tamkun JW. Modulation of ISWI function by site-specific histone acetylation. EMBO reports. 2002 Mar.;3(3):242–247.

[74] Musselman CA, Mansfield RE, Garske AL, Davrazou F, Kwan AH, Oliver SS, et al. Binding of the CHD4 PHD2 finger to histone H3 is modulated by covalent modifications. Biochem. J. 2009 Oct. 15;423(2):179–187.

[75] Mansfield RE, Musselman CA, Kwan AH, Oliver SS, Garske AL, Davrazou F, et al. Plant homeodomain (PHD) fingers of CHD4 are histone H3-binding modules with preference for unmodified H3K4 and methylated H3K9. Journal of Biological Chemistry. 2011 Apr. 1;286(13):11779–11791.

[76] Kwon SY, Xiao H, Wu C, Badenhorst P. Alternative splicing of NURF301 generates distinct NURF chromatin remodeling complexes with altered modified histone binding specificities. PLoS Genet. 2009 Jul.;5(7):e1000574.

[77] Talbert PB, Henikoff S. Histone variants--ancient wrap artists of the epigenome. Nature Reviews Molecular Cell Biology. 2010 Apr.;11(4):264–275.

[78] Nashun B, Akiyama T, Suzuki MG, Aoki F. Dramatic replacement of histone variants during genome remodeling in nuclear-transferred embryos. Epigenetics. 2011 Dec.; 6(12):1489–1497.

[79] Shechter D, Chitta RK, Xiao A, Shabanowitz J, Hunt DF, Allis CD. A distinct H2A.X isoform is enriched in Xenopus laevis eggs and early embryos and is phosphorylated in the absence of a checkpoint. Proc. Natl. Acad. Sci. U.S.A. 2009 Jan. 20;106(3):749–754.

[80] Konev AY, Tribus M, Park SY, Podhraski V, Lim CY, Emelyanov AV, et al. CHD1 motor protein is required for deposition of histone variant H3.3 into chromatin in vivo. Science. 2007 Aug. 24;317(5841):1087–1090.

[81] Luk E, Ranjan A, Fitzgerald PC, Mizuguchi G, Huang Y, Wei D, et al. Stepwise histone replacement by SWR1 requires dual activation with histone H2A.Z and canonical nucleosome. Cell. 2010 Nov. 24;143(5):725–736.

[82] Xiao A, Li H, Shechter D, Ahn SH, Fabrizio LA, Erdjument-Bromage H, et al. WSTF regulates the H2A.X DNA damage response via a novel tyrosine kinase activity. Nature. 2009 Jan. 1;457(7225):57–62.

[83] Burrage J, Termanis A, Geissner A, Myant K, Gordon K, Stancheva I. SNF2 family ATPase LSH promotes phosphorylation of H2AX and efficient repair of DNA double-strand breaks in mammalian cells. Journal of Cell Science. 2012 Sep. 3.

[84] Reddy BA, Bajpe PK, Bassett A, Moshkin YM, Kozhevnikova E, Bezstarosti K, et al. Drosophila Transcription Factor Tramtrack69 Binds MEP1 To Recruit the Chromatin Remodeler NuRD. Molecular and Cellular Biology. 2010 Oct. 11;30(21):5234–5244.

[85] Weider M, Küspert M, Bischof M, Vogl MR, Hornig J, Loy K, et al. Chromatin-remodeling factor Brg1 is required for Schwann cell differentiation and myelination. Dev. Cell. 2012 Jul. 17;23(1):193–201.

[86] Jeong KW, Lee Y-H, Stallcup MR. Recruitment of the SWI/SNF chromatin remodeling complex to steroid hormone-regulated promoters by nuclear receptor coactivator flightless-I. Journal of Biological Chemistry. 2009 Oct. 23;284(43):29298–29309.

[87] Polo SE, Kaidi A, Baskcomb L, Galanty Y, Jackson SP. Regulation of DNA-damage responses and cell-cycle progression by the chromatin remodelling factor CHD4. The EMBO Journal. Nature Publishing Group; 2010 Aug. 6;29(18):3130–3139.

[88] Ahel D, Horejsí Z, Wiechens N, Polo SE, Garcia-Wilson E, Ahel I, et al. Poly(ADP-ribose)-dependent regulation of DNA repair by the chromatin remodeling enzyme ALC1. Science. 2009 Sep. 4;325(5945):1240–1243.

[89] Hopfield JJ. Kinetic proofreading: a new mechanism for reducing errors in biosynthetic processes requiring high specificity. Proc. Natl. Acad. Sci. U.S.A. 1974 Oct.; 71(10):4135–4139.

[90] Erdel F, Schubert T, Marth C, Längst G, Rippe K. Human ISWI chromatin-remodeling complexes sample nucleosomes via transient binding reactions and become immobilized at active sites. Proc. Natl. Acad. Sci. U.S.A. 2010 Nov. 16;107(46):19873–19878.

[91] Gelbart ME, Bachman N, Delrow J, Boeke JD, Tsukiyama T. Genome-wide identification of Isw2 chromatin-remodeling targets by localization of a catalytically inactive mutant. Genes & Development. 2005 Apr. 15;19(8):942–954.

[92] Erdel F, Krug J, Längst G, Rippe K. Targeting chromatin remodelers: signals and search mechanisms. Biochim. Biophys. Acta. 2011 Sep.;1809(9):497–508.

[93] Johnson TA, Elbi C, Parekh BS, Hager GL, John S. Chromatin remodeling complexes interact dynamically with a glucocorticoid receptor-regulated promoter. Mol. Biol. Cell. 2008 Aug.;19(8):3308–3322.

[94] Li J, Längst G, Grummt I. NoRC-dependent nucleosome positioning silences rRNA genes. The EMBO Journal. 2006 Dec. 13;25(24):5735–5741.

[95] Erdel F, Rippe K. Binding kinetics of human ISWI chromatin-remodelers to DNA repair sites elucidate their target location mechanism. Nucleus. 2011 Feb.;2(2):105–112.

[96] Sif S, Stukenberg PT, Kirschner MW, Kingston RE. Mitotic inactivation of a human SWI/SNF chromatin remodeling complex. Genes & Development. 1998 Sep. 15;12(18):2842–2851.

[97] Bouazoune K, Brehm A. dMi-2 chromatin binding and remodeling activities are regulated by dCK2 phosphorylation. J. Biol. Chem. 2005 Dec. 23;280(51):41912–41920.

[98] Morrison AJ, Kim J-A, Person MD, Highland J, Xiao J, Wehr TS, et al. Mec1/Tel1 phosphorylation of the INO80 chromatin remodeling complex influences DNA damage checkpoint responses. Cell. 2007 Aug. 10;130(3):499–511.

[99] Zhou Y, Schmitz K-M, Mayer C, Yuan X, Akhtar A, Grummt I. Reversible acetylation of the chromatin remodelling complex NoRC is required for non-coding RNA-dependent silencing. Nat Cell Biol. 2009 Jul. 5;11(8):1010–1016.

[100] Charles GM, Chen C, Shih SC, Collins SR, Beltrao P, Zhang X, et al. Site-specific acetylation mark on an essential chromatin-remodeling complex promotes resistance to replication stress. Proc. Natl. Acad. Sci. U.S.A. 2011 Jun. 28;108(26):10620–10625.

[101] Ferreira R, Eberharter A, Bonaldi T, Chioda M, Imhof A, Becker PB. Site-specific acetylation of ISWI by GCN5. BMC Mol Biol. 2007;8:73.

[102] Bourachot B, Yaniv M, Muchardt C. Growth inhibition by the mammalian SWI-SNF subunit Brm is regulated by acetylation. The EMBO Journal. 2003 Dec. 15;22(24): 6505–6515.

[103] Sala A, La Rocca G, Burgio G, Kotova E, Di Gesù D, Collesano M, et al. The nucleosome-remodeling ATPase ISWI is regulated by poly-ADP-ribosylation. Plos Biol. 2008 Oct. 14;6(10):e252.

[104] Guetg C, Scheifele F, Rosenthal F, Hottiger MO, Santoro R. Inheritance of silent rDNA chromatin is mediated by PARP1 via noncoding RNA. Mol. Cell. 2012 Mar. 30;45(6):790–800.

Chapter 2

SUMO Tasks in Chromatin Remodeling

Garcia-Dominguez Mario

Additional information is available at the end of the chapter

http://dx.doi.org/10.5772/55395

1. Introduction

Post-translational modifications implicate attachment of diverse molecules to proteins after translation. These modifications are essential for many biological processes as they are involved in their regulation. From relatively simple molecules to small polypetides are common covalent modifiers of proteins. Sumoylation consists in the post-translational modification of proteins by attachment of the small polypeptide SUMO (small ubiquitin-like modifier). This post-translational modification was identified two decades ago and has been very actively investigated to date. Sumoylation has consequences on protein structure and regulation. This modification controls many processes in the eukaryotic cell and is essential for viability of all the organisms studied so far.

From the discovery of ubiquitin in 1975, a number of ubiquitin-like proteins (UBLs) have been identified in eukaryotes and it has been shown that many of them are able to covalently attach to other proteins (reviewed in [1]). Several aspects are common to most UBLs: they are small polypeptides (less than 200 amino acids) capable of attaching to other macromolecules in a covalent way, present common structural features and use similar modification pathways. These characteristics strongly support duplication and diversification during evolution as the origin of the different pathways. Ubiquitin and UBLs are characterized by the presence of the ß-grasp fold, which also appears in ubiquitin-like domains of several other proteins of the ubiquitin system and in numerous non-related proteins (reviewed in [2]). The ß-grasp fold seems to have emerged in prokaryotes as a translation-related RNA-binding module, which diversified structurally and biochemically before to dramatically expand in eukaryotes [2]. Besides ubiquitin and SUMO, examples of UBLs are NEDD8, FUBI, FAT10, ISG15, UFM1, Atg8, Atg12 and Urm1 (reviewed in [1]).

The first report of a protein being modified by SUMO occurred in the nineties and concerned the mammalian nuclear pore-associated GTPase activating protein RanGAP1 [3, 4]. Subsequently, more than a hundred proteins have been identified as SUMO substrates. Although similarities with ubiquitin are notable [5], SUMO plays many regulatory functions in the cell that significantly differ from the major role displayed by ubiquitin: labeling proteins to target them for proteasomal degradation [6]. A variety of consequences derived from protein sumoylation (new interaction surfaces, modulation of protein affinity and binding capacities to other molecules, modulation of protein activity, blocking of protein domains, steric hindrance, crosstalk or interference with other post-translational modifications) account for the many roles attributed to SUMO (reviewed in [7]). A major role of SUMO is associated with RanGAP1 and thereby with the nuclear pore complex. Thus, involvement of SUMO in nucleo-cytoplasmic transport of proteins has been well established [8]. SUMO has been also implicated in chromosome dynamics in mitosis and meiosis (condensation, cohesion, separation) and genome integrity, as many proteins involved in DNA replication, repair and recombination are modulated by SUMO modification (reviewed in [7]). Other roles attributed to SUMO are related to enzyme regulation, protein stability and cellular structure (reviewed in [9, 10]). However, the most prominent function of SUMO concerns transcriptional regulation, and specially transcription repression (reviewed in [11, 12]). The role of SUMO in transcription, in the context of chromatin structure and dynamics, is analyzed in this chapter.

2. The modification pathway

2.1. Enzymes involved

Modification by SUMO involves the ATP-dependent activation of mature SUMO (C terminus of SUMO needs to be excised by proteolysis) by the E1 enzyme, transfer to the E2 enzyme UBC9 and conjugation to the target protein, often mediated by a SUMO ligase or E3 (Figure 1 and Table 1) (reviewed in [9]). Maturation of the SUMO precursor, as well as removal of SUMO from targets is displayed by SUMO specific proteases.

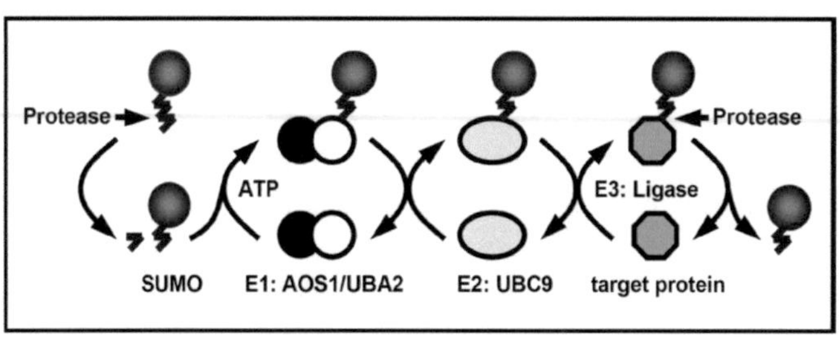

Figure 1. The sumoylation pathway. Cleavage of the SUMO C terminus enables ATP-mediated activation and binding to the E1 enzyme to be transferred to the E2 conjugating enzyme UBC9, which mediates target modification with the concourse of an E3 SUMO ligase. Recycling of SUMO is performed by the same proteases involved in maturation.

SUMO E1 activity is performed by the SAE1/UBA2 heterodimer in human, in contrast to the ubiquitination pathway where the E1 activity is displayed by a monomeric enzyme. However, the SAE1 subunit is homologous to the N-terminal part of ubiquitin E1, while the UBA2 subunit is homologous to its C terminus [13]. Both monomers work together and are not found separately [14]. E1 activation of mature SUMO involves ATP hydrolysis and formation of a thiolester bond between E1 and the C terminus of SUMO before being transferred to the E2. While several E2 have been described for ubiquitination, UBC9 is the only E2 known for sumoylation [15, 16]. Thus, UBC9 is the conjugating enzyme directly involved in attachment of SUMO to the different substrates. This second step of the sumoylation reaction involves the formation of a thiolester bond between SUMO and UBC9 upon transfer from the E1. The region surrounding the active site cysteine (C93 in mammals) in UBC9 is able to directly interact with sumoylation consensus sequence (see below) in target proteins [17-19].

Enzyme	Protein	Activity	References
E1 (activating)	AOS1/UBA2	ATP-mediated activation of SUMO	[13]
E2 (conjugating)	UBC9	SUMO conjugation to target	[15, 16]
E3 (ligase)	PIAS1-4	Facilitates transfer to target	[20, 21]
	RanBP2		[22]
	Polycomb-2 (Pc2)		[23]
	TOPORS		[24]
	Class IIa HDACs		[25]
	KAP-1		[26]
	RHES		[27]
	Krox20		[28]
protease	SENP1-3, 5-7	Maturation/recycling	[29-31]
	DeSI-1		[32]

Table 1. Enzymes involved in SUMO conjugation.

SUMO ligases are involved in facilitating the SUMO attachment to substrates (reviewed in [33]). To date, few ligases have been described for sumoylation, in contrast to ubiquitination, where lots of them are known to play an essential role and mediate substrate specificity. In fact, SUMO ligases were undervalued at the beginning, since certain substrates are sumoylated in vitro, provided that E1 and E2 are present at the adequate concentrations. Since UBC9 is able to directly interact with sumoylation consensus sequence in substrates, it is able to render sumoylation in the absence of a ligase. However, a number of proteins, which augmented the efficiency of SUMO conjugation, were identified. The list of SUMO ligases progressively increases and essential roles for these have been described in vivo (see [34]). Although mechanisms of action of SUMO ligases have not been completely elucidated, it is obvious that many ligases facilitate transfer of SUMO by bringing together SUMO-loaded UBC9 and the target protein. Thus, similar to the RING domain-containing E3 ligases involved in ubiquitination, SUMO ligases do not establish a covalent bond with SUMO. In this context, a SUMO ligase should normally i) interact with the substrate, ii) interact with UBC9, iii) facilitate SUMO transfer to the substrate. Ligases of the PIAS family (PIAS1 to 4) have been extensively studied [35]. They present a type of RING finger domain, the SP-RING (Siz/PIAS RING), for UBC9 interaction, although Ubc9 binding to a PHD domain in plant PIAS proteins has been also described [36]. Other SUMO ligases described so far are RanBP2 [22], the Polycomb-2 (Pc2) protein [23], class IIa histone deacetylases (HDACs) [25], topoisomerase I-binding RING finger protein (TOPORS) [24], the PHD containing protein KAP-1 [26], Ras homologue enriched in striatum (RHES) [27] and the transcription factor Krox20 [28]. In contrast to most ubiquitin ligases, SUMO ligases may display significant promiscuity, as many of them enhance sumoylation of a variety of substrates.

SUMO proteases are involved in maturation of the SUMO precursor by exposing two glycine residues at the C terminus for binding to E1 [37]. In addition, they are also involved in SUMO recycling by excising the SUMO moiety from substrates. Yeast Ulp1p was the first SUMO protease identified [29]. Sequence analysis revealed that it corresponded to a protease of the C48 cysteine group, not related to deubiquitylating enzymes but similar to adenovirus proteases. Mammalian SUMO proteases are represented by the SENP (sentrin-specific protease) family. It comprises six members, SENP1 to 3, and SENP5 to 7 [38]. A seventh member, initially identified as SENP4, resulted to actually correspond to SENP3. Besides SENP1 to 7, an additional family member has been reported, SENP8. However, this protease does not act on SUMO, but on another UBL, NEDD8 [39, 40]. Very recently, a new type of SUMO protease has been described, the desumoylating isopeptidase 1 (DeSI-1) [32]. The different SUMO proteases show diverse cellular localization and different specificities for the various SUMO molecules and substrates (reviewed in [38]).

2.2. SUMO molecules

Four different SUMO molecules have been described in mammals: SUMO1 to 4. SUMO1 has been implicated in regulation of many processes, while SUMO2 and SUMO3 are highly related with the response to stress. Consequently, a significant pool of free SUMO2 and SUMO3 is detected in the cell, which is rapidly mobilized after exposure to a variety of stress conditions. In contrast, most of SUMO1 appears conjugated to proteins [41]. SUMO2 and SUMO3 are usually referred as SUMO2/3, as they share 97% identity and antibodies hardly differentiate the two forms. By contrast, SUMO1 only shares about 50% identity with SUMO2/3. Despite the low similarity showed between ubiquitin and SUMO (about 18% identity with SUMO1), structurally they are quite similar, excepting the N-terminal region of SUMO not present in ubiquitin [42]. A remarkable difference between SUMO1 and SUMO2/3 is the ability of this last to form poly-SUMO chains in vitro as well as in vivo, due to the presence of a sumoylation consensus sequence in the molecule [43]. SUMO4 is the last SUMO molecule identified. It shows a restricted expression pattern [44] and several data bring into question its capacity to be conjugated to proteins [45]. However, a polymorphism found in human SUMO4 correlates with type 1 diabetes [46]. The different SUMO molecules share a common modification pathway and the existence of functional redundancy has been suggested. However, specific modification by the different SUMO paralogs has been implicated in the regulation of a variety of processes. Thus, the modification pathway is able to differentially conjugate the various SUMO molecules depending on the substrate or the regulatory process [47].

2.3. Sumoylation consensus motifs and SUMO interacting motifs

Covalent attachment of SUMO occurs through the ε-amino group of a lysine residue in target proteins. In many cases the Lys (K) residue is the core of the consensus sequence ΨKxE, being Ψ a large hydrophobic residue and x any amino acid. Extended consensus (phosphorylation-dependent SUMO motif (PDSM) and negatively charged residues-dependent SUMO motif (NDSM)) and variations have been described as well (Table 2) (reviewed in [34]). However, sumoylation also occurs at non-consensus sequences. As mentioned above, the consensus sequence is directly contacted by UBC9. Thus, it is possible that when sumoylation occurs at non-consensus sequences, certain amino acid residues, otherwise dispersed in the primary structure of the target protein, bring together in the three-dimensional structure to mimic a consensus-like environment. It is worth noting that conversely, sumoylation consensus sequences in a protein are not always substrate for SUMO attachment, indicating that additional structural features regulate and enable modification by SUMO. Besides covalent attachement of SUMO, many proteins can associate with SUMO in a different way involving a non-covalent interaction (reviewed in [48]). This occurs through SUMO interacting motifs (SIMs) in proteins. SIMs are usually characterized by the presence of a short hydrophobic region surrounded by negatively charged residues (Table 2) [49]. The non-covalent interaction of proteins with SUMO has been revealed essential in the regulation of several processes. In a variety of cases function of the system relies in the combinatorial occurrence of sumoylation sites and SIMs in a given protein or in different subunits of a complex, which determines its macromolecular architecture (Figure 2 and see below). This situation is exemplified by the promyelocytic leukaemia protein (PML), in which combination of sumoylation sites and SIMs dictates the formation of PML nuclear bodies and the recruitment of additional proteins [48].

2.4. Regulation of sumoylation

Despite that certain SUMO targets appear constitutively sumoylated, it is obvious that sumoylation, as a signaling pathway needs to be regulated. A striking feature of SUMO modification consists in the so-called "SUMO enigma" [9]. It has been observed that many SUMO targets are difficult to detect at the sumoylated state, but mutation of the acceptor lysine has severe consequences in the process involved. In other words, at the steady state, only a low proportion of the whole pool of a given target appears sumoylated, although sumoylation results essential for function of the target. Thus, sumoylation has been suggested to be a highly dynamic and transient modification that permanently marks targets for specific fates even though the SUMO moiety has been removed [9]. This can be explained by viewing sumoylation as a temporal facilitator for the establishment of protein interactions, other protein modifications, or sub-cellular localization (Figure 2).

Sumoylation can be regulated at different levels (reviewed in [34, 50]). First level of regulation in SUMO modification relies in the nature of target proteins, as target sequence, structural features, and other protein modifications affect attachment of SUMO. The other way to

SUMO binding	Type		Sequence
Sumoylation site	Consensus		ΨKxE
	Extended consensus	PDSM	ΨKxExxSP
		NDSM	ΨKxExx[D/E]$_n$
	Iverted consensus		ExKΨ
	Phosphorylated Ser		ΨKxS
SIM	ZNF198		DDDDDDD VVFI
	PIAS1		VEVI DLTI DSSSDEEEEE
	SP100		IIVI SSEDSEGSTDVD
	PML		EE R VVVI SSSEDSD
	RanBP2		SDSPSDDD VLIV
	CoREST1		EESEDELEE ANGNNP IDIEV

Table 2. Sumoylation sites and SUMO interacting motifs (SIMs). Ψ represents a large hydrophobic residue. Sumoylated Lys (K) is frequently close to a hydrophobic residue and to negatively charged environment, either acidic residues Asp/Glu (D/E) or phosphorylation sites (SP). SIMs usually consist in a stretch of 4 amino acids, containing at least 3 hydrophobic residues, close to an acidic region (Asp/Glu) (D/E) or putative phosphorylation sites (Ser/Thr) (S/T). Examples of SIMs with acidic/phosphorylation region N-terminal to the hydrophobic core (ZNF198), C-terminal (with spacer (PIAS1), without spacer (SP100)), at both sides (PML), SUMO1 specific (RanBP2) and SUMO2/3 specific (CoREST1), are shown.

regulate sumoylation depends on the modification pathway. Availability of the different SUMO paralogs when sumoylation is required, or acting on the E1 and E2 enzymes, represents a global way to regulate sumoylation. For instance, stress conditions normally leads to SUMO2/3 conjugation, as SUMO2/3 is freely available in the cell [41]. On the other hand, it has been shown that expression of the Gam1 protein by the CELO adenovirus leads to E1 and E2 degradation and thereby to inhibition of sumoylation [51]. Finally, a more selective way of regulating sumoylation is given through the activity of SUMO ligases and proteases. Thus, localization or spatiotemporal regulation of the expression of these proteins has consequences in target sumoylation.

3. SUMO in transcription

3.1. Transcription repression

It is of significance that the sumoylation consensus sequence, before being established to be the site for SUMO attachment, was initially identified as a negative regulatory sequence in several transcription factors [52]. This scenario is exemplified by the transcription factor Elk-1 (Ets (E twenty-six)-like kinase 1), where a repressive domain, the R motif, was identified as an acceptor region for SUMO attachment [53]. Targeting SUMO or the SUMO conjugation enzyme UBC9 to promoters through a Gal4-based system efficiently represses transcription [54-56],

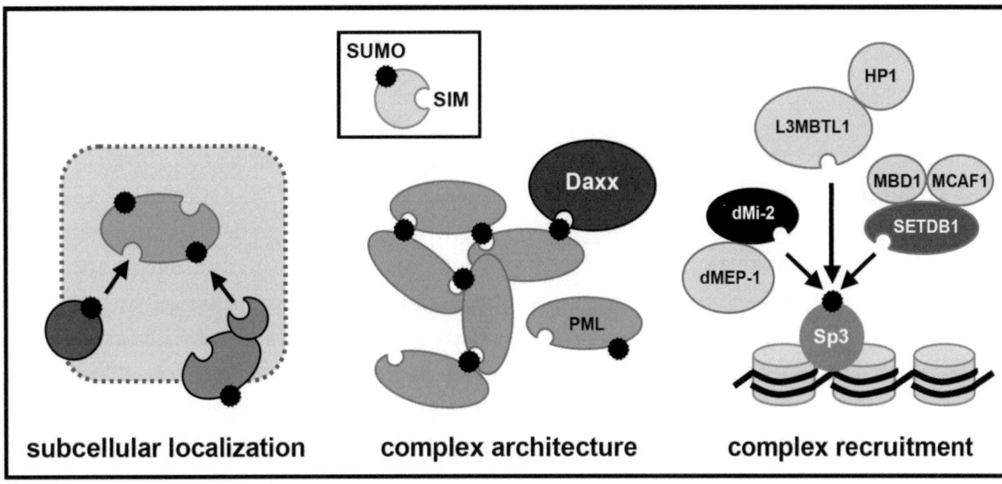

Figure 2. Sumoylation and SIMs are involved in complex architecture and function. Schematic representation of some examples for SUMO-SIM interactions involved in recruiting proteins to a particular subcellular localization, in the architecture of PML aggregates and association to Daxx, and in recruitment of different repressor complexes to the chromatin through sumoylated Sp3 for transcription repression.

indicating that sumoylation mainly associates with transcription repression. Examples from different organisms have argued in favor of such a role. A characteristic of silenced genes is that they correlate with low levels of histone acetylation, while active genes usually display high histone acetylation. It has been described in yeast that temperature-sensitive mutation in Ubc9 leads to an increase in global histone acetylation [57]. In addition, in fission yeast, it has been shown that SUMO is required for the maintenance of heterochromatin stability [58]. Early evidence of the involvement of the SUMO pathway in maintenance of the heterochromatin came from Drosophila, as a PIAS mutant was identified as a suppressor of position effect variegation, that is, as a mutant releasing heterochromatin-induced gene silencing [59]. A mechanism that clearly account for the repressive role of SUMO is explained by the ability of SUMO to recruit histone deacetylases [56]. For many transcription factors sumoylation has been linked to transcription repression. Additional examples to Elk-1 are NAB proteins [28], c-Jun [60], p53 [61], IκBα [62], C/EBP [63], Sp3 [64] and MEF2 [65]. It is worth noting that in many cases sumoylation turns activators into repressors, as it is the case of p300 and CREB binding protein (CBP) [66, 67]. However, beyond SUMO modification of transcription factors, SUMO association with architecture and function of chromatin-associated repressor complexes is recently getting increased importance. This has been reviewed in [68, 69] and is described below.

3.2. Transcription activation

Despite the clear association of SUMO with gene repression, several reports illustrate the involvement of sumoylation in transcription activation. Examples of transcription factors whose activity is stimulated by SUMO are TCF4 [70], GATA4 [71], Pax6 [72], p45 [73], Smad4

[74], Oct4 [75], p53 [76], myocardin [77], PEA3 [78], NFAT1 [79] and HSF1 and 2 [80, 81]. Intriguingly, p53 has been reported both to be activated and repressed by SUMO [76, 82]. Since sumoylation may compete other post-translational modifications, a mechanism proposed for SUMO-mediated activation of transcription consists in avoiding degradation, and thereby in stabilization, of the transcription factor, as it has been proposed for Oct4 [83]. Otherwise, SUMO modification may interfere with association of repressors with the transcription factor, as occurs for Ikaros, whose sumoylation avoid interaction with histone deacetylase complexes [84]. Recently, two publications have brought into consideration the general assumption that SUMO globally associates with transcription repression. It has been reported in yeast that SUMO is detected at all the constitutively transcribed genes tested and in inducible genes upon activation [85]. However, Ubc9 inactivation results in increased transcription of inducible genes, although sumoylation at promoters is reduced, suggesting a role for SUMO in the silencing of inducible genes. In sum, authors conclude that while SUMO associates with repression in some contexts, other properties of SUMO come into play under normal constitutive transcription [85]. More recently, a study performed in HeLa cells has revealed that from G1 to S phase of the cell cycle SUMO1 marks chromatin at the proximal promoter region on many of the most active housekeeping genes [86]. SUMO1 depletion results in reduced expression of these genes. However, this occurs for half of the active genes and the nature of the sumoylated proteins at the promoters remains unknown [86]. Taken together, all these data indicate that although SUMO may intrinsically associate with transcription repression, many other general processes, including constitutive transcription, may also depend on sumoylation, structurally or as a signaling pathway.

4. Histone modification and chromatin remodeling

4.1. Histone sumoylation

Regarding histone modification, sumoylation has been implicated in both, direct modification of histones and deposition/recognition of other histone marks, such as acetylation and methylation. Histone sumoylation has been demonstrated in both yeast and mammal cells [55, 57]. All core histones and the H2A.Z variant have been shown to be sumoylated in yeast [57, 87], while work on mammal cells has been centered on histone H4 [55]. The N-terminal tail of canonical histones is the target for sumoylation, indicating that sumoylation may interplay with other histone modifications at this region, like acetylation, methylation and phosphorylation. Interfering with the sumoylation pathway significantly reduces the level of histone sumoylation in yeast [57]. Histone sumoylation has been associated with transcription repression. Indeed, mutation of sumoylation sites in histone H2B in yeast leads to increased basal expression of several non-induced genes [57]. A more specific role in Rad51-labeling of persistent DNA double strand breaks has been attributed to sumoylation of the histone variant H2A.Z in yeast [87]. However, which is the real impact of histone sumoylation in transcription in vivo and whether it is a common feature all along the genome need to be clarified.

4.2. Involvement of SUMO in recognition of histone modifications

As explained before, sumoylation of histone tails may affect the way in which different proteins recognize other histone modifications. Conversely, sumoylation of a chromatin-associated factor may modulate its capacity to recognize a specific histone modification. For instance, it has been reported that sumoylation of the bromodomain GTE3 protein, a BET (bromodomain and extra terminal domain) family member, interferes with the capacity of this protein to associate with acetylated histone tails [36]. A surprising link between the sumoylation pathway and recognition of histone modifications is illustrated by a recent and intriguing report describing the capacity of the PHD domain of plant PIAS proteins to directly recognize histone modifications such as methylated Lys4 and Arg2 on histone H3 (methyl-H3K4 and methyl-H3R2) [88].

Polycomb group (PcG) proteins are involved in regulation of gene transcription and chromatin structure especially during development. These transcriptional repressors regulate lineage choice during development and differentiation by establishing long-term heritable gene silencing of relevant genes, for instance *Hox* genes. Thus, they are tightly linked to stem cell biology and cancer [89]. Two main complexes assembling PcG proteins have been described [90]. The polycomb repressive complex 2 (PRC2) contains the histone methyl transferase Enhancer of Zeste (EZH2) and is involved in methylation of H3K27. The PRC1 complex contains the Polycomb protein, which is involved in recognition of the repressive mark trimethyl-H3K27 through a chromodomain. Recruitment of PRC1 to the chromatin results in ubiquitination of histone H2A. Hence, coordinated action of both complexes is involved in the establishment of a compact chromatin structure, which results in gene silencing. One of the mammalian orthologs of Drosophila Polycomb is Polycomb-2 (Pc2), which has been shown to display SUMO ligase activity, as previously mentioned [23]. Interestingly, two SIMs have been described in Pc2, one of them has been shown to be relevant for the several functions attributed to Pc2 [91]. Among the SUMO substrates identified for Pc2 are the kinase HIPK2 and the corepressor CtBP1 (see also below), sumoylation of which results in enhanced transcription repression [92-94]. CtBP has been shown to colocalize with Pc2 in nuclear foci called PcG bodies, which contain several PcG proteins [95]. Other Pc2 substrates for sumoylation are ZEB2, DNMT3A and centrin-2 [96, 97]. It has been recently reported that Pc2 mediates sumoylation and recruitment of BMI1 at sites of DNA lesions, linking Pc2 ligase activity with the DNA damage response [98]. Several polycomb subunits have been shown to be sumoylated, for instance SUZ12, EZH2 and YY1, although Pc2 has not been involved in the process [99, 100]. A clear role of sumoylation in PcG proteins-mediated repression came from studies in *C. elegans*. The SOP-2 protein is related to Drosophila and vertebrate PRC1-associated PcG proteins Polyhomeotic and Sex combs on midleg (Scm). It has been shown that sumoylation of SOP-2 is required for repression of *Hox* genes in *C. elegans* [101]. Indeed, impaired sumoylation leads to ectopic *Hox* gene expression and homeotic transformations, resulting in a phenotype similar to that provoked by *sop-2* mutations. Additional evidence of SUMO involvement in PcG-mediated repression in vertebrates has been more recently reported. It was previously shown that Pc2 is a target of SUMO [23]. Later, Kang et al demonstrated that sumoylated Pc2 is a target for the SUMO protease SENP2 [102]. In *Senp2* knockout mice, sumoylated Pc2 accumulates, resulting in increased occupancy at promoters of PcG target genes, such as *Gata4* and *Gata6*. As a result, expression of these genes is reduced during development, which leads to embryonic heart defects among other disorders [102]. Chromatin occupancy by PRC2 subunits and levels of trimethyl-H3K27 seem not to be affected, suggesting that Pc2 sumoylation has a role in recognition of H3K27 methylation, which is released by SENP2.

4.3. SUMO-mediated regulation of histone modifications

As previously mentioned, the major impact of sumoylation on histone modification is linked to the role of SUMO in the architecture and function of several chromatin-associated complexes involved in histone modification. Sumoylation by itself may condition the way other histone marks are deposited. However, it has been unambiguously demonstrated that sumoylation is essential for function of a variety of complexes implicated in histone modification, which mostly associate with transcription repression [68, 69]. It has been previously indicated that SUMO is required for the maintenance of constitutive heterochromatin in fission yeast [58]. However, increased evidence of SUMO involvement in the establishment of heterochromatin-like structures in euchromatin loci (facultative heterochromatin) has emerged during the last years. Facultative heterochromatin, besides displaying significant DNA methylation, is characterized by low levels of histone acetylation and histone H3 methylated at Lys4 (H3K4), and high levels of histone H3 methylated at Lys27 (H3K27) and Lys9 (H3K9, di- or tri-methylated), and histone H4 methylated at Lys20 (H4K20, mono-, di- or tri-methylated) [103]. Some of the complexes involved in the establishment of these marks are compiled in Table 3 and described below.

4.3.1. Histone methylation

The histone methyltransferase SETDB1 is involved in tri-methylation of H3K9, a repressive histone mark. The methyl CpG binding protein MBD1 and MCAF1 associate to SETDB1 in a complex, linking DNA methylation to histone methylation. This complex is recruited to the KAP-1 (KRAB associated protein-1) corepressor in a SUMO-dependent manner [26]. In its turn, sumoylated KAP-1 recruits the SETDB1 complex to the chromatin through the zinc finger protein KRAB. This is mediated by a SIM in SETDB1 [26]. In addition, another SIM has been reported in MCAF1, and both MCAF1 and MBD1 are sumoylated [104, 105]. Interestingly, a PHD domain in KAP-1 displays an E3 ligase activity, which promotes intramolecular sumoylation of the adjacent bromodomain [26]. The SETDB1 complex, as explained below, is also recruited to the transcription factor Sp3 in a SUMO dependent manner for transcription repression [106].

Recently, the SUMO ligase PIAS1 has been involved in maintaining an epigenetic repressive state, as studied at the *Foxp3* locus, that restricts differentiation of natural occurring thymus-derived regulatory T cells [107]. Knocking down of *PIAS1* leads to reduced DNA methylation and loss of the repressive mark methyl-H3K9 on the *Foxp3* promoter. A prominent role of PIAS1 in recruitment and association to the DNA methyltransferases DNMT3A and DNMT3B is also reported. In correlation with loss of H3K9 methylation, HP1γ disappears from the *Foxp3* promoter in the absence of PIAS1 [107].

Complex (subunits)	Activity	Recruiting factor
LSD1/CoREST (LSD1, CoREST, BHC80, HDAC1/2, BRAF35, ZEB1, ZNF217/198)	H3K4 demethylation (LSD1) Histone deacetylation (HDAC1/2)	CtBP1
NurD (CHD3/4, HDAC1/2, RbAp46/48, MTA1/2, MBD3/2)	Nucleosome remodeling (CHD3) Histone deacetylation (HDAC1)	KAP-1
SETDB1 (SETDB1, MBD1, MCAF1)	H3K9 tri-methylation (SETDB1)	KAP-1 Sp3
L3MBTL1 (L3MBTL1, HP1)	Methyl-histone recognition (L3MBTL1)	Sp3
dMEC (dMi-2, dMEP-1)	Nucleosome remodeling (dMi-2)	Sp3
PCR2 (EZH2, EED, SUZ12, RbAp46/48)	H3K27 methylation (EZH2)	various
PCR1 (Pc2, PHC, RNF1/2, SCMH)	trimethyl-H3K27 recognition (Pc2)	-

Table 3. SUMO associated repressor complexes. Table summarizes some repressor complexes whose function depends on sumoylation. Examples of different transcription factors involved in recruitment of these complexes are also shown.

4.3.2. Histone demethylation

The histone demethylase LSD1 mediates gene repression by removing methyl groups from mono- or di-methyl-H3K4, which are marks of active transcription [108]. LSD1 works in a corepressor complex together with HDACs and CoREST1 [109, 110]. It has been shown that the LSD1/CoREST complex mediates SUMO-dependent repression of neuronal-specific genes, such as *SCN1A* and *SCN3A*, in non-neuronal cells [111]. Recruitment to the chromatin and repression depends on SUMO2/3 and is mediated by a specific SIM in CoREST. SUMO deconjugation by the SUMO protease SENP3 provokes increased levels of di-methyl-H3K4 and acetyl-H3, which leads to gene activation. Different subunits of the LSD1/CoREST complex have been shown to be sumoylated and/or to contain SIMs (reviewed in [68]). It has been recently shown that sumoylation of the LSD1/CoREST complex subunit BRAF35 controls neuronal differentiation [112]. Overexpression of BRAF35, but not of a sumoylation mutant, strongly impairs neuronal differentiation promoted by neurogenic factors in the vertebrate neural tube. Interestingly, iBRAF, a paralogue of BRAF35 ocasionally associated to the LSD1/CoREST complex, is not sumoylated but is able to dimerize with BRAF35, inhibiting BRAF35 sumoylation and binding to the LSD1/CoREST complex. The LSD1/CoREST complex usually associates with the corepressor CtBP (C-terminal binding protein), which in turn is recruited to the chromatin by a variety of transcription factors [113]. Two CtBPs have been reported in vertebrates, CtBP1 and CtBP2. CtBP1 mediates repression by recruiting a number of repression factors that in addition to LSD1 and HDACs, includes the H3K9 histone methyl-transferase G9a. CtBP1-mediated repression depends on sumoylation [92]. Besides direct interaction of CtBP1 with UBC9, CtBP1 sumoylation is also determined by the SUMO ligases PIAS1, PIAS2 and Pc2 [23, 92, 114]. One of the transcription factors recruiting CtBP1 to the chromatin is the Krüpel-like zinc finger DNA-binding repressor ZEB1, which is also a target for sumoylation [115]. Attachment of SUMO to ZEB1 is required for this factor to display full repression activity [94]. Another zinc finger protein that has been associated with the LSD1/CoREST complex is ZNF198. This factor is both able to be sumoylated and to non-covalently interact with SUMO through a SIM [116-118]. Altogether, these data indicate that SUMO is involved on several functional aspects of the LSD1/CoREST complex: it mediates recruitment of the complex to the chromatin, but also is involved in the architecture of the complex, as different subunits associate to the complex in a sumoylation/SIM-dependent manner.

4.3.3. Histone deacetylation

It has been indicated that repression activity of the LSD1/CoREST complex is in part displayed through HDACs. Indeed, HDAC1 and HDAC2 are components of the LSD1/CoREST complex [110]. Another complex involved in HDAC recruitment to the chromatin is the NuRD (nucleosome remodeling and deacetylation) complex [119]. The core component of the mammalian NuRD complex is the ATP-dependent nucleosome remodeling enzyme CHD3. In addition, this complex includes one or two type I HDACs, histone binding proteins RbAp46 and RbAp48, a methylated DNA-binding protein (MBD2 or MBD3), and members of the MTA and p66 families of proteins [119]. A screening in Drosophila cell cultures identified the CHD3 homologue dMi-2, as a factor required for SUMO dependent repression by Sp3 [64]. dMi-2/CHD3 both sumoylates and is able to interact with SUMO-modified transcription factors through a SIM [26, 64]. Thus, CHD3 also interacts with sumoylated KAP-1 [26]. However, it has been demonstrated that phosphorylation of Ser824 in the C terminus of KAP-1, directly impairs interaction between the CHD3 SIM and the SUMO molecule attached to KAP-1 [120]. Therefore, KAP-1 sumoylation is not affected, but recognition of SUMO by the SIM in CHD3. KAP-1 phosphorylation has a role in double-strand break repair, as displaces the chromatin barrier imposed by CHD3-dependent nucleosome-remodeling activity. Additional components of the NuRD complex have been shown to be sumoylated and/or to contain SIMs: MTA1/2, HDAC1, RbAp48 and p66 [111, 121-123]. Interestingly, phenotype of certain vulval mutants in *C. elegans*, which associate with genes coding for NuRD components [124], is quite similar to that of *SUMO* and *UBC9* mutants [125], indicating that function of the NuRD complex is linked to sumoylation.

SUMO directly associates with HDACs in a variety of ways. As previously indicated a well-established link between SUMO and HDACs is illustrated by the SIM-mediated recruitment of HDACs to sumoylated proteins [56, 121]. It was first demonstrated for HDAC2 recruitment to sumoylated Elk-1 [56], and subsequently for HDACs 1, 3, 4, 5 and 6, and class III SIRT1 deacetylases to several factors. Sumoylation of the coactivator p300 mediates recruitment of class II HDAC6 and class III SIRT1 deacetylases [66, 126]. HDAC1 recruitment to sumoylated Groucho, p68 and reptin has also been described [121, 127, 128]. Moreover, a SUMO-histone H4 fusion has been shown to precipitate HDAC1 [55]. Despite these data, it is not clear at present whether SUMO-dependent recruitment of HDACs involves direct binding of HDAC to SUMO or whether HDACs associate through cofactors recruited in a SUMO-dependent manner, as indicated for the LSD1/CoREST and NuRD complexes. Another example of SUMO-dependent recruitment of HDAC is depicted by the Daxx-mediated recruitment of HDAC2 to sumoylated CBP [67]. In this context, it is worth noting that in a variety of cases, HDAC recruitment does not account for full repression activity mediated by SUMO, as inhibition of HDACs does not relieve SUMO-dependent repression as expected. For instance, it has been shown in a reporter system that repression mediated by a Gal4-SUMO fusion is not sensitive to HDAC inhibition [56], as also occurs for SUMO-dependent Sp3-mediated repression [64, 129]. Despite HDAC2 recruitment by sumoylated Elk-1, HDAC2 knockdown only partially alleviates SUMO-dependent Elk-1-mediated repression [56]. Therefore, histone deacetylases are recruited in a SUMO-dependent manner through repressor complexes, together with additional repressor components, to account for full repression activity of the complex. Conversely, HDAC displacement by target sumoylation has been less reported, but examples have been described. Thus, sumoylation of the Prospero-related homeobox 1 (Prox1) and the de novo DNA methyltransferase DNMT3A disrupts association to HDAC3 and HDAC1/2, respectively [130, 131]. On the other hand, HDACs have also been shown to be substrates for SUMO, which regulates HDAC activity. Then, mutation of the sumoylation sites in HDAC1 has been shown to dramatically reduce its repression activity in a reporter assay [122]. It has been reported that the protease SENP1 is able to remove SUMO from sumoylated HDAC1, which leads to enhanced transcription activity by the androgen receptor [132]. Interestingly, the viral protein Gam1 interferes with HDAC1 sumoylation [133]. The RanBP2 ligase has been demonstrated to promote sumoylation of HDAC4 [134], and a relevant role for SUMO chain formation on HDAC4 has been attributed to the non-covalent interaction between SUMO and UBC9 [135]. Paradoxically, while HDAC1 sumoylation seems to be essential for its repression activity [122], SUMO attachment to HDAC1 impairs association to the CoREST repressor [116]. As previously mentioned, class IIa HDACs have been reported as SUMO ligases. HDAC4 and other class IIa HDACs promote SUMO2/3 attachment to the myocyte enhancer factor 2 family members MEF2D and MEF2C, which leads to repression of target genes [25]. Conversely, ligase activity is inhibited by HDAC4 sumoylation. HDAC4 ligase activity has been also demonstrated on liver X receptors sumoylation by SUMO2/3 [136] and on HIC1 sumoylation by SUMO1 [137], while enhanced sumoylation of PML protein has been attributed to HDAC7 [138].

4.4. Multiple complexes contribute to SUMO-dependent Sp3-mediated repression

Sp3 belongs to the specificity protein (Sp) family of transcription factors, which regulate multiple genes involved in housekeeping, development and cell cycle. Sp3 is expressed ubiquitously and can act either as an activator or a repressor depending on the promoter context [106, 139]. Sp3-mediated repression depends on Sp3 sumoylation, and as previously indicated, this repression activity is not affected by HDAC inhibitors [129, 140].

A genome-wide RNAi screen in Drosophila cell cultures revealed that multiple complexes were involved in SUMO-dependent repression by Sp3 [64]. Among the genes identified whose knockdown impaired SUMO-dependent transcription repression were genes encoding the ATP-dependent chromatin remodeler dMi-2, the Drosophila ortholog of the nematode protein MEP-1 and the polycomb protein Sfmbt. Biochemical analyses indicated that dMi-2, MEP-1 and Sfmbt interacted with each other, bound to SUMO and were recruited to the chromatin in a SUMO-dependent manner. In addition, chromatin immunoprecipitation experiments showed that sumoylated Sp3 recruits a number of heterochromatin associated proteins, including dMi-2, the H3K9 histone methyl transferase (HMT) SETDB1, the H4K20 histone methyl transferase SUV4-20H, heterochromatin protein 1 (HP1) α, ß and γ, and MBT-domain proteins [141].

It has been previously indicated that dMi-2 is the core component of NuRD complex, a complex with associated HDACs. However, Sp3-SUMO-mediated repression is not sensitive to HDACs inhibitors, indicating either that dMi-2 mediates repression outside the NuRD complex or that there is a redundancy in the mechanisms driving Sp3-SUMO-mediated repression. In fact, several data indicate that dMi-2 is also part of another complex lacking HDAC activity. This complex, dMec, is composed by dMi-2 and the Drosophila homolog of the *C. elegans* protein MEP-1 (dMEP-1), and works as a corepressor of proneural genes [142]. Knockdown of dMEP-1 leads to derepression of Sp3 target genes, which is in contrast to functional redundancy among the different repression mechanisms recruited to Sp3 [64]. It is worth noting that MEP-1 was previously shown to contribute to SUMO-dependent repression in *C. elegans* [143]. Thus, sumoylated LIN-1 recruits MEP-1 for repression and inhibition of vulval cell fate. As LIN-1 is homologous to the human Elk-1, it is tempting to speculate that a similar mechanism may account for the SUMO-mediated HDAC-independent repression by Elk-1, despite the absence of a clear MEP-1 homolog in vertebrates.

As formerly mentioned, two HMTs were also recruited to SUMO-Sp3: SETDB1 and SUV4-20H, while the HMT SUV39H1 was not associated [141]. These HMTs were shown to be recruited to the *Dhfr* promoter in a sumoylatable Sp3-dependent manner. Knocking down of *SETDB1* and *SUV4-20H* resulted in reduced trimethylation of H3K9 and H4K20 at the *Dhfr* promoter.

Finally, polycomb protein Sfmbt and the corresponding mammalian orthologs L3MBTL1 and L3MBTL2 also associate to sumoylated Sp3 [64, 141]. These proteins contain repeats of the malignant brain tumor (MBT) domain, which is structurally related to the chromodomain and the Tudor domain, and like these, is able to recognize methylated histones. However, MBTs associate with higher affinity to mono- and di- than to trimethylated histones [144]. It has been shown that L3MBTL1 binds HP1γ and compacts chromatin in a mono- and dimethylated H4K20 and H1bK26-dependent manner [145]. Therefore, this association provides a way to explain L3MBTL1-mediated repression. Binding of HP1α, ß and γ to Sp3 depends on sumoylation [141]. Sumoylated histone H4 recruits HP1γ [55], and HP1α has also been shown to preferentially bind sumoylated SP100 [146], suggesting that, as occurs for HDACs, SUMO mediates HP1 recruitment. As Sfmbt, the PRC2-associated PcG protein Scm also contains MBT repeats. In contrast to Scm, Sfmbt together with Pleiohomeotic, integrates in the polycomb complex PhoRC. Thus, different polycomb complexes include MBT-containing subunits, which might be involved in recognition of mono- and dimethylated histones to facilitate trimethylation by recruiting other subunits with histone methyltransferase activity.

In sum, Sp3 constitutes a paradigm of SUMO-dependent transcription repression through a variety of factors and chromatin-associated complexes. Clear evidence of SUMO involvement in Sp3-mediated repression came from the generation of knock-in mice with a non-sumoylatable version of Sp3 [147]. As Lys residues are targets for other modifications different of sumoylation, for instance acetylation, authors, instead of mutating core Lys551 to Arg changed the acidic residue at the sumoylation site. Interestingly, they substituted Glu by Asp, which abrogated sumoylation, despite for may authors it is assumed the consensus ΨKxE/D. Mutation did not affected Sp3 protein levels. However, spermatocyte-specific genes *Dmc1* and *Dnahc8*, and neuronal genes *Paqr6*, *Rims3* and *Robo3* appeared derepressed in non-testicular and extra-neural tissues and in mouse embryonic fibroblasts [147]. This correlated with loss of the repressive heterochromatin marks trimethyl-H3K9 and trimethyl-H4K20 and affected recruitment of repressor proteins, such as HP1, SETDB1, CHD3, and L3MBTL1/2, to the corresponding promoters. Surprisingly, homozygous knock-in mice born at expected mendelian frequency, were fertile and exhibited no obvious phenotype, in contrast to mice lacking Sp3 [148], suggesting that additional mechanisms may control protein expression from the aberrantly induced transcripts.

5. Conclusions

Sumoylation results essential for development and growth of all the investigated eukaryotes. In mice, embryos lacking the SUMO conjugating enzyme Ubc9 die at the early postimplantation stage, highlighting the relevance of SUMO conjugation during development [149]. The SUMO pathway is conserved from yeast to human and, together with ubiquitination, appears to be the most utilized pathway in post-translational modifications by UBLs. Despite similar structural features and a common evolutionary origin of SUMO and ubiquitin, they have significantly diverged from a functional point of view. In fact, a complete machinery has evolved around SUMO for specific conjugation/deconjugation of this molecule. Compared with ubiquitin, about 20 N-terminal extra amino acids are present in SUMO, which should account for the different and specific SUMO roles. From the many examples of protein modification by SUMO, structural, regulatory, signaling, and scaffold roles are inferred for this molecule. All these aspects convene to reveal SUMO modification as an important post-translational modification involved in transcription repression. Therefore, SUMO prefigures as an adaptor molecule essential for correct assembly and function of a variety of chromatin-associated repressor complexes. This does not exclude that involvement of SUMO in various systems results in transcriptional activation. A number of SUMO-dependent histone modifications and chromatin remodeling activities have been summarized in this chapter (Table 3). They include, HDACs, HMTs and histone demethylase activities, associated to the NuRD, LSD1/CoREST, SETDB1, dMec, L3MBTL1 and Polycomb complexes, which result in chromatin compaction and gene silencing. However, many questions remain open. For instance, whether proteins with intrinsic repression activity like HDACs are directly recruited by SUMO or instead, relevant repression activity in vivo results from association of HDACs to repressor complexes recruited in a SUMO-dependent manner, needs to be clarified. In addition, although HDACs have intrinsic repression activity, it has been shown that sumoylation of HDAC1 accounts for its full repression activity [122], raising the question whether SUMO modulates its activity or is recruiting additional repressors. Another intriguing aspect concerns functional redundancy among the different repressors recruited to a locus via SUMO. A number of repressors are recruited to the chromatin through a Gal4-SUMO2 fusion [123], but it has been shown that individually knocking down of these factors has little consequences in SUMO2 displayed repression, which may be explained by functional redundancy of the multiple repressors associated. In a similar way, downregulation of CHD3 (mammalian dMi-2) or L3MBTL1/2 does not impair Sp3-SUMO-mediated repression in vertebrate cells [64, 141]. However, mutation of *dMi-2* or *Sfmbt* in Drosophila has a significant impact in Sp3-SUMO-dependent repression [64], suggesting that promoter context and local features account for the level of functional redundancy of SUMO-associated repressors. In addition, an important aspect of the SUMO modification concerns the fleeting nature of the modification in many cases, which means that SUMO-SIM interactions may have permanent consequences despite they are not further detected, a notion that implies a kind of memory and that thereby links SUMO to epigenetics. Interestingly, mutation of the SUMO2 SIM in CoREST is sufficient to abrogate repression of some neuronal specific genes in non-neuronal cells [111], highlighting the relevance of the non-covalent interaction of proteins with SUMO in regulating SUMO-dependent repression. In this context, SIMs and sumoylation sites have been described in many subunits within a repressor complex (reviewed in [68]), which rises the question about how the appropriate connections are established.

Abbreviations

CBP, CREB binding protein

DeSI-1, desumoylating isopepyidase-1

EZH2, Enhancer of Zeste

HDAC, histone deacetylase

HMT, histone methyl transferase

KAP-1, KRAB associated protein-1

NDSM, negatively charged residues-dependent SUMO motif

Pc2, polycomb-2

PcG, polycomb group

PCR1/2, polycomb repressive complex 1/2

PDSM, phosphorylation-dependent SUMO motif

PIAS, protein inhibitor of activated STAT

PML, promyelocytic leukaemia protein

SENP, sentrin-specific protease

SIM, SUMO interacting motif

Sp3, specificity protein 3

SP-RING, Siz/PIAS-RING

SUMO, small ubiquitin-like modifier

UBLs, ubiquitin-like proteins

Acknowledgements

Work in the Garcia-Dominguez laboratory is supported by the Spanish National Ministry of Economy and Competitiveness grant BFU2012-37304/BFI. I thank JC Reyes, P Garcia-Gutierrez and F Juarez-Vicente for critical reading of this chapter.

Author details

Garcia-Dominguez Mario

Address all correspondence to: mario.garcia@cabimer.es

Stem Cells Department. Andalusian Center for Molecular Biology and Regenerative Medicine (CABIMER) & High Council for Scientific Research (CSIC), Seville, Spain

References

[1] Hochstrasser M (2009) Origin and function of ubiquitin-like proteins. *Nature* 458: 422-429.

[2] Burroughs AM, Iyer LM, Aravind L (2012) The natural history of ubiquitin and ubiquitin-related domains. *Frontiers in Bioscience* 17: 1433-1460.

[3] Mahajan R, Delphin C, Guan T, Gerace L, Melchior F (1997) A small ubiquitin-related polypeptide involved in targeting RanGAP1 to nuclear pore complex protein RanBP2. *Cell* 88: 97-107.

[4] Matunis MJ, Coutavas E, Blobel G (1996) A novel ubiquitin-like modification modulates the partitioning of the Ran-GTPase-activating protein RanGAP1 between the cytosol and the nuclear pore complex. *The Journal of Cell Biology* 135: 1457-1470.

[5] Muller S, Hoege C, Pyrowolakis G, Jentsch S (2001) SUMO, ubiquitin's mysterious cousin. *Nature Reviews* 2: 202-210.

[6] Weissman AM (2001) Themes and variations on ubiquitylation. *Nature Reviews* 2: 169-178.

[7] Seeler JS, Dejean A (2003) Nuclear and unclear functions of SUMO. *Nature Reviews* 4: 690-699.

[8] Palancade B, Doye V (2008) Sumoylating and desumoylating enzymes at nuclear pores: underpinning their unexpected duties? *Trends in Cell Biology* 18: 174-183.

[9] Hay RT (2005) SUMO: a history of modification. *Molecular Cell* 18: 1-12.

[10] Johnson ES (2004) Protein modification by SUMO. *Annual Review of Biochemistry* 73: 355-382.

[11] Gill G (2005) Something about SUMO inhibits transcription. *Current Opinion in Genetics & Development* 15: 536-541.

[12] Lyst MJ, Stancheva I (2007) A role for SUMO modification in transcriptional repression and activation. *Biochemical Society Transactions* 35: 1389-1392.

[13] Johnson ES, Schwienhorst I, Dohmen RJ, Blobel G (1997) The ubiquitin-like protein Smt3p is activated for conjugation to other proteins by an Aos1p/Uba2p heterodimer. *The EMBO Journal* 16: 5509-5519.

[14] Azuma Y, Tan SH, Cavenagh MM, Ainsztein AM, Saitoh H, Dasso M (2001) Expression and regulation of the mammalian SUMO-1 E1 enzyme. *Faseb Journal* 15: 1825-1827.

[15] Desterro JM, Thomson J, Hay RT (1997) Ubch9 conjugates SUMO but not ubiquitin. *FEBS Letters* 417: 297-300.

[16] Johnson ES, Blobel G (1997) Ubc9p is the conjugating enzyme for the ubiquitin-like protein Smt3p. *The Journal of Biological Chemistry* 272: 26799-26802.

[17] Sampson DA, Wang M, Matunis MJ (2001) The small ubiquitin-like modifier-1 (SUMO-1) consensus sequence mediates Ubc9 binding and is essential for SUMO-1 modification. *The Journal of Biological Chemistry* 276: 21664-21669.

[18] Tatham MH, Chen Y, Hay RT (2003) Role of two residues proximal to the active site of Ubc9 in substrate recognition by the Ubc9.SUMO-1 thiolester complex. *Biochemistry* 42: 3168-3179.

[19] Tatham MH, Kim S, Yu B, Jaffray E, Song J, Zheng J, Rodriguez MS, Hay RT, Chen Y (2003) Role of an N-terminal site of Ubc9 in SUMO-1, -2, and -3 binding and conjugation. *Biochemistry* 42: 9959-9969.

[20] Kotaja N, Karvonen U, Janne OA, Palvimo JJ (2002) PIAS proteins modulate transcription factors by functioning as SUMO-1 ligases. *Molecular and Cellular Biology* 22: 5222-5234.

[21] Sachdev S, Bruhn L, Sieber H, Pichler A, Melchior F, Grosschedl R (2001) PIASy, a nuclear matrix-associated SUMO E3 ligase, represses LEF1 activity by sequestration into nuclear bodies. *Genes & Development* 15: 3088-3103.

[22] Pichler A, Gast A, Seeler JS, Dejean A, Melchior F (2002) The nucleoporin RanBP2 has SUMO1 E3 ligase activity. *Cell* 108: 109-120.

[23] Kagey MH, Melhuish TA, Wotton D (2003) The polycomb protein Pc2 is a SUMO E3. *Cell* 113: 127-137.

[24] Weger S, Hammer E, Heilbronn R (2005) Topors acts as a SUMO-1 E3 ligase for p53 in vitro and in vivo. *FEBS Letters* 579: 5007-5012.

[25] Gregoire S, Yang XJ (2005) Association with class IIa histone deacetylases upregulates the sumoylation of MEF2 transcription factors. *Molecular and Cellular Biology* 25: 2273-2287.

[26] Ivanov AV, Peng H, Yurchenko V, Yap KL, Negorev DG, Schultz DC, Psulkowski E, Fredericks WJ, White DE, Maul GG, Sadofsky MJ, Zhou MM, Rauscher FJ, 3rd (2007) PHD domain-mediated E3 ligase activity directs intramolecular sumoylation of an adjacent bromodomain required for gene silencing. *Molecular Cell* 28: 823-837.

[27] Subramaniam S, Sixt KM, Barrow R, Snyder SH (2009) Rhes, a striatal specific protein, mediates mutant-huntingtin cytotoxicity. *Science* 324: 1327-1330.

[28] Garcia-Gutierrez P, Juarez-Vicente F, Gallardo-Chamizo F, Charnay P, Garcia-Dominguez M (2011) The transcription factor Krox20 is an E3 ligase that sumoylates its Nab coregulators. *EMBO Reports* 12: 1018-1023.

[29] Li SJ, Hochstrasser M (1999) A new protease required for cell-cycle progression in yeast. *Nature* 398: 246-251.

[30] Li SJ, Hochstrasser M (2000) The yeast ULP2 (SMT4) gene encodes a novel protease specific for the ubiquitin-like Smt3 protein. *Molecular and Cellular Biology* 20: 2367-2377.

[31] Nishida T, Tanaka H, Yasuda H (2000) A novel mammalian Smt3-specific isopeptidase 1 (SMT3IP1) localized in the nucleolus at interphase. *European Journal of Biochemistry / FEBS* 267: 6423-6427.

[32] Shin EJ, Shin HM, Nam E, Kim WS, Kim JH, Oh BH, Yun Y (2012) DeSUMOylating isopeptidase: a second class of SUMO protease. *EMBO Reports* 13: 339-346.

[33] Melchior F, Schergaut M, Pichler A (2003) SUMO: ligases, isopeptidases and nuclear pores. *Trends in Biochemical Sciences* 28: 612-618.

[34] Gareau JR, Lima CD (2010) The SUMO pathway: emerging mechanisms that shape specificity, conjugation and recognition. *Nature Reviews* 11: 861-871.

[35] Rytinki MM, Kaikkonen S, Pehkonen P, Jaaskelainen T, Palvimo JJ (2009) PIAS proteins: pleiotropic interactors associated with SUMO. *Cellular and Molecular Life Sciences* 66: 3029-3041.

[36] Garcia-Dominguez M, March-Diaz R, Reyes JC (2008) The PHD domain of plant PIAS proteins mediates sumoylation of bromodomain GTE proteins. *The Journal of Biological Chemistry* 283: 21469-21477.

[37] Yeh ET (2009) SUMOylation and De-SUMOylation: wrestling with life's processes. *The Journal of Biological Chemistry* 284: 8223-8227.

[38] Mukhopadhyay D, Dasso M (2007) Modification in reverse: the SUMO proteases. *Trends in Biochemical Sciences* 32: 286-295.

[39] Gan-Erdene T, Nagamalleswari K, Yin L, Wu K, Pan ZQ, Wilkinson KD (2003) Identification and characterization of DEN1, a deneddylase of the ULP family. *The Journal of Biological Chemistry* 278: 28892-28900.

[40] Wu K, Yamoah K, Dolios G, Gan-Erdene T, Tan P, Chen A, Lee CG, Wei N, Wilkinson KD, Wang R, Pan ZQ (2003) DEN1 is a dual function protease capable of processing the C terminus of Nedd8 and deconjugating hyper-neddylated CUL1. *The Journal of Biological Chemistry* 278: 28882-28891.

[41] Saitoh H, Hinchey J (2000) Functional heterogeneity of small ubiquitin-related protein modifiers SUMO-1 versus SUMO-2/3. *The Journal of Biological Chemistry* 275: 6252-6258.

[42] Bayer P, Arndt A, Metzger S, Mahajan R, Melchior F, Jaenicke R, Becker J (1998) Structure determination of the small ubiquitin-related modifier SUMO-1. *Journal of Molecular Biology* 280: 275-286.

[43] Tatham MH, Jaffray E, Vaughan OA, Desterro JM, Botting CH, Naismith JH, Hay RT (2001) Polymeric chains of SUMO-2 and SUMO-3 are conjugated to protein substrates by SAE1/SAE2 and Ubc9. *The Journal of Biological Chemistry* 276: 35368-35374.

[44] Bohren KM, Nadkarni V, Song JH, Gabbay KH, Owerbach D (2004) A M55V polymorphism in a novel SUMO gene (SUMO-4) differentially activates heat shock transcription factors and is associated with susceptibility to type I diabetes mellitus. *The Journal of Biological Chemistry* 279: 27233-27238.

[45] Owerbach D, McKay EM, Yeh ET, Gabbay KH, Bohren KM (2005) A proline-90 residue unique to SUMO-4 prevents maturation and sumoylation. *Biochemical and Biophysical Research Communications* 337: 517-520.

[46] Wang CY, She JX (2008) SUMO4 and its role in type 1 diabetes pathogenesis. *Diabetes/Metabolism Research and Reviews* 24: 93-102.

[47] Zhu J, Zhu S, Guzzo CM, Ellis NA, Sung KS, Choi CY, Matunis MJ (2008) Small ubiquitin-related modifier (SUMO) binding determines substrate recognition and paralog-selective SUMO modification. *The Journal of Biological Chemistry* 283: 29405-29415.

[48] Kerscher O (2007) SUMO junction-what's your function? New insights through SUMO-interacting motifs. *EMBO Reports* 8: 550-555.

[49] Minty A, Dumont X, Kaghad M, Caput D (2000) Covalent modification of p73alpha by SUMO-1. Two-hybrid screening with p73 identifies novel SUMO-1-interacting proteins and a SUMO-1 interaction motif. *The Journal of Biological Chemistry* 275: 36316-36323.

[50] Bossis G, Melchior F (2006) SUMO: regulating the regulator. *Cell Div* 1: 13.

[51] Boggio R, Colombo R, Hay RT, Draetta GF, Chiocca S (2004) A mechanism for inhibiting the SUMO pathway. *Molecular Cell* 16: 549-561.

[52] Iniguez-Lluhi JA, Pearce D (2000) A common motif within the negative regulatory regions of multiple factors inhibits their transcriptional synergy. *Molecular and Cellular Biology* 20: 6040-6050.

[53] Yang SH, Jaffray E, Hay RT, Sharrocks AD (2003) Dynamic interplay of the SUMO and ERK pathways in regulating Elk-1 transcriptional activity. *Molecular Cell* 12: 63-74.

[54] Holmstrom S, Van Antwerp ME, Iniguez-Lluhi JA (2003) Direct and distinguishable inhibitory roles for SUMO isoforms in the control of transcriptional synergy. *Proceedings of the National Academy of Sciences* USA 100: 15758-15763.

[55] Shiio Y, Eisenman RN (2003) Histone sumoylation is associated with transcriptional repression. *Proceedings of the National Academy of Sciences* USA 100: 13225-13230.

[56] Yang SH, Sharrocks AD (2004) SUMO promotes HDAC-mediated transcriptional repression. *Molecular Cell* 13: 611-617.

[57] Nathan D, Ingvarsdottir K, Sterner DE, Bylebyl GR, Dokmanovic M, Dorsey JA, Whelan KA, Krsmanovic M, Lane WS, Meluh PB, Johnson ES, Berger SL (2006) Histone sumoylation is a negative regulator in Saccharomyces cerevisiae and shows dynamic interplay with positive-acting histone modifications. *Genes & Development* 20: 966-976.

[58] Shin JA, Choi ES, Kim HS, Ho JC, Watts FZ, Park SD, Jang YK (2005) SUMO modification is involved in the maintenance of heterochromatin stability in fission yeast. *Molecular Cell* 19: 817-828.

[59] Hari KL, Cook KR, Karpen GH (2001) The Drosophila Su(var)2-10 locus regulates chromosome structure and function and encodes a member of the PIAS protein family. *Genes & Development* 15: 1334-1348.

[60] Muller S, Berger M, Lehembre F, Seeler JS, Haupt Y, Dejean A (2000) c-Jun and p53 activity is modulated by SUMO-1 modification. *The Journal of Biological Chemistry* 275: 13321-13329.

[61] Wu SY, Chiang CM (2009) Crosstalk between sumoylation and acetylation regulates p53-dependent chromatin transcription and DNA binding. *The EMBO journal*.

[62] Desterro JM, Rodriguez MS, Hay RT (1998) SUMO-1 modification of IkappaBalpha inhibits NF-kappaB activation. *Molecular Cell* 2: 233-239.

[63] Kim J, Cantwell CA, Johnson PF, Pfarr CM, Williams SC (2002) Transcriptional activity of CCAAT/enhancer-binding proteins is controlled by a conserved inhibitory domain that is a target for sumoylation. *The Journal of Biological Chemistry* 277: 38037-38044.

[64] Stielow B, Sapetschnig A, Kruger I, Kunert N, Brehm A, Boutros M, Suske G (2008) Identification of SUMO-dependent chromatin-associated transcriptional repression components by a genome-wide RNAi screen. *Molecular Cell* 29: 742-754.

[65] Shalizi A, Gaudilliere B, Yuan Z, Stegmuller J, Shirogane T, Ge Q, Tan Y, Schulman B, Harper JW, Bonni A (2006) A calcium-regulated MEF2 sumoylation switch controls postsynaptic differentiation. *Science* 311: 1012-1017.

[66] Girdwood D, Bumpass D, Vaughan OA, Thain A, Anderson LA, Snowden AW, Garcia-Wilson E, Perkins ND, Hay RT (2003) P300 transcriptional repression is mediated by SUMO modification. *Molecular Cell* 11: 1043-1054.

[67] Kuo HY, Chang CC, Jeng JC, Hu HM, Lin DY, Maul GG, Kwok RP, Shih HM (2005) SUMO modification negatively modulates the transcriptional activity of CREB-binding protein via the recruitment of Daxx. *Proceedings of the National Academy of Sciences* USA 102: 16973-16978.

[68] Garcia-Dominguez M, Reyes JC (2009) SUMO association with repressor complexes, emerging routes for transcriptional control. *Biochimica et Biophysica Acta* 1789: 451-459.

[69] Ouyang J, Gill G (2009) SUMO engages multiple corepressors to regulate chromatin structure and transcription. *Epigenetics* 4: 440-444.

[70] Yamamoto H, Ihara M, Matsuura Y, Kikuchi A (2003) Sumoylation is involved in beta-catenin-dependent activation of Tcf-4. *The EMBO Journal* 22: 2047-2059.

[71] Wang J, Feng XH, Schwartz RJ (2004) SUMO-1 modification activated GATA4-dependent cardiogenic gene activity. *The Journal of Biological Chemistry* 279: 49091-49098.

[72] Yan Q, Gong L, Deng M, Zhang L, Sun S, Liu J, Ma H, Yuan D, Chen PC, Hu X, Liu J, Qin J, Xiao L, Huang XQ, Zhang J, Li DW (2010) Sumoylation activates the transcrip-

tional activity of Pax-6, an important transcription factor for eye and brain development. *Proceedings of the National Academy of Sciences* USA 107: 21034-21039.

[73] Shyu YC, Lee TL, Ting CY, Wen SC, Hsieh LJ, Li YC, Hwang JL, Lin CC, Shen CK (2005) Sumoylation of p45/NF-E2: nuclear positioning and transcriptional activation of the mammalian beta-like globin gene locus. *Molecular and Cellular Biology* 25: 10365-10378.

[74] Lin X, Liang M, Liang YY, Brunicardi FC, Feng XH (2003) SUMO-1/Ubc9 promotes nuclear accumulation and metabolic stability of tumor suppressor Smad4. *The Journal of Biological Chemistry* 278: 31043-31048.

[75] Wei F, Scholer HR, Atchison ML (2007) Sumoylation of Oct4 enhances its stability, DNA binding, and transactivation. *The Journal of Biological Chemistry* 282: 21551-21560.

[76] Gostissa M, Hengstermann A, Fogal V, Sandy P, Schwarz SE, Scheffner M, Del Sal G (1999) Activation of p53 by conjugation to the ubiquitin-like protein SUMO-1. *The EMBO Journal* 18: 6462-6471.

[77] Wang J, Li A, Wang Z, Feng X, Olson EN, Schwartz RJ (2007) Myocardin sumoylation transactivates cardiogenic genes in pluripotent 10T1/2 fibroblasts. *Molecular and Cellular Biology* 27: 622-632.

[78] Guo B, Sharrocks AD (2009) Extracellular signal-regulated kinase mitogen-activated protein kinase signaling initiates a dynamic interplay between sumoylation and ubiquitination to regulate the activity of the transcriptional activator PEA3. *Molecular and Cellular Biology* 29: 3204-3218.

[79] Terui Y, Saad N, Jia S, McKeon F, Yuan J (2004) Dual role of sumoylation in the nuclear localization and transcriptional activation of NFAT1. *The Journal of Biological Chemistry* 279: 28257-28265.

[80] Goodson ML, Hong Y, Rogers R, Matunis MJ, Park-Sarge OK, Sarge KD (2001) Sumo-1 modification regulates the DNA binding activity of heat shock transcription factor 2, a promyelocytic leukemia nuclear body associated transcription factor. *The Journal of Biological Chemistry* 276: 18513-18518.

[81] Hong Y, Rogers R, Matunis MJ, Mayhew CN, Goodson ML, Park-Sarge OK, Sarge KD (2001) Regulation of heat shock transcription factor 1 by stress-induced SUMO-1 modification. *The Journal of Biological Chemistry* 276: 40263-40267.

[82] Wu SY, Chiang CM (2009) Crosstalk between sumoylation and acetylation regulates p53-dependent chromatin transcription and DNA binding. *The EMBO Journal* 28: 1246-1259.

[83] Zhang Z, Liao B, Xu M, Jin Y (2007) Post-translational modification of POU domain transcription factor Oct-4 by SUMO-1. *Faseb Journal* 21: 3042-3051.

[84] Gomez-del Arco P, Koipally J, Georgopoulos K (2005) Ikaros SUMOylation: switching out of repression. *Molecular and Cellular Biology* 25: 2688-2697.

[85] Rosonina E, Duncan SM, Manley JL (2010) SUMO functions in constitutive transcription and during activation of inducible genes in yeast. *Genes & Development* 24: 1242-1252.

[86] Liu HW, Zhang J, Heine GF, Arora M, Gulcin Ozer H, Onti-Srinivasan R, Huang K, Parvin JD (2012) Chromatin modification by SUMO-1 stimulates the promoters of translation machinery genes. *Nucleic Acids Research*.

[87] Kalocsay M, Hiller NJ, Jentsch S (2009) Chromosome-wide Rad51 spreading and SUMO-H2A.Z-dependent chromosome fixation in response to a persistent DNA double-strand break. *Molecular Cell* 33: 335-343.

[88] Shindo H, Suzuki R, Tsuchiya W, Taichi M, Nishiuchi Y, Yamazaki T PHD finger of the SUMO ligase Siz/PIAS family in rice reveals specific binding for methylated histone H3 at lysine 4 and arginine 2. *FEBS Letters* 586: 1783-1789.

[89] Bracken AP, Helin K (2009) Polycomb group proteins: navigators of lineage pathways led astray in cancer. *Nature Reviews Cancer* 9: 773-784.

[90] Lanzuolo C, Orlando V (2012) Memories from the Polycomb Group Proteins. *Annual Review of Genetics* 46: 559-587.

[91] Yang SH, Sharrocks AD The SUMO E3 ligase activity of Pc2 is coordinated through a SUMO interaction motif. *Molecular and Cellular Biology* 30: 2193-2205.

[92] Lin X, Sun B, Liang M, Liang YY, Gast A, Hildebrand J, Brunicardi FC, Melchior F, Feng XH (2003) Opposed regulation of corepressor CtBP by SUMOylation and PDZ binding. *Molecular Cell* 11: 1389-1396.

[93] Roscic A, Moller A, Calzado MA, Renner F, Wimmer VC, Gresko E, Ludi KS, Schmitz ML (2006) Phosphorylation-dependent control of Pc2 SUMO E3 ligase activity by its substrate protein HIPK2. *Molecular Cell* 24: 77-89.

[94] Wang J, Scully K, Zhu X, Cai L, Zhang J, Prefontaine GG, Krones A, Ohgi KA, Zhu P, Garcia-Bassets I, Liu F, Taylor H, Lozach J, Jayes FL, Korach KS, Glass CK, Fu XD, Rosenfeld MG (2007) Opposing LSD1 complexes function in developmental gene activation and repression programmes. *Nature* 446: 882-887.

[95] van der Vlag J, Otte AP (1999) Transcriptional repression mediated by the human polycomb-group protein EED involves histone deacetylation. *Nat Genet* 23: 474-478.

[96] Klein UR, Nigg EA (2009) SUMO-dependent regulation of centrin-2. *Journal of Cell Science* 122: 3312-3321.

[97] Wotton D, Merrill JC (2007) Pc2 and SUMOylation. *Biochemical Society Transactions* 35: 1401-1404.

[98] Ismail IH, Gagne JP, Caron MC, McDonald D, Xu Z, Masson JY, Poirier GG, Hendzel MJ CBX4-mediated SUMO modification regulates BMI1 recruitment at sites of DNA damage. *Nucleic Acids Research* 40: 5497-5510.

[99] Deng Z, Wan M, Sui G (2007) PIASy-mediated sumoylation of Yin Yang 1 depends on their interaction but not the RING finger. *Molecular and Cellular Biology* 27: 3780-3792.

[100] Riising EM, Boggio R, Chiocca S, Helin K, Pasini D (2008) The polycomb repressive complex 2 is a potential target of SUMO modifications. *PLoS ONE* 3: e2704.

[101] Zhang H, Smolen GA, Palmer R, Christoforou A, van den Heuvel S, Haber DA (2004) SUMO modification is required for in vivo Hox gene regulation by the Caenorhabditis elegans Polycomb group protein SOP-2. *Nature Genetics* 36: 507-511.

[102] Kang X, Qi Y, Zuo Y, Wang Q, Zou Y, Schwartz RJ, Cheng J, Yeh ET (2010) SUMO-specific protease 2 is essential for suppression of polycomb group protein-mediated gene silencing during embryonic development. *Molecular Cell* 38: 191-201.

[103] Trojer P, Reinberg D (2007) Facultative heterochromatin: is there a distinctive molecular signature? *Molecular Cell* 28: 1-13.

[104] Lyst MJ, Nan X, Stancheva I (2006) Regulation of MBD1-mediated transcriptional repression by SUMO and PIAS proteins. *The EMBO Journal* 25: 5317-5328.

[105] Uchimura Y, Ichimura T, Uwada J, Tachibana T, Sugahara S, Nakao M, Saitoh H (2006) Involvement of SUMO modification in MBD1- and MCAF1-mediated heterochromatin formation. *The Journal of Biological Chemistry* 281: 23180-23190.

[106] Valin A, Gill G (2007) Regulation of the dual-function transcription factor Sp3 by SUMO. *Biochemical Society Transactions* 35: 1393-1396.

[107] Liu B, Tahk S, Yee KM, Fan G, Shuai K (2010) The ligase PIAS1 restricts natural regulatory T cell differentiation by epigenetic repression. *Science* 330: 521-525.

[108] Shi Y, Lan F, Matson C, Mulligan P, Whetstine JR, Cole PA, Casero RA (2004) Histone demethylation mediated by the nuclear amine oxidase homolog LSD1. *Cell* 119: 941-953.

[109] Lee MG, Wynder C, Cooch N, Shiekhattar R (2005) An essential role for CoREST in nucleosomal histone 3 lysine 4 demethylation. *Nature* 437: 432-435.

[110] Shi YJ, Matson C, Lan F, Iwase S, Baba T, Shi Y (2005) Regulation of LSD1 histone demethylase activity by its associated factors. *Molecular Cell* 19: 857-864.

[111] Ouyang J, Shi Y, Valin A, Xuan Y, Gill G (2009) Direct binding of CoREST1 to SUMO-2/3 contributes to gene-specific repression by the LSD1/CoREST1/HDAC complex. *Molecular Cell* 34: 145-154.

[112] Ceballos-Chavez M, Rivero S, Garcia-Gutierrez P, Rodriguez-Paredes M, Garcia-Dominguez M, Bhattacharya S, Reyes JC (2012) Control of neuronal differentiation

by sumoylation of BRAF35, a subunit of the LSD1-CoREST histone demethylase complex. *Proceedings of the National Academy of Sciences* USA 109: 8085-8090.

[113] Chinnadurai G (2007) Transcriptional regulation by C-terminal binding proteins. *The International Journal of Biochemistry and Cell Biology* 39: 1593-1607.

[114] Kagey MH, Melhuish TA, Powers SE, Wotton D (2005) Multiple activities contribute to Pc2 E3 function. *The EMBO Journal* 24: 108-119.

[115] Kuppuswamy M, Vijayalingam S, Zhao LJ, Zhou Y, Subramanian T, Ryerse J, Chinnadurai G (2008) Role of the PLDLS-binding cleft region of CtBP1 in recruitment of core and auxiliary components of the corepressor complex. *Molecular and Cellular Biology* 28: 269-281.

[116] Gocke CB, Yu H (2008) ZNF198 stabilizes the LSD1-CoREST-HDAC1 complex on chromatin through its MYM-type zinc fingers. *PLoS ONE* 3: e3255.

[117] Gocke CB, Yu H, Kang J (2005) Systematic identification and analysis of mammalian small ubiquitin-like modifier substrates. *The Journal of Biological Chemistry* 280: 5004-5012.

[118] Kunapuli P, Kasyapa CS, Chin SF, Caldas C, Cowell JK (2006) ZNF198, a zinc finger protein rearranged in myeloproliferative disease, localizes to the PML nuclear bodies and interacts with SUMO-1 and PML. *Experimental Cell Research* 312: 3739-3751.

[119] Denslow SA, Wade PA (2007) The human Mi-2/NuRD complex and gene regulation. *Oncogene* 26: 5433-5438.

[120] Goodarzi AA, Kurka T, Jeggo PA (2011) KAP-1 phosphorylation regulates CHD3 nucleosome remodeling during the DNA double-strand break response. *Nature Structural & Molecular Biology* 18: 831-839.

[121] Ahn JW, Lee YA, Ahn JH, Choi CY (2009) Covalent conjugation of Groucho with SUMO-1 modulates its corepressor activity. *Biochemical and Biophysical Research Communications* 379: 160-165.

[122] David G, Neptune MA, DePinho RA (2002) SUMO-1 modification of histone deacetylase 1 (HDAC1) modulates its biological activities. *The Journal of Biological Chemistry* 277: 23658-23663.

[123] Rosendorff A, Sakakibara S, Lu S, Kieff E, Xuan Y, DiBacco A, Shi Y, Shi Y, Gill G (2006) NXP-2 association with SUMO-2 depends on lysines required for transcriptional repression. *Proceedings of the National Academy of Sciences* USA 103: 5308-5313.

[124] Solari F, Ahringer J (2000) NURD-complex genes antagonise Ras-induced vulval development in Caenorhabditis elegans. *Current Biology* 10: 223-226.

[125] Poulin G, Dong Y, Fraser AG, Hopper NA, Ahringer J (2005) Chromatin regulation and sumoylation in the inhibition of Ras-induced vulval development in Caenorhabditis elegans. *The EMBO Journal* 24: 2613-2623.

[126] Bouras T, Fu M, Sauve AA, Wang F, Quong AA, Perkins ND, Hay RT, Gu W, Pestell RG (2005) SIRT1 deacetylation and repression of p300 involves lysine residues 1020/1024 within the cell cycle regulatory domain 1. *The Journal of Biological Chemistry* 280: 10264-10276.

[127] Jacobs AM, Nicol SM, Hislop RG, Jaffray EG, Hay RT, Fuller-Pace FV (2007) SUMO modification of the DEAD box protein p68 modulates its transcriptional activity and promotes its interaction with HDAC1. *Oncogene* 26: 5866-5876.

[128] Kim JH, Choi HJ, Kim B, Kim MH, Lee JM, Kim IS, Lee MH, Choi SJ, Kim KI, Kim SI, Chung CH, Baek SH (2006) Roles of sumoylation of a reptin chromatin-remodelling complex in cancer metastasis. *Nature Cell Biology* 8: 631-639.

[129] Ross S, Best JL, Zon LI, Gill G (2002) SUMO-1 modification represses Sp3 transcriptional activation and modulates its subnuclear localization. *Molecular Cell* 10: 831-842.

[130] Ling Y, Sankpal UT, Robertson AK, McNally JG, Karpova T, Robertson KD (2004) Modification of de novo DNA methyltransferase 3a (Dnmt3a) by SUMO-1 modulates its interaction with histone deacetylases (HDACs) and its capacity to repress transcription. *Nucleic Acids Research* 32: 598-610.

[131] Shan SF, Wang LF, Zhai JW, Qin Y, Ouyang HF, Kong YY, Liu J, Wang Y, Xie YH (2008) Modulation of transcriptional corepressor activity of prospero-related homeobox protein (Prox1) by SUMO modification. *FEBS Letters* 582: 3723-3728.

[132] Cheng J, Wang D, Wang Z, Yeh ET (2004) SENP1 enhances androgen receptor-dependent transcription through desumoylation of histone deacetylase 1. *Molecular and Cellular Biology* 24: 6021-6028.

[133] Colombo R, Boggio R, Seiser C, Draetta GF, Chiocca S (2002) The adenovirus protein Gam1 interferes with sumoylation of histone deacetylase 1. *EMBO Reports* 3: 1062-1068.

[134] Kirsh O, Seeler JS, Pichler A, Gast A, Muller S, Miska E, Mathieu M, Harel-Bellan A, Kouzarides T, Melchior F, Dejean A (2002) The SUMO E3 ligase RanBP2 promotes modification of the HDAC4 deacetylase. *The EMBO Journal* 21: 2682-2691.

[135] Knipscheer P, van Dijk WJ, Olsen JV, Mann M, Sixma TK (2007) Noncovalent interaction between Ubc9 and SUMO promotes SUMO chain formation. *The EMBO Journal* 26: 2797-2807.

[136] Ghisletti S, Huang W, Ogawa S, Pascual G, Lin ME, Willson TM, Rosenfeld MG, Glass CK (2007) Parallel SUMOylation-dependent pathways mediate gene- and signal-specific transrepression by LXRs and PPARgamma. *Molecular Cell* 25: 57-70.

[137] Stankovic-Valentin N, Deltour S, Seeler J, Pinte S, Vergoten G, Guerardel C, Dejean A, Leprince D (2007) An acetylation/deacetylation-SUMOylation switch through a phylogenetically conserved psiKXEP motif in the tumor suppressor HIC1 regulates transcriptional repression activity. *Molecular and Cellular Biology* 27: 2661-2675.

[138] Gao C, Ho CC, Reineke E, Lam M, Cheng X, Stanya KJ, Liu Y, Chakraborty S, Shih HM, Kao HY (2008) Histone deacetylase 7 promotes PML sumoylation and is essential for PML nuclear body formation. *Molecular and Cellular Biology* 28: 5658-5667.

[139] Li L, He S, Sun JM, Davie JR (2004) Gene regulation by Sp1 and Sp3. *Biochemistry and Cell Biology* 82: 460-471.

[140] Sapetschnig A, Rischitor G, Braun H, Doll A, Schergaut M, Melchior F, Suske G (2002) Transcription factor Sp3 is silenced through SUMO modification by PIAS1. *The EMBO Journal* 21: 5206-5215.

[141] Stielow B, Sapetschnig A, Wink C, Kruger I, Suske G (2008) SUMO-modified Sp3 represses transcription by provoking local heterochromatic gene silencing. *EMBO Reports* 9: 899-906.

[142] Kunert N, Wagner E, Murawska M, Klinker H, Kremmer E, Brehm A (2009) dMec: a novel Mi-2 chromatin remodelling complex involved in transcriptional repression. *The EMBO Journal* 28: 533-544.

[143] Leight ER, Glossip D, Kornfeld K (2005) Sumoylation of LIN-1 promotes transcriptional repression and inhibition of vulval cell fates. *Development* 132: 1047-1056.

[144] Kim J, Daniel J, Espejo A, Lake A, Krishna M, Xia L, Zhang Y, Bedford MT (2006) Tudor, MBT and chromo domains gauge the degree of lysine methylation. *EMBO Reports* 7: 397-403.

[145] Trojer P, Li G, Sims RJ, 3rd, Vaquero A, Kalakonda N, Boccuni P, Lee D, Erdjument-Bromage H, Tempst P, Nimer SD, Wang YH, Reinberg D (2007) L3MBTL1, a histone-methylation-dependent chromatin lock. *Cell* 129: 915-928.

[146] Seeler JS, Marchio A, Losson R, Desterro JM, Hay RT, Chambon P, Dejean A (2001) Common properties of nuclear body protein SP100 and TIF1alpha chromatin factor: role of SUMO modification. *Molecular and Cellular Biology* 21: 3314-3324.

[147] Stielow B, Kruger I, Diezko R, Finkernagel F, Gillemans N, Kong-a-San J, Philipsen S, Suske G (2010) Epigenetic silencing of spermatocyte-specific and neuronal genes by SUMO modification of the transcription factor Sp3. *PLoS Genetics* 6: e1001203.

[148] Bouwman P, Gollner H, Elsasser HP, Eckhoff G, Karis A, Grosveld F, Philipsen S, Suske G (2000) Transcription factor Sp3 is essential for post-natal survival and late tooth development. *The EMBO Journal* 19: 655-661.

[149] Nacerddine K, Lehembre F, Bhaumik M, Artus J, Cohen-Tannoudji M, Babinet C, Pandolfi PP, Dejean A (2005) The SUMO pathway is essential for nuclear integrity and chromosome segregation in mice. *Developmental Cell* 9: 769-779.

Section 2

Chromatin Remodeling in Regulating Gene Expression

Chapter 3

SWI/SNF Chromatin Remodeling Complex Involved in RNA Polymerase II Elongation Process in *Drosophila melanogaster*

Nadezhda E. Vorobyeva, Marina U. Mazina and
Semen A. Doronin

Additional information is available at the end of the chapter

http://dx.doi.org/10.5772/55877

1. Introduction

After more than a decade of studying the chromatin remodeling, better view of the function mechanisms of the chromatin remodeling complexes has been developed. It was found that chromatin remodeling complexes facilitate transcription of genes by reducing the nucleosome density on specific genomic regions, such as enhancers and promoters, and increasing their affinity to activators and activator-binding complexes. Moreover, the importance of the chromatin remodeling complexes for transcriptional repression has been shown recently [1, 2]. Therefore chromatin remodeling complexes appear to be involved in nearly all aspects of transcription regulation [3].

At present, the SWI/SNF chromatin remodeling complex is considered to be a significant player in the process of RNA Polymerase II transcription initiation. Recruitment of the complex precedes other transcriptional events and is important for the binding of the general transcriptional machinery [4]. The interplay between chromatin remodeling and general transcriptional factors is so close, that these complexes may unite into physically stable formations termed supercomplexes [5]. An example of such cooperation has been demonstrated for the *Drosophila* SWI/SNF (dSWI/SNF) and TFIID complexes with the SAYP coactivator as a linchpin unit [6].

Recently, abundant evidence concerning SWI/SNF participation in the process of RNA Polymerase II elongation has been reported. It has been demonstrated that the SWI/SNF complex does not leave the promoter after general transcriptional factors recruitment but is involved in transcription elongation and co-transcriptional events. In addition SWI/SNF direct influence on alternative splicing has been revealed in several studies. Using the human *CD44* gene as a model it has been shown that SWI/SNF decreases the elongation rate of RNA Polymerase II and facilitates the alternative exons incorporation. Moreover, biochemical interaction of human SWI/SNF (hSWI/SNF) complex with splicing machinery including both protein factor Sam68 and snRNAs of sliceosome has been demonstrated [7]. Later, a protein complex containing $p54^{nrb}$ and PSF factors of mRNA splicing and one of the hSWI/SNF ATPase subunit hBrg1 has been biochemically purified. The influence of the hBrg1 subunit knockdown on the alternative exons incorporation in the *TERT* gene transcripts has been demonstrated. It has been shown that hBrg1 knockdown leads to growth arrest and senescence of the human cells [8].

Further the several evidences concerning SWI/SNF complex role in mRNP processing in insects have been published. The knockdown of core *Drosophila melanogaster* SWI/SNF (dSWI/SNF) subunits has been shown to facilitate the alternative splicing of several *Drosophila* genes both in culturing cells and in the larvae [9]. Recently, physical association of the SWI/SNF complex with pre-mRNP of *Chironomus tentans* was demonstrated both biochemically and by immune-electron microscopy [10]. Thus participation of SWI/SNF complex in RNA Polymerase II elongation coupled events is not the distinctive feature of mammals but the evolutionary conserved phenomenon.

The participation in other important steps of the RNA Polymerase II elongation process has been described for the SWI/SNF complex in addition to its significance for the alternative pre-mRNP splicing. The accumulation of the SWI/SNF complex in the coding region of the genes during active transcription has been demonstrated for the yeast. Yeast genes, tested in that study, do not have introns. So, the presence of the SWI/SNF complex inside the coding region of yeast genes could not be explained by its interaction with splicing machinery. ySWI/SNF complex is rather important for the RNA Polymerase II elongation process. It has been shown, that the swi2Δ mutant (the ATPase subunit of the yeast SWI/SNF) possesses heightened sensitivity to the drugs that inhibit RNA Polymerase II elongation [11].

Similar data has been obtained for the human *hsp70* gene which, like the yeast genes, contains no introns at all. The SWI/SNF but not ISWI complex (another type of chromatin remodeling complex) binding to the coding region of the mouse *hsp70* during active transcription has been shown. Like the yeast counterpart, the homologous SWI/SNF complex of the human has demonstrated sensitivity to the drug (α-amanitin) which suppresses RNA Polymerase II elongation. Amanitin treatment led to a dramatic decrease in the level of SWI/SNF binding to the coding region of the *hsp70* gene during active transcription. It has been shown that point mutations of the HSF1 factor, which disrupts transcription elongation but not initiation of *hsp70* transcription, also causes a dramatic decrease in the SWI/SNF complex binding to the gene [12].

Participation of the SWI/SNF complex in RNA Polymerase II elongation process on the intronless genes like yeast genes and human *hsp70* indicates, that its function during transcription is not limited to splicing events. Moreover, importance of the SWI/SNF for the RNA Polymerase II elongation process itself has been demonstrated.

Furthermore, the evidence concerning SWI/SNF complex participation in RNA Polymerase II transition from the initiation to the productive elongation state has been described in the last two years. *Drosophila melanogaster* developmental *ftz-f1* gene was used as a model gene to demonstrate the role of dSWI/SNF in RNA Polymerase II pausing process. It has been demonstrated that dSWI/SNF complex participates in the organization of the repressed gene state via the pausing of the RNA Polymerase II. Moreover dSWI/SNF has been revealed to be important for the transient pausing of RNA Polymerase II during active transcription. So, the significance of the dSWI/SNF for the proper elongation and Ser2 CTD phosphorylation marker loading has been demonstrated for the same gene during the active transcription state [13]. Furthermore, the influence of the SWI/SNF complex on the RNA Polymerase II transition to the elongation state has been reported for the human. It has been shown that human SWI/SNF stimulates the occasional transcriptional elongation of the HIV-1 provirus in the absence of the Tat activator thus disrupting the early termination of the short viral transcripts [14]. There are a number of studies that indicate association of SWI/SNF with the process of RNA Polymerase II elongation but the exact function of the complex during the process remains to be seen.

The first and simplest model of SWI/SNF function during elongation that comes to mind is that SWI/SNF assists RNA Polymerase II in overcoming the nucleosome barriers during elongation. This idea complies with the general view on SWI/SNF functions but is not in a good correlation with the results of the splicing studies. According to that studies the SWI/SNF complex slows down RNA Polymerase II elongation rate rather than stimulates it. This conclusion has been made by investigators on the base of the mutation and knockdown experiments where the incorporation rate of longer exons during transcription processing decreased upon SWI/SNF complex disruption. One more evidence could be concluded from these splicing studies: the RNA Polymerase II complex does not require the SWI/SNF complex for the productive elongation on the intron-containing genes. The SWI/SNF complex knock-down performed in the experiments impaired splicing of the genes transcripts but had no effect on the total transcription level [7]. On the other hand, it has been demonstrated recently that RNA Polymerase II complex alone could overcome the nucleosome barrier, suggesting that there is no urgent need for the special remodeling enzymes [15]. Thus, SWI/SNF functions during transcription elongation are not completely clear and still need to be investigated.

The *Drosophila melanogaster* (d) dSWI/SNF chromatin remodeling complex is comprised of the two types of the subcomplexes PBAP and BAP (in mammals, PBAF and BAF respectively). These subcomplexes share several common subunits and Brahma ATPase, but also contain several specific subunits: OSA in the BAP complex and Polybromo, Bap170 and SAYP in PBAP [16][17]. These subcomplexes control the expression of different, but partially overlapping gene patterns and are involved in different functions of the dSWI/SNF complex. For example, BAP but not the PBAP subcomplex is important for proper cell cycle progression [18]. However one question still remains uninvestigated: are there differences in the molecular mechanisms of the subcomplexes functioning, e.g., in the way they remodel histones or in the specific actions they perform.

The main idea of this work is to clarify the next issue: which of the two dSWI/SNF subcomplex-es is involved in the new function of the dSWI/SNF complex and accompanies RNA Polymerase II during transcription elongation. For that goal we have generated and characterized antibodies against the BAP170 and OSA subunits of the PBAP and BAP subcomplexes of the dSWI/SNF complex respectively. Using them we have investigated the changes in distribution of the subcomplexes along the *ftz-f1* and *hsp70* genes upon activation of transcription.

2. Results

2.1. Polyclonal antibodies against PBAP and BAP subcomplexes specific subunits generation and purification

Plasmids, containing two different fragments of BAP170 protein tagged with a 6xHis, for expression in prokaryotic system were generously provided by P. Verrijzer and Y. Moshkin (Erasmus University Medical Center, Rotterdam, The Netherlands)[16]. Expressed antigens were purified on Ni-NTA agarose. The quality of the purified antigens was examined by PAGE with subsequent Coomassie blue staining (Figure1A). Specific antibodies against BAP170 protein were raised in rabbits by series of immunization with both of the antigens. Antibodies were affinity purified from the obtained sera by the column with the antigens immobilized. The quality of the generated antibody was analyzed by Western blot (Figure1B). *Drosophila melanogaster* embryonic nuclear extract (from 0-12h embryo) were loaded on the Western blot for the analysis. Thus the affinity purified antibodies are effective against Bap170.

Antibodies against OSA specific subunit of BAP subcomplex were generated by the same scheme as BAP170 antibodies was. Sequence coding 108-330 aa of OSA were subcloned into pET system for the antigen expression in *E.coli*. Purified OSA antigen was used for the immunization (Figure1C). After series of immunization sera was affinity purified by OSA antigen immobilized on the sepharose column. The sera and purified antibodies were analyzed on Western blot with *Drosophila* embryonic nuclear extract loaded (Figure1D).

2.2. Antibodies against PBAP and BAP-specific subunits precipitate the common subunit but do not precipitate each other

The SWI/SNF chromatin remodeling complex of *Drosophila* is comprised of two different subclasses of remodeling complexes: PBAP and BAP. These subcomplexes reveal different targeting through the *Drosophila* genome and possess different functions. But the main divergence between the subcomplexes is their ability to form protein complexes, which could be separated biochemically. The specific subunits of the subcomplexes interact with the common subunits of dSWI/SNF (like BRM, MOR, BAP111, SNR1 etc.) but fail to precipitate the specific subunits of another subcomplex.

To confirm the specificity of antibodies generated against specific subunits of dSWI/SNF complex the immunoprecipitation experiment was performed (Figure2). The subcomplexes of the dSWI/SNF complex were precipitated from the crude lysate of the S2 Schneider cells by the generated antibodies against BAP170 and OSA subunits. S2 Schneider cells are the most widely used cells for the investigation of *Drosophila* proteins [19]. Both generated antibodies successfully

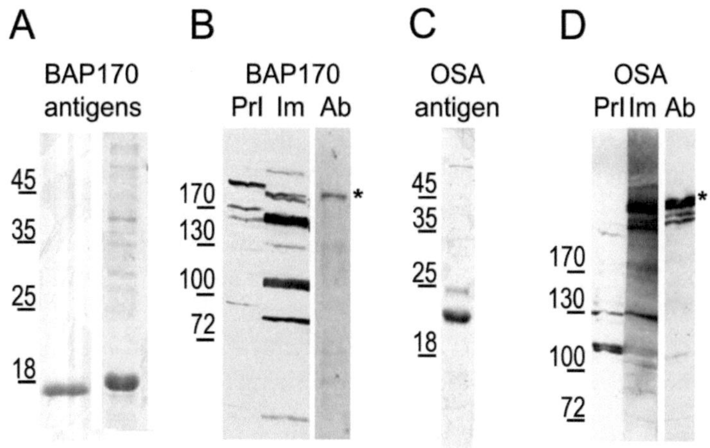

Figure 1. Polyclonal antibodies against PBAP and BAP subcomplexes specific subunits generation and purification A) The antigens, used for the antibodies against BAP170 subunit generation, were purified and loaded on the PAGE (Coomassie blue staining) B) The *Drosophila* embryonic nuclear extract was loaded on the Western blot and stained with the serum of rabbit immunized with BAP170 antigens (Im), the serum before immunization (Prl) and affinity purified antibodies against BAP170 protein. The BAP170 protein recognized with the antibodies is marked with asterisk. C) The antigen, used for the antibodies against OSA subunit generation, was purified and loaded on the PAGE (Coomassie blue staining) D) The Drosophila embryonic nuclear extract was loaded on the Western blot and stained with the serum of rabbit immunized with OSA antigen (Im), the serum before immunization (Prl) and affinity purified antibodies against OSA protein. The OSA protein recognized with the antibodies is marked with asterisk.

precipitated the corresponding proteins and completely depleted them from the cell lysate. Both specific subunits of the PBAP and BAP subcomplexes (BAP170 and OSA correspondingly) successfully co-precipitated the common MOR subunit of dSWI/SNF but failed to precipitate the specific subunits of other subcomplex. Therefore the generated antibodies against BAP170 and OSA could specifically precipitate the corresponding subcomplex.

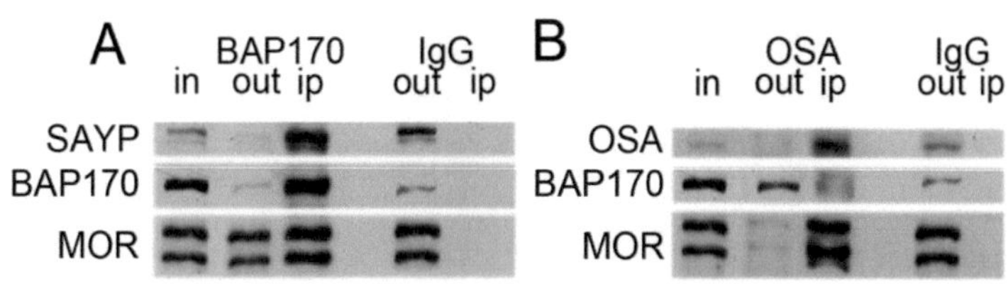

Figure 2. The immunoprecipitation of the dSWI/SNF protein complex from the S2 Schneider cells lysate by antibodies against BAP170 and OSA subunits (in – input; out – output; ip – immunoprecipitation) A) The immunoprecipitation of the dSWI/SNF complex with the anti-BAP170 antibodies. The Western blot was stained with the antibodies against SAYP, BAP170 and MOR subunits of the dSWI/SNF complex. As a negative control for the immunoprecipitation serum of non-immunized rabbits (IgG fraction) was taken. B) The immunoprecipitation of the dSWI/SNF complex with the anti-OSA antibodies. The Western blot was stained with the antibodies against OSA, BAP170 and MOR subunits of the dSWI/SNF complex. As a negative control for the immunoprecipitation serum of non-immunized rabbits (IgG fraction) was taken.

2.3. Both PBAP and BAP subcomplexes of dSWI/SNF chromatin remodeling complex are detected on the promoter of the ftz-f1 gene

The generated antibodies were tested in the chromatin immunoprecipitation experiment on S2 Schneider cells. According to our previous studies, the promoter of the *ftz-f1* ecdysone cascade gene with a high affinity binds the PBAP subcomplex of the dSWI/SNF [13]. It was demonstrated for the PB- and SAYP-specific subunits of PBAP subcomplex. Therefore, BAP170 is expected to bind the promoter of the *ftz-f1* gene. There are no published results about the BAP subcomplex binding to the target genes. But there are some data which represents the PBAP and BAP subcomplexes overlapping targeting across the *Drosophila* genome. These data were obtained from the experiments with the polythene chromosome staining [18]. So, we expected both the BAP and PBAP subcomplexes binding to the *ftz-f1* gene promoter.

Two types of negative controls were used in chromatin immunoprecipitation experiment: PrA resin without any antibody bound (to demonstrate that there is no non-specific binding of *ftz-f1* promoter) and secondly, primers for the 28S rDNA region amplification for analysis the specificity of binding to *ftz-f1* promoter region but not throughout the genome. The locus of rDNA was chosen as a negative control because in our previous studies it did not bind the common subunits of the dSWI/SNF complex [13]. The results of chromatin immunoprecipitation are shown on Figure 3. As expected, both generated antibodies against the PBAP and BAP subcomplexes successfully precipitated the promoter region of *ftz-f1* gene ("0" primer pair in the description) while showed no affinity to the 28S rDNA locus.

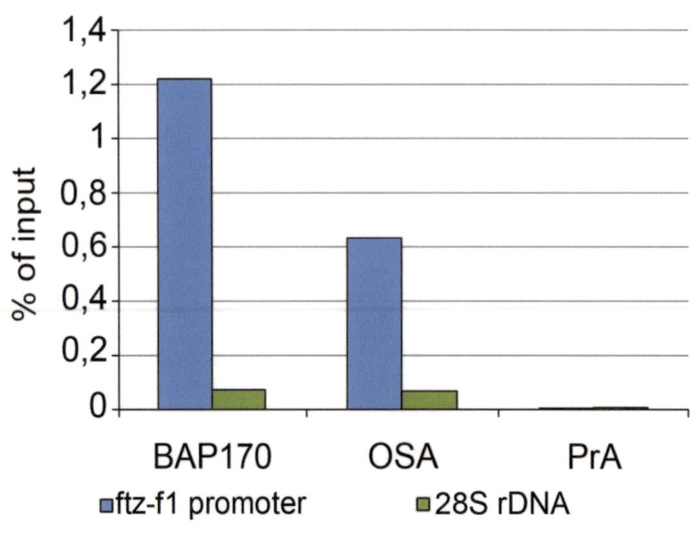

Figure 3. The immunoprecipitation of the chromatin (ChIP) from the S2 Schneider cells with antibodies against BAP170 and OSA subunits of dSWI/SNF complex. The blue bar represents the RT-PCR analysis of the ChIP experiment with the primers to the *ftz-f1* promoter region ("0" point in the description). The green bar represents the analysis with the primers to the 28S rDNA locus (negative control). The results of the chromatin immunoprecipitation experiment were calculated as a % of precipitated chromatin relative to input fraction.

Therefore we have proved the fact of simultaneous PBAP and BAP recruitment on the promoter region of the same gene. The *ftz-f1* gene is an example of the target gene for both of the subcomplexes.

2.4. PBAP but not BAP subcomplex of the dSWI/SNF complex is accumulated at the coding region of the ftz-f1 gene after transcription activation

In our previous studies we have described in details the scheme which makes possible to activate the *Drosophila* developmental *ftz-f1* gene in S2 Schneider cells [13]. A simultaneous recruitment of the BAP170 and OSA subunits to the promoter of this gene in a non-activated stage (in normal S2 Schneider cells) was demonstrated above. To evaluate which one of the dSWI/SNF subcomplexes assists RNA Polymerase II in elongation process we have studied the re-distribution of the subunits on the *ftz-f1* gene upon transcription activation.

Earlier, we have described the multistep scheme of the *ftz-f1* gene activation by the addition and subsequent withdrawal of the 20 hydroxyecdysone (below, referred to simply as ecdysone) hormone into the S2 Schneider cells culturing medium [13]. The main steps of the induction system are schematically presented in the Figure 4. The ecdysone is the main regulator of the ecdysone cascade and its addition to the cell medium induces the expression of the DHR3 nuclear receptor, the activator protein for the *ftz-f1* gene. In spite of DHR3 activator recruitment on the *ftz-f1* promoter soon after DHR3 protein expression, the activation of the *ftz-f1* transcription does not start until the level of the ecdysone in the medium decreases close to basal level. Previously, we have shown that at the high ecdysone concentration, the DHR3 receptor settles on the promoter region of the *ftz-f1* gene and stimulates the formation of the PIC complex by increasing the level of TFIID and dSWI/SNF complexes and as a consequence RNA Polymerase II binding to the promoter. But transcription of the *ftz-f1* gene at this stage does not start because recruited RNA Polymerase II is not in fully active state. It bears the Ser5 phosphorylation marker on its CTD domain but lacks the Ser2 phosphorylation marker which is an illustrator of a RNA Polymerase II elongation-competent state. So, the *ftz-f1* gene in our scheme of activation has preliminary activation state with pre-recruited activator and with RNA Polymerase II poised for the transcription elongation. This phenomenon is called RNA Polymerase II pausing. The ecdysone withdrawal from the culturing medium causes removing of the repressive signal and disturbs the RNA Polymerase II complex pausing state. That leads to the productive transcription elongation and synthesis of the *ftz-f1* gene full-length transcripts.

Two steps, required to verify the *ftz-f1* activation scheme were performed: the 1 μM ecdysone addition (overnight) and subsequent triple washing with the fresh Schneider medium. The level of the *ftz-f1* gene transcription was measured in all activation stages: in the ecdysone-free medium (–), after overnight cultivation in the ecdysone-containing medium (+), and finally 4 hours after ecdysone withdrawal from the culturing medium (+;–). As expected, the *ftz-f1* was not transcribed during (–) and (+) stages and significantly activated 4 hours after the ecdysone removal in (+;–) stage (see Figure 5).

Next, the distribution of the BAP170 and OSA subunits of the dSWI/SNF complex along the *ftz-f1* gene on different stages of activation was analyzed by the chromatin immunoprecipitation technique (see Figure 6A and B). Both of the proteins were readily bound to the promoter

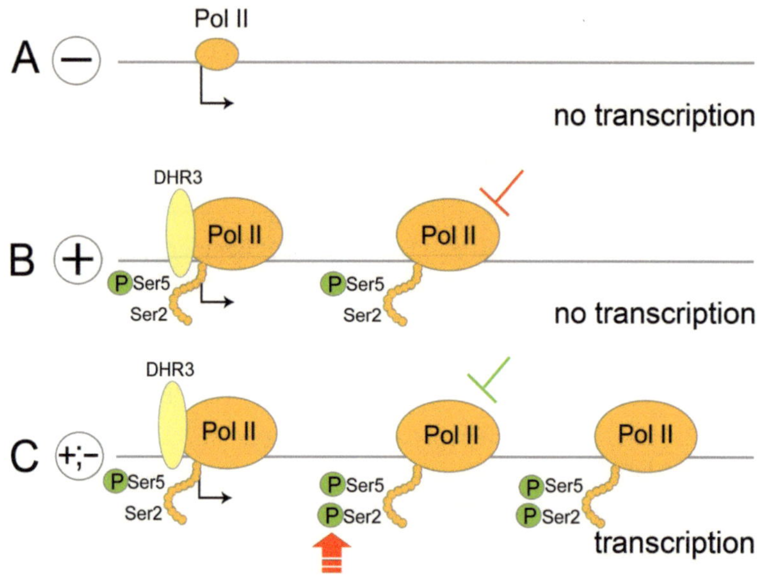

Figure 4. The scheme representation of the *Drosophila* developmental *ftz-f1* gene transcription induction by the ecdysone hormone in S2 Schneider cells. A) The *ftz-f1* gene is not expressed in the normal S2 Schneider cells. The promoter of the gene is not bound with the DHR3 activator and contains few RNA Polymerase II. The (-) mark on the scheme represents low ecdysone titer in the medium of the culturing cells. B) After ecdysone addition (represented with the (+) mark) the DHR3 activator is recruited on the *ftz-f1* promoter region. The DHR3 binding to the promoter stimulates RNA Polymerase II loading. Transcription of the *ftz-f1* gene is initiated but the RNA Polymerase II complex pauses close to the promoter. The RNA Polymerase II at (+) stage is not in the state competent for the elongation and is not phosphorylated on Ser2 of the CTD domain. The *ftz-f1* gene is not transcribed at (+) stage. C) After ecdysone withdrawal from the culturing medium the block on the RNA Polymerase II elongation is disposed. At the point of transient pausing (it completely coincides with the region of pausing at (+) stage) the RNA Polymerase II is phosphorylated on Ser2 of the CTD domain and continues the moving into the coding region of the gene. A few hours after ecdysone titer decreasing the *ftz-f1* gene is actively transcribed.

region of the studied gene with a high affinity in all stages of activation. The level of the promoter binding of the BAP170 protein increased twice in (+;-) stage after the *ftz-f1* transcription activation. The amount of OSA subunit bound to the *ftz-f1* promoter was increased in (+) stage during the stage of RNA Polymerase II recruitment and was not changed significantly after the withdrawal of the transcriptional block. Thus both of the dSWI/SNF subcomplexes bind the promoter region of the *ftz-f1* gene in all stages of activation.

The patterns of the PBAP and BAP subcomplexes distribution in the coding region of the *ftz-f1* gene during active transcription differ distinctly. The significant increase in the BAP170 subunit binding at the coding region of the *ftz-f1* gene during (+;-) stage of active transcription was detected. At that stage the binding level of the BAP170 subunit in the coding region exceeded by a factor of several times the negative control region of the 28S rDNA, while in all other stages was close to the background. At the same time, the binding level of the OSA subunit of the BAP subcomplex was close to the background throughout the coding region of the *ftz-f1* gene during all transcriptional stages.

http://dx.doi.org/10.5772/55877

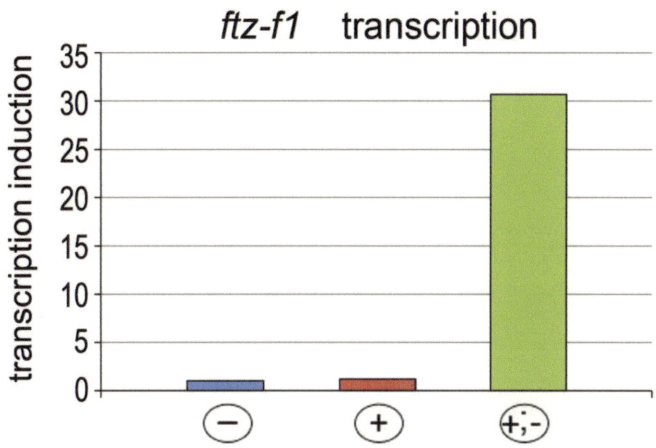

Figure 5. The *ftz-f1* gene transcription induction in the S2 Schneider cells with the ecdysone hormone addition ("+" state) and sequential removing ("+;-" state). The cells of the all states were collected for the analysis at the same time. The ecdysone was added overnight to the cells of (+) and (+;-) states and in (+;-) state it was removed from the cells medium 4 hours before analysis. The Y – axis represents the level of transcription induction relative to non-induced conditions.

Thus the accumulation of the BAP170-specific subunit of the PBAP subcomplex in the coding region of the *ftz-f1* gene during the active stage of the transcription was demonstrated. Thereby the participation of the PBAP but not the BAP subcomplex of the dSWI/SNF chromatin remodeling complex in the elongation process of the RNA Polymerase II was shown.

2.5. PBAP subcomplex of the dSWI/SNF complex is accumulated at the coding region of the hsp70 gene after transcription activation

To prove the wideness of the observation and non-specificity of the finding to the model of gene activation the recruitment of the PBAP subcomplex on the coding region of the active gene was studied in another system (on the model of *hsp70* gene).

The *hsp70* gene model system is widely used in transcriptional machinery studies. The model uses *Drosophila* cells treatment with heat shock conditions (37 °C for 20 min) for induction while the normal temperature for culturing is 25-28 °C [20]. In those stress conditions the transcriptional system of the *Drosophila* cell is drastically changed. Almost all of the genes stop being transcribed while several genes (called heat shock genes) exhibit very fast and high level of transcriptional activation. It should be taken into account that in such stress and non-physiological conditions the transcriptional machinery could not function by the same mechanisms as in the normal cell. But nevertheless the *hsp70* gene represents the system with the highest induction level which was ever being described for the *Drosophila*. Therefore these genes are a good model for the investigation of the subtle changes on the coding region of the gene during transcription activation.

To verify the induction scheme the S2 Schneider cells were exposed to the heat shock conditions (37°C) and the *hsp70* gene transcription was measured before and after the heat shock. The

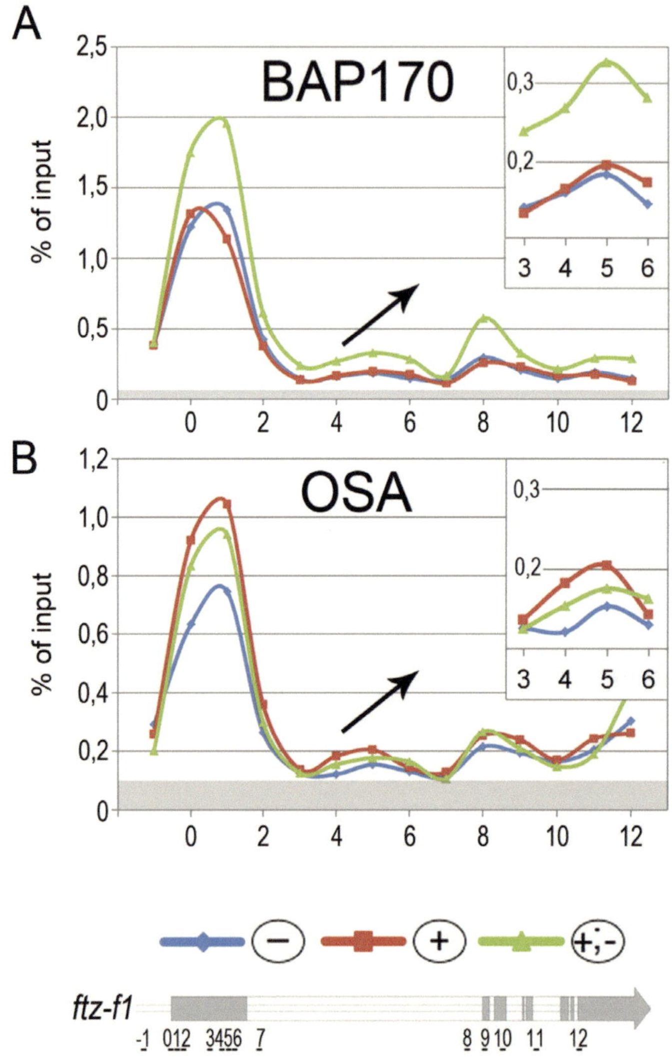

Figure 6. The BAP170 (A) and OSA (B) subunits distribution along the *ftz-f1* gene at different stages of transcription activation. The analysis was performed by chromatin immunoprecipitation technique on the S2 Schneider cells which was growing in the ecdysone-free medium (–), after overnight cultivation in the ecdysone-containing medium (+), and finally 4 hours after ecdysone withdrawal from the culturing medium (+;–). The positions of primer pairs which were used for the RT-PCR analysis of the *ftz-f1* gene are shown on the scheme of the gene. The precipitation level of the negative control (28S rDNA region) is shown on the graphs as a grey line. The results of the chromatin immunoprecipitation experiment were calculated as a % of precipitated chromatin relative to input fraction.

fifty fold increase in *hsp70* gene transcription was detected after the heat shock. The *hsp70* transcription induction was measured by Real-Time PCR using primer "7" from the description list.

To prove the involvement of the PBAP subcomplex in the process of RNA Polymerase II elongation the BAP170 subunit distribution was analyzed along the *hsp70* gene before and after

http://dx.doi.org/10.5772/55877

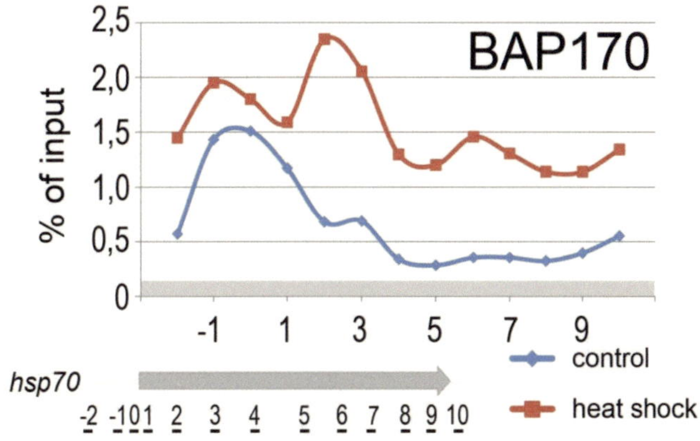

Figure 7. The BAP170 subunit distribution along the *hsp70* gene at heat shock (red) and non-heat shock (blue) conditions. The analysis was performed by chromatin immunoprecipitation technique on the S2 Schneider cells treated with the heat shock conditions (37°C) and harvested at room temperature (presented as "heat shock" and "control" line on the graph). The positions of primer pairs which were used for the RT-PCR analysis of the *hsp70* are shown on the scheme of the gene. The results of the chromatin immunoprecipitation experiment were calculated as a % of precipitated chromatin relative to input fraction.

heat shock (Figure 7). The BAP170 subunit of the PBAP subcomplex binding to the promoter region was detected both in the repressed and active state of the gene. But several times increase in the level of the BAP170 subunit binding inside the *hsp70* coding region was observed after transcription activation.

Thus the accumulation of the PBAP subcomplex inside the coding region upon transcription activation was demonstrated not only for the *ftz-f1*, but also for the *hsp70* gene.

3. Conclusions

Several pieces of evidence concerning SWI/SNF participation in the elongation process of RNA Polymerase II have emerged during the last few years [21]. These data describe SWI/SNF complex participation both in elongation process of RNA Polymerase II and in transcription elongation coupled events like pre-mRNP splicing [22]. There have been a few studies to date but there can be no doubt that the SWI/SNF complex travels with the RNA Polymerase II along the gene during active transcription. This research area is only starting to be investigated and attracts much attention because the participation in transcription elongation represents a novel function of the SWI/SNF complex.

The properties of the SWI/SNF complex is under extensive study because subunits of the complex are indispensable for the living organism [23][24]. The ability to possess all types of nucleosome remodeling activities distinguishes it from other chromatin remodeling complexes [24]. The recent studies concerning the significance of SWI/SNF complex for the cell reprogramming and association of the SWI/SNF subunits mutations with cancer susceptibility have made this complex interesting for a wide circle of investigators [25][26].

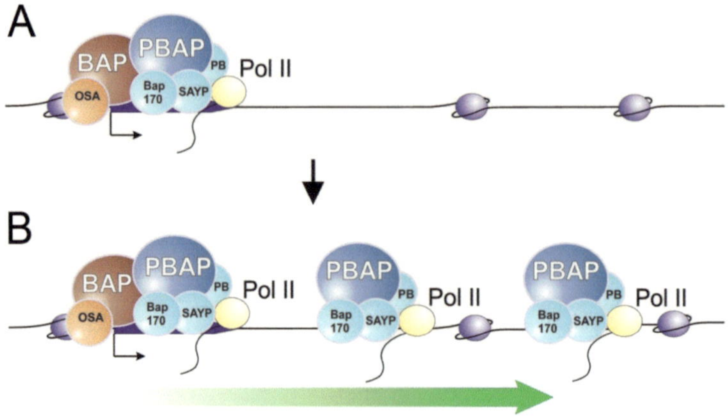

Figure 8. The descriptive model of the PBAP and BAP subcomplexes of the dSWI/SNF chromatin remodeling complex re-distribution along the gene before and after transcription activation. Both of the subcomplexes are bound to the promoter region before transcription induction (A). At the active transcription state the PBAP subcomplex of dSWI/SNF complex is detected on the coding region of the gene (B). The PBAP subcomplex of the dSWI/SNF assists the RNA Polymerase II in the process of transcription elongation.

It has been known for a few years that the SWI/SNF complex is comprised of PBAP and BAP types of subcomplexes (in mammals, PBAF and BAF respectively) [16]. The subcomplexes have partially overlapping but mostly distinct targeting throughout the genome [27]. These subcomplexes possess different functions. Thus, the BAP but not the PBAP complex is working in the cell cycle regulating pathway [18]. For the BAF250/ARID1-specific subunit of the BAP subcomplex an activity of the E3 ligase and ability to ubiquitinylate histone H2B has been demonstrated [28]. The capabilities of these subcomplexes to possess different functions obviously lie in their specific subunits.

The main idea of the current study was to investigate which one of the subcomplexes participates in the new functions of SWI/SNF during transcription elongation. The model describing results of this study is presented in Figure 8 A and B.

The drosophila developmental *ftz-f1* gene was chosen as a model for the investigation. The *ftz-f1* gene transcription induction was performed by developmental ecdysone hormone (so conditions were close to natural). This system of induction has advantages both in terms of the physiological non-stress conditions of gene activation and the simplicity of performing chromatin immunoprecipitation experiments on the culturing cells. The accumulation of the PBAP but not BAP subcomplex inside the coding region upon transcription activation was observed by chromatin immunoprecipitation with antibodies against specific subunits of the subcomplexes. Thus, for the *Drosophila melanogaster* it was demonstrated that the PBAP subcomplex of dSWI/SNF is not only important for the transcriptional initiation events but also assists the RNA Polymerase II in transcription elongation.

The discovered effect was confirmed in another inducible gene system. The *hsp70* gene is induced by subjecting the cell to the stress heat shock conditions and the transcription level after induction is characterized by the extremely high rate. In the inducible system of the *hsp70* gene the significant accumulation of the PBAP subcomplex inside the coding region upon transcription activation was observed. Thus PBAP subcomplex participation in RNA Polymerase II elongation is not restricted to the solitary gene, but is realized at least on two inducible genes of *Drosophila melanogaster*.

The specification of the SWI/SNF subcomplex participation in the functions during the RNA Polymerase II elongation process will make easier further investigations of these functions.

The presence of the SWI/SNF complex inside the coding region of the intron-less genes testifies to the existence of some other functions during elongation in addition to the participation in the splicing process. The nature of these functions is not fully understood yet. But the functional link of the SWI/SNF complex with the process of RNA Polymerase II elongation definitely exists. It was shown for the yeast that mutants of the SWI/SNF subunit display heightened sensitivity to the drugs, inhibitors of transcription elongation [11]. The participation of the PBAP subcomplex in regulation of the RNA Polymerase II elongation rate has been described for the *Drosophila* using the *ftz-f1* gene as a model system. It was demonstrated that knockdown of the PBAP subcomplex subunit causes decrease in the level of the elongated RNA Polymerase II on the coding region, but at the same time it does not reduce the level of the promoter-bound RNA Polymerase II complex. Moreover, the PBAP subunit knockdown leads to a considerable decrease in level of the RNA Polymerase II CTD Ser2 phosphorylation state but does not change the Ser5 phosphorylation. The participation of the SWI/SNF complex in the process of CTD Ser2 phosphorylation could be one of the chromatin remodeling complex functions during elongation. This marker of active transcription is loaded close to the promoter area and increases towards the 3′ end of the gene. The new kinase which is responsible for the Ser2 CTD phosphorylation RNA Polymerase II elongation through the coding region of the gene has been described recently [29]. The participation of SWI/SNF in this process could explain the observed accumulation of the complex inside the coding region of the gene upon transcription activation.

Experimental procedures

Drosophila embryonic nuclear extract purification

The Method of the *Drosophila* embryonic nuclear extract purification was described earlier in [30].

Experiments with S2 Schneider cell

The protocol of the *Drosophila* Schneider line 2 (S2) cells cultivation and *ftz-f1* gene induction was in the details described in [13]. For the *hsp70* gene transcription induction cells were incubated at the 37°C in water bath for the 20 min and briefly cooled to the RT. To extract proteins for IP, S2 Schneider cells were lysed in 10 mM Hepes (pH 7.9) buffer containing 5 mM MgCl2, 0.5% Nonidet P-40, 0.45 M NaCl, 1 mM DTT, and complete protease inhibitor mixture (Roche). IP was performed as described earlier [31].

Chromatin immunoprecipitation

For one ChIP experiment $3x10^6$ of S2 Schneider cells were taken. Crosslinking was made by 15 min incubation with 1,5% formaldehyde and was stopped by addition of 1/20 volume of the

2,5M glycine. Cells were triple washed with cold (4°C) PBS and resuspended in SDS-containing buffer (50 mM HEPES-KOH pH 7.9, 140 mM NaCl, 1 mM EDTA, 1% Triton X-100, 0,1% deoxycholate Na, 0,1% SDS, Protease inhibitors cocktail (Roche)). Chromatin was sheared to DNA size of appr. 700 b.p. and centrifuged (16 rcf, 20 min). For the one chromatin immunoprecipitation were taken: 10 μg of antibodies, 15 μl of PrA sepharose (Sigma), ssDNA and BSA up to 1 mg/ml. The precipitated chromatin was sequentially washed by buffers: SDS-containing buffer, SDS-containing buffer with 0,5M NaCl, LiCl-containing buffer (20mM Tris-HCl pH 8,0, 1mM EDTA, 250 mM LiCl, 0,5% NP40, 0,5% Deoxycholate Na) and TE buffer (20mM Tris-HCl pH 8,0, 1mM EDTA). Precipitated complexes were eluted by incubation in buffer (50mM Tris-HCl pH 8,0, 1mM EDTA, 1% SDS) at RT. Eluted chromatin was de-crosslinked for the 16 h at 65°C (16 μl of 5M NaCl was added) and treated with the 3 units of proteinase K for 4 h at 55°C (5 μl of 0,5 M EDTA was added to each sample). DNA was purified with the phenol/chloroform extraction and precipitated with the isopropanol. The precipitate was dissolved in TE buffer and subjected to the Real-Time PCR (RT PCR) analysis. The result of the chromatin immunoprecipitation experiment was calculated as a rate of precipitated fraction relative to the input chromatin fraction (presented as a percent). Each point was measured in at least five experiments and the mean value was calculated.

RNA purification and cDNA synthesis

The RNA purifications were performed as described in [13].

Primers for qPCR

ftz-f1 gene fragments:

Region	Forward primer	Reverse primer
–1	ACAAAAAACTGCTGAAGAAGAGACC	ACTGTGGGTATGGCATTATGAAAG
0	GAGGCAGAGGCAGCGACG	GCTTTGTCATCTATGTGTGTGTTGTTG
1	AGTCAATCGAGATACGTGGTTGATG	GTAACGCTTTGTCATCTATGTGTGT
2	GTTCTCTTGCTGCGTTGCG	GAAAGTGGGTCACGAATTTATTGC
3	ACCGCAACCTATTTTACTACC	TTAGAAGACCGAAGAGTTATCC
4	ACAACAACAATAACAACGACAATGATGC	CTGATTGCCGCTGCCACTCC
5	CAGCAGCAACAGCAACAGAATATC	GCGAGTGTGAGGAGGTGGTG
6	CTCCTCACACTCGCAACAGAGC	AGCAGCATGTAGCCACCGC
7	CTCCGTAAGAGTCAGCTTTAAC	CAGGGACATCACACATACG
8	CAACGCTTCACAGAAACAAACG	GTTGTACAAAGCGGCGTATGC
9	GTTCGAGCGGATAGAATGCGT	GATATGCTTGCTGGTAGCCCG
10	GAGGAGGAGGTGGCAATAATGC	GATCCTATTCCAGCCTCGTGG
11	TTCAATGCACATTCTGCCG	GCAGCAACATGGTTCAAAGC
12	AACATCTTACCGGAAATCCATGC	ATCTCCATGAGCAGCGTTTGG

Table 1. Primers for the amplification of the *ftz-f1* gene fragments.

http://dx.doi.org/10.5772/55877

hsp70 gene fragments:

Region	Forward primer	Reverse primer
-2	GCAACTAAATTCTAATACACTTCTC	TGCTGCGTTTCTAAAGATTAAAG
-1	GTGACAGAGTGAGAGAGCATTAGTG	ATTGTGGTAGGTCATTTGTTTGGC
0	TTGAATTGAATTGTCGCTCCGTAG	ACATACTGCTCTCGTTGGTTCG
1	GCAGTTGATTTACTTGGTTG	AACAAGCAAAGTGAACACG
2	ATGAGGCGTTCCGAGTCTGTG	CTACTCCTGCGTGGGTGTCTAC
3	CGCTGAGAGTCGTTGAAGTAAG	GTGCTGACCAAGATGAAGGAG
4	GCTGTTCTGAGGCGTCGTAGG	TTGGGCGGCGAGGACTTTG
5	CCTCCAGCGGTCTCAATTCCC	GACGAGGCAGTGGCATACGG
6	GGGTGTGCCCCAGATAGAAG	TGTCGTTCTTGATCGTGATGTTC
7	CTTCTCGGCGGTGGTGTTG	GTAAAGCAGTCCGTGGAGCAG
8	AGCTAAAATCAATTTGTTGCTAACTT	AGGTCGACTAAAGCCAAATAGA
9	GCTGTTTAATAGGGATGCCAAC	TATTGTCAGGGAGTGAGTTTGC
10	GTTGTTGAACTCCGTAACCATTCTG	GCCCCGCTAAGTGAGTCCTG

Table 2. Primers for the amplification of the *hsp70* gene fragments.

28S rDNA:

Forward primer	Reverse primer
AGAGCACTGGGCAGAAATCACATTG	AATTCAGAACTGGCACGGACTTGG

Table 3. Primers for the amplification of the 28S rDNA locus fragment.

Acknowledgements

We thanks S.G. Georgieva for her critical reading of the manuscript; P. Verrijzer and Y. Moshkin (Erasmus University Medical Center, Rotterdam) for the constructs with sequences coding BAP170 antigens and for the antibodies against MOR (described in [16]). This work was supported by the program "Molecular and Cell Biology" of the Russian Academy of Sciences, N.V. were supported by the RF Presidential Program in Support of Young Scientists, MK-5961.2012.4 and MD-4874.2011.4. N.V. acknowledges a fellowship from Dmitry Zimin Dynasty Foundation.

Author details

Nadezhda E. Vorobyeva[1*], Marina U. Mazina[1] and Semen A. Doronin[2]

*Address all correspondence to: nvorobyova@gmail.com

1 Group of Transcription and mRNA Transport, Institute of Gene Biology, Russian Academy of Sciences, Moscow, Russia

2 Department of Regulation of Gene Expression, Institute of Gene Biology, Russian Academy of Sciences, Moscow, Russia

References

[1] Rendina, R, Strangi, A, Avallone, B, & Giordano, E. Bap170, a subunit of the Drosophila PBAP chromatin remodeling complex, negatively regulates the EGFR signaling.," *Genetics*, Sep. (2010). , 186(1), 167-181.

[2] Baig, J, Chanut, F, Kornberg, T. B, & Klebes, A. The chromatin-remodeling protein Osa interacts with CyclinE in Drosophila eye imaginal discs.," *Genetics*, Mar. (2010). , 184(3), 731-744.

[3] Wu, J, Lessard, J, & Crabtree, G. Understanding the Words of Chromatin Regulation," *Cell*, (2009). , 136(2), 200-206.

[4] Métivier, R, Penot, G, Hübner, M. R, Reid, G, Brand, H, Kos, M, & Gannon, F. Estrogen receptor-alpha directs ordered, cyclical, and combinatorial recruitment of cofactors on a natural target promoter.," *Cell*, Dec. (2003). , 115(6), 751-763.

[5] Nakamura, T, Mori, T, Tada, S, Krajewski, W, Rozovskaia, T, Wassell, R, Dubois, G, Mazo, A, Croce, C. M, & Canaani, E. ALL-1 is a histone methyltransferase that assembles a supercomplex of proteins involved in transcriptional regulation.," *Molecular Cell*, Nov. (2002). , 10(5), 1119-1128.

[6] Vorobyeva, N. E, Soshnikova, N. V, Nikolenko, J. V, Kuzmina, J. L, Nabirochkina, E. N, Georgieva, S. G, & Shidlovskii, Y. V. Transcription coactivator SAYP combines chromatin remodeler Brahma and transcription initiation factor TFIID into a single supercomplex.," *Proceedings of the National Academy of Sciences of the United States of America*, Jul. (2009). , 106(27), 11049-11054.

[7] Batsché, E, Yaniv, M, & Muchardt, C. The human SWI/SNF subunit Brm is a regulator of alternative splicing.," *Nature Structural & Molecular Biology*, Jan. (2006). , 13(1), 22-29.

[8] Ito, T, Watanabe, H, Yamamichi, N, Kondo, S, Tando, T, Haraguchi, T, Mizutani, T, Sakurai, K, Fujita, S, Izumi, T, Isobe, T, & Iba, H. Brm transactivates the telomerase

reverse transcriptase (TERT) gene and modulates the splicing patterns of its transcripts in concert with p54(nrb).," *The Biochemical Journal,* Apr. (2008). , 411(1), 201-209.

[9] Waldholm, J, Wang, Z, Brodin, D, Tyagi, A, Yu, S, Theopold, U, Farrants, A. K. Ö, & Visa, N. SWI/SNF regulates the alternative processing of a specific subset of pre-mRNAs in Drosophila melanogaster.," *BMC Molecular Biology,* Jan. (2011). , 12(46), 1-12.

[10] Tyagi, A, Ryme, J, Brodin, D, & Ostlund, A. K. Farrants, and N. Visa, "SWI/SNF associates with nascent pre-mRNPs and regulates alternative pre-mRNA processing.," *PLoS Genetics,* May (2009). , 5(5), e1000470.

[11] Schwabish, M, & Struhl, K. The Swi/Snf complex is important for histone eviction during transcriptional activation and RNA polymerase II elongation in vivo.," *Molecular and Cellular Biology,* Oct. (2007). , 27(20), 6987-6995.

[12] Corey, L. L, Weirich, C. S, Benjamin, I. J, & Kingston, R. E. Localized recruitment of a chromatin-remodeling activity by an activator in vivo drives transcriptional elongation, *Genes and Development,* (2003). , 17, 1392-1401.

[13] Vorobyeva, N. E, Nikolenko, J. V, Nabirochkina, E. N, Krasnov, A. N, Shidlovskii, Y. V, & Georgieva, S. G. SAYP and Brahma are important for 'repressive' and 'transient' Pol II pausing.," *Nucleic Acids Research,* May (2012). , 40(15), 7319-7331.

[14] Mizutani, T, Ishizaka, A, Tomizawa, M, Okazaki, T, Yamamichi, N, Kawana-tachikawa, A, Iwamoto, A, & Iba, H. Loss of the Brm-type SWI/SNF chromatin remodeling complex is a strong barrier to the Tat-independent transcriptional elongation of human immunodeficiency virus type 1 transcripts.," *Journal of Virology,* Nov. (2009). , 83(22), 11569-11580.

[15] Kulaeva, O. I, Hsieh, F. -K, & Studitsky, V. M. RNA polymerase complexes cooperate to relieve the nucleosomal barrier and evict histones.," *Proceedings of the National Academy of Sciences of the United States of America,* Jun. (2010). , 107(25), 11325-11330.

[16] Mohrmann, L, Langenberg, K, Krijgsveld, J, Kal, A. J, Heck, A. J. R, & Verrijzer, C. P. Differential Targeting of Two Distinct SWI / SNF-Related Drosophila Chromatin-Remodeling Complexes," *Molecular and Cellular Biology,* (2004). , 24(8), 3077-3088.

[17] Vorobyeva, N. E, Soshnikova, N. V, Kuzmina, J. L, Kopantseva, M. R, Nikolenko, J. V, Nabirochkina, E. N, Georgieva, S. G, & Shidlovskii, Y. V. The novel regulator of metazoan development SAYP organizes a nuclear coactivator supercomplex.," *Cell Cycle,* Jul. (2009). , 8(14), 2152-2156.

[18] Moshkin, Y. M, Mohrmann, L, Van Ijcken, W. F. J, & Verrijzer, C. P. Functional differentiation of SWI/SNF remodelers in transcription and cell cycle control.," *Molecular and cellular biology,* Jan. (2007). , 27(2), 651-661.

[19] Schneider, I. Cell lines derived from late embryonic stages of Drosophila melanogaster," *J Embryol Exp Morphol*, Apr. (1972). , 27(2), 353-365.

[20] Brien, T, & Lis, J. T. RNA Polymerase II pauses at the 5′ end of the transcriptionally Induced Drosophila hsp70 Gene," *Molecular and Cellular Biology*, (1991). , 11(10), 5285-5290.

[21] Subtil-rodríguez, A, & Reyes, J. C. To cross or not to cross the nucleosome, that is the elongation question…," *RNA Biology*, May (2011). , 8(3), 389-393.

[22] Kornblihtt, A. R. Chromatin, transcript elongation and alternative splicing.," *Nature Structural & Molecular Biology*, Jan. (2006). , 13(1), 5-7.

[23] Shidlovskii, Y. V, Krasnov, A. N, Nikolenko, J. V, Lebedeva, L. a, Kopantseva, M, Ermolaeva, M. a, Ilyin, Y. V, Nabirochkina, E. N, Georgiev, P. G, & Georgieva, S. G. A novel multidomain transcription coactivator SAYP can also repress transcription in heterochromatin.," *The EMBO Journal*, Jan. (2005). , 24(1), 97-107.

[24] Hargreaves, D. C, & Crabtree, G. R. ATP-dependent chromatin remodeling: genetics, genomics and mechanisms.," *Cell Research*, Mar. (2011). , 21(3), 396-420.

[25] He, L, Liu, H, & Tang, L. SWI/SNF chromatin remodeling complex: a new cofactor in reprogramming.," *Stem Cell Reviews*, Mar. (2012). , 8(1), 128-136.

[26] Brownlee, P. M, Chambers, A. L, Oliver, A. W, & Downs, J. a. Cancer and the bromodomains of BAF180.," *Biochemical Society Transactions*, Apr. (2012). , 40(2), 364-369.

[27] Mohrmann, L, & Verrijzer, C. P. Composition and functional specificity of SWI2/SNF2 class chromatin remodeling complexes.," *Biochimica et Biophysica Acta*, Jan. (2005). , 1681(2-3), 59-73.

[28] Li, X. S, Trojer, P, Matsumura, T, Treisman, J. E, & Tanese, N. Mammalian SWI/SNF--a subunit BAF250/ARID1 is an E3 ubiquitin ligase that targets histone H2B.," *Molecular and Cellular Biology*, Apr. (2010). , 30(7), 1673-1688.

[29] Bartkowiak, B, Liu, P, Phatnani, H. P, Fuda, N. J, Cooper, J. J, Price, D. H, Adelman, K, Lis, J. T, & Greenleaf, A. L. CDK12 is a transcription elongation- associated CTD kinase, the metazoan ortholog of yeast Ctk1," *Genes and Development*, (2007). , 24, 2303-2316.

[30] Blank, T. A, Sandaltzopoulos, R, & Becker, P. B. Biochemical analysis of chromatin structure and function using Drosophila embryo extracts.," *Methods*, May (1997). , 12(1), 28-35.

[31] Georgieva, S, Kirschner, D. B, Jagla, T, Nabirochkina, E, Hanke, S, Schenkel, H, De Lorenzo, C, Sinha, P, Jagla, K, Mechler, B, & Tora, L. Two novel Drosophila TAF(II)s have homology with human TAF(II)30 and are differentially regulated during development.," *Molecular and Cellular Biology*, Mar. (2000). , 20(5), 1639-1648.

Chapter 4

Condensins, Chromatin Remodeling and Gene Transcription

Laurence O. W. Wilson and Aude M. Fahrer

Additional information is available at the end of the chapter

http://dx.doi.org/10.5772/55732

1. Introduction

Condensin complexes condense chromosomes during mitosis, turning the diffuse interphase chromosomes into the familiar X-shaped compact chromosomes that segregate during cell division. More recently a second role for condensins has emerged, in the epigenetic regulation of interphase gene transcription. This second fascinating role is very difficult to study since defects in condensin will usually interfere with mitosis and result in cell death. While several excellent reviews of condensin function have recently been published (see [1-3]), in this article we concentrate on the epigenetic functions of condensins and how they can be studied. We also provide the first summary of condensin protein splice forms, a largely overlooked contributor to condensin variation.

The DNA within a cell is too large to fit inside if left in its unwound state. In order to accommodate the genetic material, a cell packages this DNA as chromati:, a combination of DNA bound to protein. The DNA is wound around protein complexes known as histones to form nucleosomes, which form a "beads-on-a-string" structure. These nucleosomes can be compacted further to produce a highly condensed structure that fits inside the nucleus of a cell.

The regulation of this structure is vital for cell growth and survival. During mitosis, chromatin must be unwound so that it can be properly replicated and then repackaged into sister chromosomes that must then be segregated into the dividing cells. Defects in any of these processes can result in cell death. Additionally, the compact nature of the chromatin limits the cell's transcription machinery from properly interacting with its targets, preventing gene transcription. In order to counter this, selected regions of chromatin must be unwound during interphase to allow the genes present to be transcribed. The chromatin structure of the cell is therefore under tight control. Changes in chromatin structure are thought to occur via three broad mechanisms; 1. methylation of DNA; 2. covalent modification of histones; 3. at a "higher level" by tethering distant regions of DNA.

The condensin protein complexes, originally identified in Xenopus egg extracts [4], function through the third pathway: inducing condensation in chromatin structure through the introduction of positive super-coils, and by tethering together distinct regions of DNA [5, 6]. This ability to condense chromatin has been found to be central to the compaction of chromosomes during mitosis.

Vertebrates possess two condensins, known as condensin I and condensin II, each consisting of 5 proteins. A dimer of Structural Maintenance of Chromosome (SMC) proteins 2 and 4 forms the core of both condensin I and II. SMC proteins are large proteins (1000 – 1300 amino acid long) which fold so that their amino and carboxy termini join to form an ATPase [7]. SMC2 and 4 form a dimer with a V-shape, with the ATPase domains of each protein localized to the tips of the V. This dimer of SMC proteins then associates with either Ncaph, Ncapg and Ncapd2 to form condensin I or with Ncaph2, Ncapg2 and Ncapd3 to form condensin II (Figure 1) [8, 9].

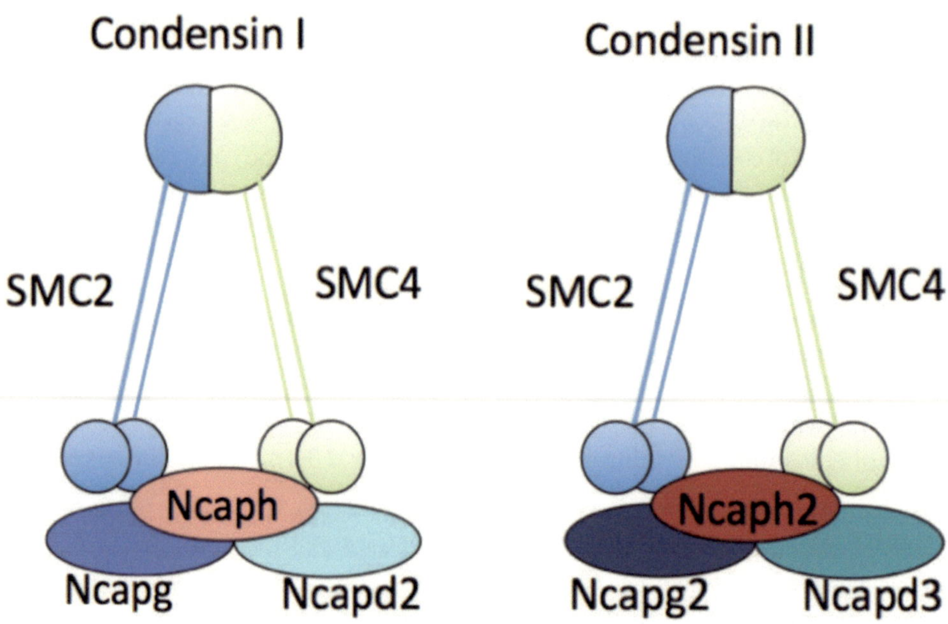

Figure 1. Schematic representation of the condensin complexes. A heterodimer of SMC2 and SMC4 combines with either Ncaph, Ncapg and Ncapd2 to form condensin I or with Ncaph2, Ncapg2 and Ncapd3 to form condensin II.

Condensins were initially studied in the context of mitotic chromosomes. Mutations interfering with the function of either condensin complex results in aberrant chromosome formation, and a complete loss of function of either complex is lethal [9, 10]. The emerging evidence for chromatin structure's role in gene transcription however has lead to idea that condensins may play roles beyond mitosis, acting in interphase to influence gene transcription through the reorganization of chromatin [11-13]. Subsequently, evidence has begun to emerge which shows that condensins are much more than architects of chromatin structure, they are also important regulators of gene transcription.

The vital role condensins play in mitosis makes their study difficult; disruption of their function through means such as mutations or transcriptional interference often fatally disrupts cell division. A variety of methods of study have therefore been employed in order to gain insight into the complexes' roles in mitosis and gene regulation.

2. The study of condensin homologs

An alternative to studying a protein directly is to study functionally and structurally similar homologs. Such homologs may provide insight into a protein of interest through shared mechanisms, but prove easier to study. Such an approach has been used to study condenins and provided great insight into how they might regulate gene transcription.

One of the first examples of condenins regulating gene expression was the discovery of a condensin homolog in *C. elegans* known as the Dosage Compensation Complex (DCC) [14]. In most species, the sexes are determined by a difference in the presence of specific chromosomes (such as the X and Y chromosomes in human). In *C. elegans* the population is divided into males, which possess a single X chromosome, and hermaphrodites, which possess two copies of the X chromosome. The increased number of X chromosome present in hermaphrodites would lead to a two-fold increase in X-linked gene expression with potentially dire consequences unless properly regulated [15]. To counter this, hermaphrodite *C. elegans* can reduce the expression of their X-linked genes by half, resulting in normal levels of transcription [15].

The DCC is comprised of SMC proteins DPY-27 and MIX-1 as well as DPY-26, DPY-28 and Capg1 [16-20]. The DCC then associates with a second 5-protein complex consisting of SDC-1, SDC-2, SDC-3, DPY-21 and DPY-30. The structure of the DCC differs from the worm condensin I complex only in the presence of DPY-27, which is replaced by SMC-4 in condensin I, yet despite the similarities has a different function.

Studies have shown that the DCC is directed towards the X chromosome by a combination of histone modifications and specific DNA motifs. The histone variant H2A.Z (called HTZ-1 in *C. elegans*) is found on the X chromosome of *C. elegans.* Disrupting the expression of this histone using RNAi's was shown to disrupt DCC binding. The disruption was not caused by a decrease in DCC protein levels, which suggests the histone assists in the binding/recruitment of the complex to the X chromosome [21, 22]. Once recruited to the correct chromosome, the complex binds to the DNA through the recognition of specific sequence motifs in what is now known to be a two-step process. First, the DCC recognizes and binds to recruitment elements on X (or *rex*) sites. Once bound, the DCC is then distributed along the X chromosome by migrating to dependent-on-X (or *dox*) sites. The result is the distribution of the DCC along the full length of the X chromosome, allowing it to exert its effects over the entire chromosome [23].

A second, less widely known example of a condensin- related protein was identified in a mouse study looking for epigenetic regulators. Blewitt *et al.* identified the gene SMC Hinge domain containing 1 (SMCHD1) [24]. While not a full homolog of SMC, it does bear similarities and further investigation showed that it plays a crucial role in X-inactivation in mice, similar to the DCC in *C. elegans* [25]. Further study of this protein may provide insights into the function of SMC complexes such as condensin.

3. The study of condensins through knock-outs

Removal of a gene of interest, and study of the resulting phenotype, is a common method for studying the function of a gene. The vital role condensins play in mitosis prevents such an approach, as knock-outs are often lethal. Knockouts in SMC2, SMC4, Ncapd2, Ncapg and Ncaph have all proven to be lethal [26-34]. The majority of the knock-out work has been conducted in yeast, bacteria, *Drosophila,* and *C. elegans*. A study in 2004 generated the only reported mammalian phenotype for a condensin knockout: a mouse strain with a deletion of the condensin II Ncapg2 protein [35]. The resulting knock-outs were embryonic lethal, with the mice fetuses dying almost immediately after implantation due to a catastrophic disruption in cell growth and division.

An alternative to the use of full knock-outs is the generation of conditional knock-outs. Cell lines can be engineered to turn-off expression of target genes when exposed to specific signals (such as the addition of doxycylcin). Expression of the gene is then lost over time and a resulting phenotype emerges. Chicken cell lines have now been created that stop expression of select condensin genes upon exposure to doxycycline [36]. Whereas a normal knock-out of these genes would likely prove lethal and prevent any sort of study, the gradual emergence of the phenotype in these conditional knock-outs can be studied. Such an approach has been used to investigate the different contributions of condensin I and condensin II to mitotic-chromosome formation, showing differences in phenotype between knock-outs of the two complexes. The results suggest that condensin II is required for the formation of the chromosome scaffold and for providing rigidity, while condensin I acts to compact the chromatin around the scaffold. While only used so far to study the role of these complexes in mitosis, their use could be expanded to investigate the role condensins play during interphase. Gene expression profiling of these cell lines could be carried out to look for evidence of the direct regulation of transcription by condensins.

4. Knock-down and overexpression studies

Altering the expression of target proteins, either through over- or under-expression can provide an alternative to knock-out studies, producing informative phenotypes while avoiding the lethal side-effects often associated with complete removal of a protein. Such approaches have been used in *Drosophila* to great effect, providing insights into the functions of Condensins.

The *Drosophila* Barren protein, a homolog of Ncaph and component of the *Drosophila* Condensin I complex, was investigated using a knock-down approach [37]. The study showed that fly Ncaph interacts directly with the Polycomb group protein polyhomeotic. Polycomb group proteins are a group of proteins responsible for repressing transcription in various regions across the genome and for maintaining this silenced state through the life of the fly. This is achieved by the binding of these proteins to specific elements within the genome and the compaction of neighboring DNA. The physical interaction with Ncaph suggests that this compaction is achieved through the recruitment of Condensin via the polycomb group proteins to the target region of the genome. The authors demonstrated a specific instance of this, showing the fly requires Ncaph to silence the *abdominal-B* gene by inducing its binding to an upstream silencer. Reducing the levels of Ncaph through knock-downs greatly diminished the silencing of this gene, highlighting the role of condensin I in transcriptional regulation.

A similar approach was used in a second *Drosophila* study [38]. The authors noted that *Drosophila* larvae with mutations in retinoblastoma family protein RBF1 often showed defects in chromsome condensation during mitosis. Further investigation showed a direct interaction between RBF1 and the *Drosophila* Ncapd3 protein. The authors showed that this interaction was required for proper loading of condensin II onto the chromosome. A reduction in the levels of RBF1 greatly diminished the capacity of condensin II to bind to the chromatin, but could be compensated by over-expression of Ncapd3.

Over-expression was also used to explore the role of murine Ncapg2/MTB in erythropoiesis [39]. Ncapg2 was found to be upregulated in erythroid cell lines. Further investigation found the protein was capable of inhibiting SCL/E12 mediated transcription. Over-expression of the protein was also shown to be sufficient to induce terminal differentiation of erythroleukemia cell lines. While the precise mechanism of Ncapg2-mediated differentiation is still poorly understood, the authors proposed two non-exclusive hypotheses. During erythroid cell development, the chromatin becomes progressively more compacted as the cell matures and the nucleus is ultimately ejected [40]. An increased level of Ncapg2 could result in a higher level of condensin II, in turn leading to a higher level of chromatin compaction. Alternatively, the authors proposed that Ncapg2 may act independently of the Condensin complex, cooperating with additional enzymes to induce red blood cell development.

5. Mutation studies

In 2007, our laboratory reported the first viable mammalian mutant of a condensin protein; the *Nessy* mouse, with a point mutation in the Ncaph2 (kleisinβ) gene [41]. The mutant was identified as part of an ENU-mutagenesis screen for immunological phenotypes, and has a partial block in T-cell development. The mutation was mapped to a region in mouse chromosome 15 and ultimately identified as a T to A substitution in exon 1 of the Ncaph2 gene. The mice are viable and appear otherwise normal. The phenotype therefore is not due to impairment of cell division. Indeed, evidence was obtained that at one stage of T-cell development (the $CD4^{+}CD8^{+}$ double positive stage) *Nessy* thymocytes undergo more cell divisions than their wild-type counterparts. No defects were identified in the B-cell lineage. These studies provide the first evidence for a cell-type specific role of a condensin complex component. A subsequent study pinpointed functional deficiencies in mature Nessy T-cells [42]. More recently a study by Rawlings *et al.* presented evidence suggesting that the point mutation in the Nessy mouse prevents Condensin II from condensing the chromatin at a key stage during thymocyte development, resulting in aberrant gene transcription [43].

Another ENU mutagenesis screen, this time conducted on zebrafish, identified a mutation in condensin I subunit Ncapg which caused a reduction in the number of retinal cells [44]. In addition, the animals displayed a high incidence of polyploidy suggesting defects in cell division.

6. Study of alternative splice forms

Until recently, it has been assumed that the genes encoding the components of the condensin complexes each produce only a single protein. Recently however, it has emerged that this may not be the case. In the same study that described the mutant mouse model, our laboratory also showed that mouse Ncaph2 can undergo alternative splicing to produce multiple distinct protein isoforms [41]. We have since studied this in more detail, showing that the mouse Ncaph2 gene is capable of encoding at least 6 unique protein isoforms [45]. The first exon of the gene can be translated into one of three forms. In addition, we detailed the inclusion of an additional alanine residue between exons 15 and 16 resulting from NAGNAG variation. Our data show that the amino-termini variants are ubiquitous throughout the mouse, expressed at similar levels in all tissues tested.

The remaining components of the condensin complexes have never been studied to see if they undergo alternative splicing despite annotated instances existing in the NCBI and ENSEMBL database. We recently completed a large scale study into alternative splicing that identified additional instances of splice variation in Ncaph2 and Ncapd2. A comprehensive summary of the splice variants of all condensin subunits is presented in Table 1. None of the splice variants have been characterized yet, so it remains to be seen if they are functionally unique. Their existence however, raises the possibility that these distinct isoforms may regulate the different functions of condensins. Inclusion of one splice form over another may switch the complex from an architect of chromosomes to a regulator of gene function, providing an elegant method to regulate function.

http://dx.doi.org/10.5772/55732

Mouse			
Protein	**Splice Type**	**Description of splicing**	**Reference**
SMC2	Partial transcription	Transcription of only the first 11 exons, resulting in a truncated protein	ENSEMBL
SMC4	Partial transcription	Transcription of only the first 8 exons, resulting in a truncated protein	ENSEMBL
	Alternate splice site	Alternate in frame splice site at the start of exon 3, resulting in the deletion of 25 amino-acids from the beginning of the exon	ENSEMBL
Ncapd2	Cryptic exon	Inclusion of a cryptic exon between exons 20 and 21 and initiating translation at an alternate start codon produces a truncated protein with a unique amino-terminus	Wilson et al (submitted)
Ncapd3	Exon skipping	Skipping of exons 25 – 28, resulting in the deletion of 283 amino-acids	ENSEMBL
Ncaph2	Alternate splicing of exon 1	The protein can splice the first coding exon in one of three ways, producing proteins with distinct amino-termini	Theodoratos et al, 2012
	Cryptic exon	Inclusion of a cryptic exon between exons 5 and 6, as well as initiating translation from an alternate start site produces a protein with a unique amino-terminus	Wilson et al (submitted)
	NAG-NAG variation	Potential choice of a second splice site can introduce an extra residue between exons 15 and 16	Theodoratos et al, 2012
Human			
Protein	**Splice Type**	**Description of splicing**	**Reference**
SMC2	Cryptic exon	Inclusion of a cryptic exon after exon 23 introduces an alternate stop codon	ENSEMBL
SMC4	Alternate splice site	Alternate in frame splice site at the start of exon 3, resulting in the deletion of 25 amino-acids	ENSEMBL
	Exon skipping	Skipping of exon 19, resulting in the deletion of 58 amino-acids	ENSEMBL
Ncaph	Exon skipping	Skipping of exon 2, resulting in the deletion of 136 amino-acids	ENSEMBL
	Alternate splice site	Alternate in frame splice site at the start of exon 2, resulting in the deletion of 11 amino-acids	ENSEMBL
Ncapd2	Alternate splice site of exon 1	Alternate splice site at the end of exon 1 and initiating translation at an alternate start codon	Wilson et al (submitted)
	Exon skipping	Skipping of exon 4, resulting in the deletion of 45 amino-acids	ENSEMBL
Ncapd3	Alternate exon	Can be transcribed with one of two first exons	ENSEMBL
	Cryptic exon	Inclusion of a cryptic exon after exon 12, creating an alternate stop-codon	ENSEMBL
Ncaph2	Alternate splice site of exon 9	Alternate splice site of exon 9 creating an alternate stop-codon, resulting in a truncated protein with an alternate carboxy-terminus	NCBI
	NAG-NAG variation	Potential choice of a second splice site can introduce an extra residue between exons 15 and 16	Theodoratos et al, 2012

Table 1. Splice variations of the condensin components

7. Separation of function

The separation of the condensin complexes' functions in mitosis and gene regulation remains an inherently difficult process. The *Nessy* mouse represents the first true separation of function in a vertebrate model, the point mutation disrupting the cell-specific role of condensin II while leaving its mitotic role unperturbed. A previous study in bacteria reported a similar separation. Mutations in the kleisin protein ScpA in *Bacillius subtillis* were found to disrupt the DNA repair pathways as well as resulting in the deregulation of specific genes while leaving the mitotic function intact [46].

Such results show that the functions of condensin can be separated, but is still unknown how this occurs. The alternative splice forms may play a role in the regulation of condensin function. Inclusion of alternate isoforms may influence weather the complex acts as a compacter of chromosomes or as a regulator of gene transcription. In our original 2007 paper, we showed that the *Nessy* mutation could be rescued by reintroduction of only one splice variant (designated as the Long-form). The rescue was of the peripheral phenotype ($CD44^{hi}$ T-cells in the spleen). Technical limitations meant that rescue of the thymus phenotype could not be confirmed. Rescue with different splice forms, may have provided additional insight.

Condensins have also been shown to interact with additional proteins capable of regulating their function. Once such protein is protein phosphatase 2A (PP2A), which is capable of dephosphorylating the Ncapg subunit of condensin I, inhibiting its function [47]. This activity has been shown to be important for gene-bookmarking. During cell division, individual cells must "remember" their lineage. Promoters of select genes remain un-compacted during the process of division, allowing for rapid expression of the genes after mitosis [48, 49]. PP2A was found to be important for leaving these genes un-compacted. PP2A interacts with the TATA-binding protein (TBP) which binds to the promoter regions of active genes during mitosis. The combination of the two proteins then dephosphorylate nearby condensin, preventing condensation of chromatin and allowing the genes to become active shortly after division [50].

Additionally, condensin II has been shown to bind to specific histone markers. Ncapg2 and Ncapd3 were found to recognize mono-methylation of H4K20, inducing condensin II to bind to the DNA whereas di-methylation of the histone was found to lead to dissociation of the complex [51]. Based on this finding, the authors suggested a model for chromosome condensation during mitosis; once the cell progresses into mitosis, a demethlyase converts H4K20me2 to H4K20me1, inducing condensin II to bind and compact the chromatin into chromosomes. Upon proper separation of the chromosomes, H4K20me1 is converted back to H4K20me2 causing condensin II to separate from the chromatin, resulting in the DNA returning to an open state. This mechanism also provides a possible explanation for how condensins could be targeted to distinct locations along the genome during interphase. Modification of histones at specific loci could recruit the condensin II complex, inducing compaction of the surrounding chromatin and repression of transcription.

Most studies have assumed that the function of condensins in mitosis and gene regulation is similar: the compaction of chromatin through the tethering of distinct regions. However, this has never been experimentally demonstrated. In fact, despite its similarities to the condensin complex, the *C. elegans* DCC is thought to regulate gene expression through the modification of histones [52], and/or through the recruitment of secondary proteins to the X chromosome [53] rather than by physically restructuring chromatin. Thus, while condensins may exert their epigenetic/ transcriptional regulation function by compacting DNA, it is also entirely possible that they use a different mechanism. Separation of function mutants, such as the condensin II Nessy mutant mouse, are likely to be the key to answering this fundamental question.

8. Concluding remarks

It has become clear that condensins have a role in epigenetic/transcriptional regulation in addition to their better-studied role in chromosome compaction during mitosis. The vital role of condensins makes the study of these complexes difficult, with presently only 3 vertebrate models studied, one of which is embryonic lethal. However, numerous studies using a variety of methods have managed to glean insights into the function of these complexes. Despite the progress of the last decade, there is still much left to be discovered about the condensins and especially how they regulate gene transcription.

Author details

Laurence O. W. Wilson and Aude M. Fahrer

Research School of Biology, College of Medicine, Biology and Environment, The Australian National University, Canberra, Australia

References

[1] Hirano T: Condensins: universal organizers of chromosomes with diverse functions *Genes Dev* (2012).

[2] Hudson, D. F, & Marshall, K. M. Earnshaw WC: Condensin: Architect of mitotic chromosomes. *Chromosome Res* (2009).

[3] Wood, A. J, & Severson, A. F. Meyer BJ: Condensin and cohesin complexity: the expanding repertoire of functions. *Nat Rev Genet* (2010).

[4] Hirano, T, & Mitchison, T. J. A heterodimeric coiled-coil protein required for mitotic chromosome condensation in vitro. *Cell* (1994).

[5] Bazett-jones, D. P, & Kimura, K. Hirano T: Efficient supercoiling of DNA by a single condensin complex as revealed by electron spectroscopic imaging. *Mol Cell* (2002).

[6] Kimura, K. Hirano T: ATP-dependent positive supercoiling of DNA by 13S condensin: a biochemical implication for chromosome condensation. *Cell* (1997).

[7] Hirano T: The ABCs of SMC proteins: two-armed ATPases for chromosome condensationcohesion, and repair. *Genes Dev* (2002).

[8] Hirano, T, & Kobayashi, R. Hirano M: Condensins, chromosome condensation protein complexes containing XCAP-C, XCAP-E and a Xenopus homolog of the Drosophila Barren protein. *Cell* (1997).

[9] Ono, T, Losada, A, Hirano, M, Myers, M. P, & Neuwald, A. F. Hirano T: Differential contributions of condensin I and condensin II to mitotic chromosome architecture in vertebrate cells. *Cell* (2003).

[10] Ono, T, Fang, Y, & Spector, D. L. Hirano T: Spatial and temporal regulation of Condensins I and II in mitotic chromosome assembly in human cells. *Mol Biol Cell* (2004).

[11] Legagneux, V, & Cubizolles, F. Watrin E: Multiple roles of Condensins: a complex story. *Biol Cell* (2004).

[12] Cobbe, N, & Savvidou, E. Heck MM: Diverse mitotic and interphase functions of condensins in Drosophila. *Genetics* (2006).

[13] Hagstrom, K. A. Meyer BJ: Condensin and cohesin: more than chromosome compactor and glue. *Nat Rev Genet* (2003).

[14] Chuang, P. T, & Lieb, J. D. Meyer BJ: Sex-specific assembly of a dosage compensation complex on the nematode X chromosome. *Science* (1996).

[15] Meyer, B. J. Casson LP: Caenorhabditis elegans compensates for the difference in X chromosome dosage between the sexes by regulating transcript levels. *Cell* (1986).

[16] Chuang, P. T, & Albertson, D. G. Meyer BJ: DPY-27:a chromosome condensation protein homolog that regulates C. elegans dosage compensation through association with the X chromosome. *Cell* (1994).

[17] Hsu, D. R. Meyer BJ: The dpy-30 gene encodes an essential component of the Caenorhabditis elegans dosage compensation machinery. *Genetics* (1994).

[18] Lieb, J. D, Capowski, E. E, & Meneely, P. Meyer BJ: DPY-26, a link between dosage compensation and meiotic chromosome segregation in the nematode. *Science* (1996).

[19] Lieb, J. D, Albrecht, M. R, & Chuang, P. T. Meyer BJ: MIX-1: an essential component of the C. elegans mitotic machinery executes X chromosome dosage compensation. *Cell* (1998).

[20] Csankovszki, G, Collette, K, Spahl, K, Carey, J, Snyder, M, Petty, E, Patel, U, Tabuchi, T, Liu, H, Mcleod, I, et al. Three distinct condensin complexes control C. elegans chromosome dynamics. *Curr Biol* (2009).

[21] Petty, E. L, Collette, K. S, Cohen, A. J, & Snyder, M. J. Csankovszki G: Restricting dosage compensation complex binding to the X chromosomes by H2A.Z/HTZ-1. *PLoS Genet* (2009). e1000699.

[22] Petty, E, & Laughlin, E. Csankovszki G: Regulation of DCC localization by HTZ-1/ H2A.Z and DPY-30 does not correlate with H3K4 methylation levels. *PLoS One* (2011). e25973.

[23] Mcdonel, P, Jans, J, & Peterson, B. K. Meyer BJ: Clustered DNA motifs mark X chromosomes for repression by a dosage compensation complex. *Nature* (2006).

[24] Blewitt, M. E, Vickaryous, N. K, Hemley, S. J, Ashe, A, Bruxner, T. J, Preis, J. I, & Arkell, R. Whitelaw E: An N-ethyl-N-nitrosourea screen for genes involved in variegation in the mouse. *Proc Natl Acad Sci U S A* (2005).

[25] Blewitt, M. E, Gendrel, A. V, Pang, Z, Sparrow, D. B, Whitelaw, N, Craig, J. M, Apedaile, A, Hilton, D. J, Dunwoodie, S. L, Brockdorff, N, et al. SmcHD1, containing a structural-maintenance-of-chromosomes hinge domain, has a critical role in X inactivation. *Nat Genet* (2008).

[26] Freeman, L, & Aragon-alcaide, L. Strunnikov A: The condensin complex governs chromosome condensation and mitotic transmission of rDNA. *J Cell Biol* (2000).

[27] Lavoie, B. D, & Hogan, E. Koshland D: In vivo dissection of the chromosome condensation machinery: reversibility of condensation distinguishes contributions of condensin and cohesin. *J Cell Biol* (2002).

[28] Lavoie, B. D, Tuffo, K. M, Oh, S, & Koshland, D. Holm C: Mitotic chromosome condensation requires Brn1p, the yeast homologue of Barren. *Mol Biol Cell* (2000).

[29] Steffensen, S, Coelho, P. A, Cobbe, N, Vass, S, Costa, M, Hassan, B, Prokopenko, S. N, Bellen, H, Heck, M. M, & Sunkel, C. E. A role for Drosophila SMC4 in the resolution of sister chromatids in mitosis. *Curr Biol* (2001).

[30] Britton, R. A, & Lin, D. C. Grossman AD: Characterization of a prokaryotic SMC protein involved in chromosome partitioning. *Genes Dev* (1998).

[31] Biggins, S, Bhalla, N, Chang, A, & Smith, D. L. Murray AW: Genes involved in sister chromatid separation and segregation in the budding yeast Saccharomyces cerevisiae. *Genetics* (2001).

[32] Strunnikov, A. V, & Hogan, E. Koshland D: SMC2, a Saccharomyces cerevisiae gene essential for chromosome segregation and condensation, defines a subgroup within the SMC family. *Genes Dev* (1995).

[33] Strunnikov, A. V, & Larionov, V. L. Koshland D: SMC1: an essential yeast gene encoding a putative head-rod-tail protein is required for nuclear division and defines a new ubiquitous protein family. *J Cell Biol* (1993).

[34] Saka, Y, Sutani, T, Yamashita, Y, Saitoh, S, Takeuchi, M, & Nakaseko, Y. Yanagida M: Fission yeast cut3 and cut14, members of a ubiquitous protein family, are required for chromosome condensation and segregation in mitosis. *EMBO J* (1994).

[35] Smith, E. D, Xu, Y, Tomson, B. N, Leung, C. G, Fujiwara, Y, & Orkin, S. H. Crispino JD: More than blood, a novel gene required for mammalian postimplantation development. *Mol Cell Biol* (2004).

[36] Green, L. C, Kalitsis, P, Chang, T. M, Cipetic, M, Kim, J. H, Marshall, O, Turnbull, L, Whitchurch, C. B, Vagnarelli, P, Samejima, K, et al. Contrasting roles of condensin I and condensin II in mitotic chromosome formation. *J Cell Sci* (2012).

[37] Lupo, R, Breiling, A, & Bianchi, M. E. Orlando V: Drosophila chromosome condensation proteins Topoisomerase II and Barren colocalize with Polycomb and maintain Fab-7 PRE silencing. *Mol Cell* (2001).

[38] Longworth, M. S, Herr, A, & Ji, J. Y. Dyson NJ: RBF1 promotes chromatin condensation through a conserved interaction with the Condensin II protein dCAP-D3. *Genes Dev* (2008).

[39] Xu, Y, Leung, C. G, Lee, D. C, & Kennedy, B. K. Crispino JD: MTB, the murine homolog of condensin II subunit CAP-G2, represses transcription and promotes erythroid cell differentiation. *Leukemia* (2006).

[40] Rothmann, C, & Cohen, A. M. Malik Z: Chromatin condensation in erythropoiesis resolved by multipixel spectral imaging: differentiation versus apoptosis. *J Histochem Cytochem* (1997).

[41] Gosling, K. M, Makaroff, L. E, Theodoratos, A, Kim, Y. H, Whittle, B, Rui, L, Wu, H, Hong, N. A, Kennedy, G. C, Fritz, J. A, et al. A mutation in a chromosome condensin II subunit, kleisin beta, specifically disrupts T cell development. *Proc Natl Acad Sci U S A* (2007).

[42] Gosling, K. M, Goodnow, C. C, & Verma, N. K. Fahrer AM: Defective T-cell function leading to reduced antibody production in a kleisin-beta mutant mouse. *Immunology* (2008).

[43] Rawlings, J. S, Gatzka, M, & Thomas, P. G. Ihle JN: Chromatin condensation via the condensin II complex is required for peripheral T-cell quiescence. *EMBO J* (2011).

[44] Seipold, S, Priller, F. C, Goldsmith, P, Harris, W. A, & Baier, H. Abdelilah-Seyfried S: Non-SMC condensin I complex proteins control chromosome segregation and survival of proliferating cells in the zebrafish neural retina. *BMC Dev Biol* (2009).

[45] Theodoratos, A, Wilson, L. O, & Gosling, K. M. Fahrer AM: Splice variants of the condensin II gene Ncaph2 include alternative reading frame translations of exon 1. *FEBS J* (2012).

[46] Dervyn, E, Noirot-gros, M. F, Mervelet, P, Mcgovern, S, Ehrlich, S. D, & Polard, P. Noirot P: The bacterial condensin/cohesin-like protein complex acts in DNA repair and regulation of gene expression. *Mol Microbiol* (2004).

[47] Yeong, F. M, Hombauer, H, Wendt, K. S, Hirota, T, Mudrak, I, Mechtler, K, Loregger, T, Marchler-bauer, A, Tanaka, K, & Peters, J. M. Ogris E: Identification of a subunit of a novel Kleisin-beta/SMC complex as a potential substrate of protein phosphatase 2A. *Curr Biol* (2003).

[48] Larsen, A. Weintraub H: An altered DNA conformation detected by S1 nuclease occurs at specific regions in active chick globin chromatin. *Cell* (1982).

[49] Michelotti, E. F, & Sanford, S. Levens D: Marking of active genes on mitotic chromosomes. *Nature* (1997).

[50] Xing, H, & Vanderford, N. L. Sarge KD: The TBP-mitotic complex bookmarks genes by preventing condensin action. *Nat Cell Biol* (2008). , 2A.

[51] Liu, W, Tanasa, B, Tyurina, O. V, Zhou, T. Y, Gassmann, R, Liu, W. T, Ohgi, K. A, Benner, C, Garcia-bassets, I, Aggarwal, A. K, et al. PHF8 mediates histone H4 lysine 20 demethylation events involved in cell cycle progression. *Nature* (2010).

[52] Wells, M. B, Snyder, M. J, & Custer, L. M. Csankovszki G: Caenorhabditis elegans dosage compensation regulates histone H4 chromatin state on X chromosomes. *Mol Cell Biol* (2012).

[53] Jans, J, Gladden, J. M, Ralston, E. J, Pickle, C. S, Michel, A. H, Pferdehirt, R. R, Eisen, M. B, & Meyer, B. J. A condensin-like dosage compensation complex acts at a distance to control expression throughout the genome. *Genes Dev* (2009).

Chapter 5

The Role of Id2 in the Regulation of Chromatin Structure and Gene Expression

Elena R. García-Trevijano, Luis Torres,
Rosa Zaragozá and Juan R. Viña

Additional information is available at the end of the chapter

http://dx.doi.org/10.5772/54969

1. Introduction

1.1. The helix-loop-helix Id2 proteins

Cell function and tissue homeostasis are dependent on the precise regulation of multiple and converging pathways that ultimately will control a variety of biological processes such as cell proliferation, growth arrest, differentiation or apoptosis. Frequently these pathways share one or several steps in the signal cascade resulting in either redundant or opposing responses.

Chromatin structure is an essential part of the regulatory mechanisms for gene transcription. Moreover, chromatin has been revealed as a dynamic structure exquisitely regulated through multiple mechanisms including histone modifications and chromatin remodeling complexes that finally, will give rise to an open or closed structure changing the accessibility of specific transcription factors to nucleosomal DNA. Therefore, the protein complexes involved in the modulation of chromatin remodelers and histone acetyltransferases (HAT) or deacetylases (HDAC) could be somehow considered as part of a previous sensitization process necessary for a full and specific biological response.

In the recent literature there is a number of papers describing a variety of biological processes in which cells from different tissues need to be previously sensitized or "primed" to achieve a full response to either a chemical or a biological signal. This concept has been extensively studied in the experimental model of liver regeneration after 2/3 partial hepatectomy (PHx). Hepatocytes in normal liver are quiescent, resting at the G0 phase of the cell cycle, and exhibit a poor response to potent *in vitro* mitogens. Once hepatocytes reach the early G1 phase, cells respond to those mitogens and can progress through the cell cycle. Consequently, it is generally accepted that hepatocytes need to be previously sensitized to overcome the G1 restriction point and become competent for DNA replication [1]. On the other hand, it has been long known that apoptosis-inducing cytokines such as TNF-α are not able to trigger apoptosis in hepatocytes unless they are accompanied by chemicals such as actinomycin D or cycloheximide [2].

Accordingly, unveiling the nature of those signals participating in the cell priming events would be crucial to understand the molecular mechanisms mediating, not only the physiology of different biological processes, but also the pathogenesis of many diseases. We propose here that the helix-loop-helix (HLH) protein Id2 has an important role in the process of cell sensitization by a mechanism affecting chromatin structure of selected genes.

Id2 belongs to a family of HLH proteins identified and named over two decades ago for its dual role as both, inhibitors of the differentiation process and inhibitors of DNA binding. Id proteins were initially found during a screen for determination of factors from the family of basic-helix-loop-helix (bHLH) proteins. Paradoxically, Id proteins lack the basic region adjacent to the HLH domain [3]. This region rich in basic aminoacids, has been shown to be essential for specific binding to DNA: It binds to a hexanucleotide E box sequence on the DNA of target genes (CANNTG) [4].

The HLH proteins are classified into seven groups of factors according to their DNA-binding motif. The seven classes of HLH proteins share highly conserved amphipatic helices connected by a loop of variable sequence and length.

Class-I (or class-A) bHLH proteins are also known as the E proteins since they are encoded by spliced variants from the EA2 gene. This group includes proteins that are ubiquitously expressed. Class-II (or class-B) bHLH proteins, includes members such as MyoD, NeuroD, or Hes with a tissue-restricted pattern of gene expression. Class-I and class-II proteins can form either homo- or heterodimers. Binding of these dimers to "E box" in the promoters of tissue-specific genes will regulate a number of developmental processes [for review see reference 5]. Id proteins belong to the class-V of HLH factors including four members going from Id1 to Id4 [3-6]. Id proteins can dimerize with either class-I or class-II proteins but since they do not contain the DNA-binding motif, this dimerization will inhibit class-I and class-II factor-activity in a dominant-negative fashion [3]. Consequently, the developmental processes modulated by Class-I and-II factors will be blocked by Id proteins [6-10]

Over the past few years among all members of Id family of proteins, Id2 has been shown to be essential for the modulation of biological processes other than its first described function during cell differentiation and development. Among these functions, Id2 has been found to be involved in the regulation or coordination of cell proliferation, cell cycle control, senescence, apoptosis or angiogenesis and metastasis [6,11-16]. Moreover, data in the literature describing the role of Id2 in different cell types suggest that Id2 function is highly dependent on the cell microenvironment and that its molecular mechanism of action is far more complicated than it was thought at first. Since the expression of individual genes is induced in response to a variety of stimuli and frequently, the same signal participates in so many different biological processes, the study of all Id2 functions turns out to be extremely complex. In this review we discuss some of the potential mechanisms by which Id2 has been proposed to modulate cell prolifer-

http://dx.doi.org/10.5772/54969

ation under both, physiological and pathological conditions. We also present the newest findings of the signaling network leading to the modulation of Id2 activity

2. Role of Id2 in cell proliferation

In addition to other functions described for Id2, it seems that its role as a proliferative factor is now recognized as one of the most significant. In fact, there is a growing number of evidences derived from both, *in vitro* and *in vivo* experiments in support of this notion. Ectopic over-expression of Id2 in different cell types enhances proliferation [17,18] and cells acquire some features of transformation [19]. More importantly, in some human cancers such as pancreatic, neuroblastoma or colon carcinoma among others, Id2 is over-expressed [20-22]. Partial ablation of Id2 by antisense oligonucleotides in these tumors decreases cell proliferation. Indeed, Id2 has been proposed as a prognostic factor and a potential therapeutical target for cancer treatment [15,20, 23].

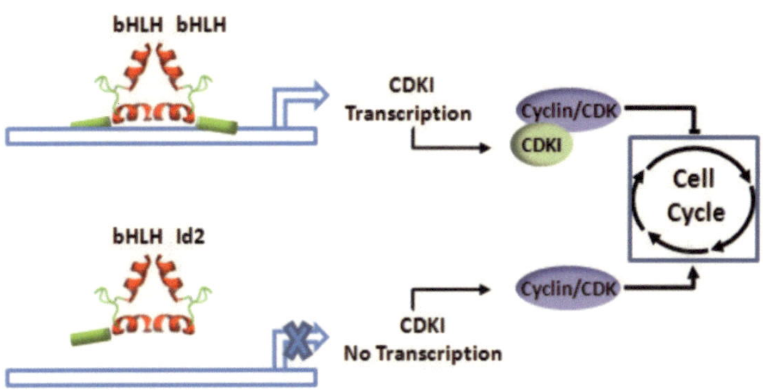

Figure 1. Model of Id2 as a dominant-negative factor for the cell cycle control. (*Upper*) Proteins of the bHLH family dimerize and bind to the promoter of *cdki* genes by their basic domain. Transcription of *cdki* is up-regulated. CDKI binds to the cyclin/CDK complex and blocks its activity. Cell cycle will be blocked. (*Lower*) bHLH proteins dimerize with Id2. Since Id2 lacks a basic domain, the dimer bHLH/Id2 cannot bind to gene promoters. CDKI transcription is down-regulated. Cyclin/CDK complex is active and cell cycle will progress.

2.1. Molecular mechanisms

From the classical point of view, the role of Id2 as a proliferative factor was thought to be dependent only on its ability to dimerize with bHLH proteins as a dominant-negative factor (Figure 1). In this model, Id2 would control cell proliferation by repressing the expression of cell cycle inhibitors such as $p21^{Cip1}$ or $p57^{Kip2}$ [24-26]. Nevertheless, later was demonstrated that Id2 could bind to proteins different from bHLH factors such as the tumor suppressor pRB and the pRb-related proteins p130 and p107 [20]. In this sense, it is largely known that RB (referred to pRb or the pocket proteins) directly associates with E2F on E2F-responsive promoters to restrain gene expression of cell cycle-related genes [for review see reference 27]. Therefore, these data ultimately connect Id2 and E2F-target genes.

E2Fs contribution to cell proliferation and the molecular signaling network that converges on RB proteins has been extensively documented. Although all RB proteins bind to E2F and are modulated by a cell-cycle dependent mechanism, their pattern of expression is different. Whereas p130 is most prominent in arrested cells and preferentially binds to E2F4/5, p107 is mainly expressed in proliferating cells. Finally, pRB is expressed in both proliferating and quiescent cells. The phosphorylation of RB proteins by specific cyclin/CDK complexes will render the subsequent waves of E2F-dependent transcription that will guarantee the sequential transition of cells through the cell cycle (figure 2):

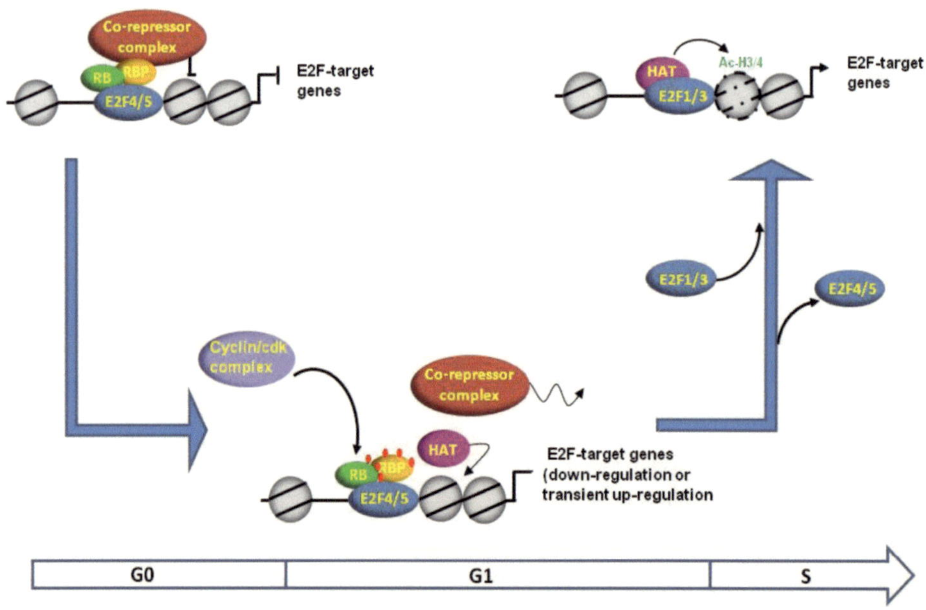

Figure 2. Cell cycle control of E2F-target genes. In G0 cells, E2F4/5 associates with RB proteins and RBP. RBP connects RB to co-repressors (HDAC). E2F-target genes are repressed at this phase. Upon stimulation, sequential phosphorylation of both, RB and RBP will release the co-repressors and transition G0-G1 will take place. HATs could have access to chromatin as G1 progress. At late G1 phase cumulative phosphorylation of RB and RBP will result in the loss of RB function, release of E2F4/5 and the accumulation of newly synthesized E2F1,-2 and -3. These events will drive cells into the S phase.

In quiescent or differentiated cells, ubiquitously expressed E2F4/5 and p130 can bind simultaneously to various co-repressors such as DNA methyltransferase 1 (DNMT1) or histone deacetylases (HDAC) complexes. p130 will inhibit E2F4/5 transcriptional activity by two mechanisms, including binding and inhibition of the E2F transactivation domain, and by recruiting co-repressors such as those mentioned above. These events will lead to chromatin compaction and transcriptional inhibition of genes necessary to entry into the S phase of the cell cycle.

Upon a mitogenic stimulus, during G1 phase, phosphorylation of RB binding proteins (RBP) by cyclinD/CDK4/6 and cyclin E/A/CDK2 will dissociate the transcriptional co-repressors from E2F allowing the access of acetyltransferases (HATs) to gene promoters [28].

At the late G1 phase of the cell cycle, the concurrent and cumulative CDK-mediated phosphorylation of pRb and/or p107 will result in the loss of RB function.

Finally, during G1 to S phase transition, newly synthesized E2F1, -2 and -3 will substitute E2F4/5 and, HATs will be recruited to gene promoters. These two events will drive cells into the S phase.

In this context Id2 seems to take part in a crucial checkpoint for cell proliferation since it can bind to each of the pocket proteins of the RB family in a cell cycle-regulated fashion [20]. Importantly, Id2 is the only member of Id family of proteins that can bind to hypophosphorylated pRB, p107 or p130 [26]. Furthermore, Id2 has been shown to disrupt the growth suppressive activity of RB when the latter is unphosphorylated [17,20,26].

The observation of the pattern of Id2 expression following a mitogenic stimulus suggests different functional roles for this protein during cell cycle progression. The first peak of Id2 expression takes place during the transition from G0-G1[13]. Id2 could have a role in the modulation of p130-E2F4/5 complex activity and in the priming events that occur during this reversible phase of the cell cycle. The second peak of Id2 expression takes place at late G1 phase, where Id2 could disrupt the repressor activity of p107 and/or pRb facilitating the entry into the S phase. The link between Id2 and RB has been further confirmed in animal experiments with double knockout mice for both RB and Id2 [20]. The early lethal phenotype shown in Rb -/- embryos was rescued by Id2 ablation. Several mechanisms not mutually exclusive, have been proposed to explain the physiological role of Id2 on the RB pathway (figure 3):

1. Id2 binding to tumor suppressor protein RB would interfere with its anti-proliferative functions. Expression of Id2 is induced as a response to mitogenic stimuli in a variety of cell types. Therefore, a stoichiometric excess of Id2 would block RB by direct binding to this tumor suppressor [9,12, 29]. E2F is an important factor involved in RB function. Although the direct binding of Id2 to RB proteins have been demonstrated, the relationship between cellular RB-E2F and RB-Id2 complexes is poorly understood. Immunoprecipitation experiments have shown that E2F, RB and Id2 take part of the same complex in rat liver, most probably bound to gene promoters [30]. These data suggests that Id2 and E2F can bind simultaneously to the same molecule of RB (figure 3a). Nevertheless, it cannot be exclude the possibility that Id2 and E2F would compete for binding to RB (figure 3b). In this model, the cellular excess of pocket proteins is the main safeguard mechanism of negative control on cell cycle progression.

2. In addition to RB, the targets of Id2 could be the effectors of RB-mediated cell cycle arrest (figure 3c). These effectors could be either, bHLH or non-bHLH proteins that can also modulate the expression or activity of important proteins controlling the cell-cycle.

CDK inhibitors (CDKIs) enhance the suppressor activity of RB proteins blocking cell cycle progression. Therefore, proteins involved in the modulation of CDKI expression or activity could be considered as part of the RB effectors. As mentioned above, Id2 blocks the expression of cell cycle inhibitors such as $p21^{Cip1}$ or $p57^{Kip2}$. Over-expression of Id2 was able to reverse $p57^{Kip2}$- and $p21^{Cip1}$-induced cell cycle arrest [24,25] The expression of these inhibitors is modulated by bHLH transcription factors. Id2 heterodimerization with these factors will lead to CDKI repression and activation of CDKs. Moreover, MyoD a class II

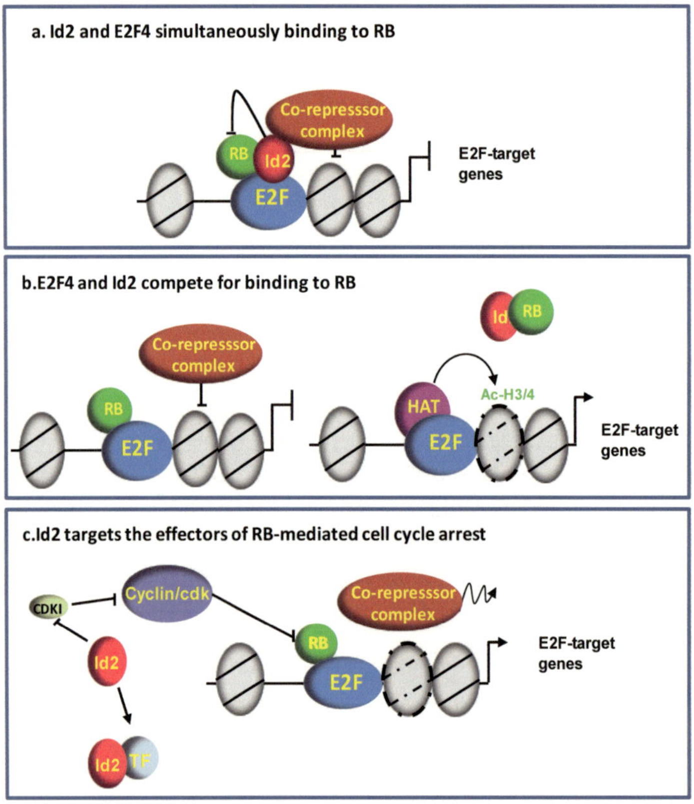

Figure 3. Models for Id2 function associated to RB proteins.(a) Id2 and E2F4 simultaneously bind to the same molecule of RB on gene promoters. Id2 excess gets restrain the repressive activity of RB. (b).E2F4 and Id2 compete for binding to RB. When RB is in excess prevents binding of Id2 to E2F and keeps its repressive activity. An excess of Id2 prevents binding of RB to E2F and restrains its repressive activity recruiting HATs to gene promoters. (c) Id2 targets the effectors of RB-mediated cell cycle arrest. Id2 dimerization with bHLH factors down-regulates the expression of CDKIs. RB hyperphosphorylation by free cyclin/CDKs will lead to the transcription of E2F-target genes. In addition, Id2 dimerization with non-bHLH transcription factors will block their DNA-binding activity necessary to modulate transcription of E2F-target genes.

bHLH protein known to induce p21 ^{Cip1} transcription, has been shown to act by itself as a CDKI. MyoD binds to and inhibits CDK4 [31]. Therefore, Id2 heterodimerization with MyoD would block MyoD function as a CDKI.

In addition to bHLH proteins, Id2 (and other members of the Id family of proteins) also binds to other classes of transcription factors. A brief example of these non-bHLH factors includes Pax [32] or factors from the ternary complex (TCF) sub-family of ETS-domain proteins. TCF proteins such as Elk-1, SAP-1 and SAP-2 modulate the expression of immediate-early genes following a mitogenic stimulus by binding to serum response factor (SRF). Id2 binding to the

http://dx.doi.org/10.5772/54969

ETS DNA binding domain of TCFs prevents the interaction TCF/SRF and disrupts binding of this complex to the serum responsive element on gene promoters [33].

In all these models, Id2 activity could be restrained by RB to keep its anti-proliferative function as shown by Lasorella [20]. The negative role of RB proteins on Id2 could be essential to keep cell cycle arrest for two reasons: First RB would be free to bind to and to restrain the expression of E2F-target genes, and second it would prevent Id2 binding to other targets. On the other hand, a high concentration of Id2, as it occurs in neoplastic transformation, may relieve E2F-driven transcription from the repressive influence of RB. In addition, Id2 would enhance cell proliferation modulating the expression and/or activity of other targets.

2.2. Id2 in cancer: Increased cell proliferation and survival

The role of Id proteins in cancer has been of much interest in the last decade. Variations in expression levels of Id proteins have to be integrated into the whole cellular equilibrium. An upstream deregulation of Id activity, going from Id gene transcription to Id protein, can result in the downstream deregulation of diverse genes. The first evidence connecting Id2 expression and cancer came from the observation that Id2 is a transcriptional target of both N-Myc and c-Myc [20]. Id2 transcription is induced by Myc via binding to E-boxes on Id2 promoter. It has been suggested that Myc increases Id2 expression to bypass the inhibitory activity of RB. TGF-β, a cytokine known to induce a cytostatic program, inhibits Id2 expression in epithelial cells and in human keratinocytes by induction of the Myc antagonistic repressors Mad2 and Mad4. Replacement of Myc-Max complexes with Mad-Max complexes on the Id2 promoter drives Id2 downregulation [34].

Additional evidence for the oncogenic role of Id2 came from studies in which ectopic over-expression of Id2 in developing thymocytes caused a rapid development of lymphomas [35]. On the other hand, aberrant Id2 expression has been reported in squamous cell carcinoma, primary human colorectal adenocarcinomas, pancreatic and prostate cancer or neuroblastoma [11-16]. Id2 has also been related to cancer progression, showing that Id2 expression was higher in high-grade astrocytic tumors than in low-grade tumors [36].

Data in the literature point out to the transcriptional control of Id2 as a key event in the modulation of its function. In this sense, a highly expressed Id2 is not only involved in cell proliferation, but it also promotes cell survival in different cell types. Over-expression of Id2 blocks the TGF-β-induced apoptosis [37]. The role for Id2 as a survival factor in mammary gland development has also been demonstrated [38]. On the other hand, IGF-I known to be a survival growth factor, induces Id2 expression in murine hematopoietic cells [39]. Furthermore, knockdown of Id1 and Id2 gene expression have been shown to induce apoptosis in gut epithelial cells [37]. These observations, together with the fact that ectopic over-expression of Id2 enhances cell proliferation, would suggest that a highly expressed Id2 could confer a proliferative advantage to tumor cells through the modulation of both, growth and survival pathways.

Although it is generally accepted that deregulated expression of Id2 maintains a highly proliferative state and/or extends the half-life of cells in culture [13], Id2 over-expression is not sufficient for cell transformation. Actually, we must be careful to distinguish between events in cell culture and in animals, because the requirements for the modulation and role of Id2 in culture may be mainly related to its requirements in a transformed state more than the requirements in a normal physiological situation. Finally, even though Id2 over-expression has been detected in the above mentioned cancer types and its oncogenic activities cannot be denied, its deregulation is relatively rare. In contrast, Id1 over-expression has been detected in a larger number of cancer types [23] and seems to have a more prominent role during cancer progression.

2.3. Id2 during G0-G1 transition

Since Id2 appears to facilitate and not to support cell cycle progression, it is possible that Id2 could have a role in the process of cell priming, sensitizing cells to a proliferative stimulus. This priming events take place during the G0 to G1 transition and, as already mentioned, are needed to obtain a fully proliferative response to mitogenic stimuli. The pattern of Id2 expression during the priming events support this hypothesis: During G0-G1 transition there is a transient increase of Id2 mRNA levels [13,30].

Liver regeneration after PHx is a unique model to study cell cycle events that take place in a synchronized manner *in vivo*. The protein c-Myc, proposed as part of the priming events in liver regeneration, modulates the expression of proteins important to progress into the cell cycle. The expression of very-early genes such as *c-fos, c-jun,* or *c-myc* takes places in a coordinated and sequential way. The up-regulation of some genes will trigger the next wave of gene expression. c-Myc was suggested to use Id2 as a mediator to bypass the suppressive activity of RB [19,20]. During G0-G1 transition after PHx in rat liver there is a concomitant and short up-regulation of both Id2 and c-myc mRNA.

In the last decades, c-Myc has been the object of intense study in an attempt to unveil the molecular mechanism behind the control of its abundance [review in ref 40]. c-Myc levels can be subject to several modes of regulation, going from posttranslational control to mRNA stability and transcriptional regulation [41-44]. The c-myc gene, although it contains a dual promoter, is predominantly transcribed from the P2 promoter [45]. It is shown to harbor a promoter-paused RNApol II [46] In addition to other important regulatory sites upstream of P2 promoter, an E2F binding site at position -58 from the P2 transcription start site has been identified [45,47]. This E2F site has been demonstrated to be essential for c-myc transcription. It negatively controls c-myc transcription by recruitment of pocket proteins such as p130 that will function as a scaffold for HDAC complexes [48]. Overlapping with the E2F site there is an element essential to remodel nucleosome structure and to open c-myc promoter [45].

c-Myc expression, like Id2 expression, is induced in two stages following PHx. The first induction during G0-G1 phase, takes place at the onset of liver regeneration and the second peak is observed during the transition into the S phase. However, both peaks of c-myc expression are the result of different modes of regulation. While the first increase of c-myc expression is caused by a transcriptional and posttranscriptional up-regulation of the gene, the second peak results as a consequence of enhanced mRNA stability [49]. During G0-G1, c-myc transcriptional initiation increases at 1h after PHx in mice liver. Strikingly, this transcrip-

http://dx.doi.org/10.5772/54969

tional initiation has been shown to be compensated by a concomitant block of transcriptional elongation [46,49]. Elongation blockage of c-myc transcription has been considered as a mechanism to prevent over-expression of the mRNA [50].

The puzzling observation that both pausing and transcriptional initiation of c-myc are enhanced in the regenerating liver lead to hypothesize that increased transcriptional initiation of c-myc in this growth process might be driven by a component of a more general response [49]. Several genes that share common target sequences could be simultaneously activated by a common mechanism, but only additional and specific factors will render the final pattern of gene expression. Indeed, there are hundreds of E2F-target genes that, although transcriptionally dependent on RB proteins, do not show the same gene expression profile. This suggestive idea make us wonder about the identity of that "component of a more general response" involved in transcription initiation.

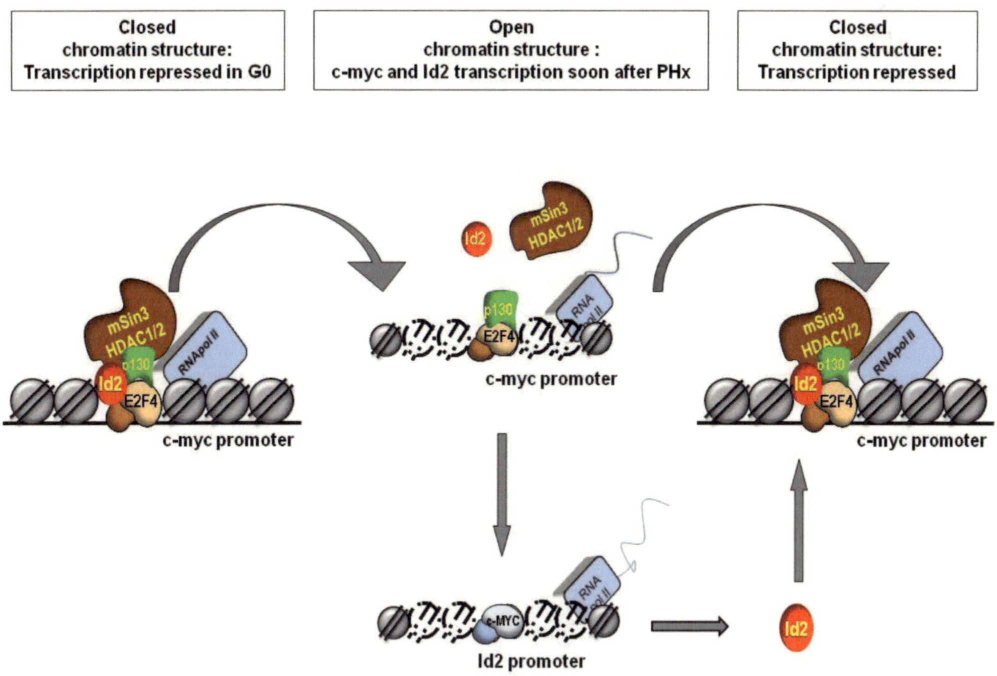

Figure 4. Model for the role of Id2 on c-myc expression in rat liver after PHx. In liver under basal conditions hepatocytes rest at G0. E2F4, p130, Id2 and the HDAC complex are bound on the c-myc promoter. RNApol II is paused on gene promoter. Since chromatin is deacetylated and closed, paused RNApol II cannot progress and c-myc transcription is repressed. Soon early after PHx, Id2 and the HDAC complex are released. Chromatin will be acetylated and opened. This chromatin structure will allow paused RNApol II to progress. c-myc transcription will be transiently up-regulated. c-Myc protein will bind to Id2 promoter inducing its expression. High levels of Id2 will favor its reassemble on c-myc promoter together with the HDAC complex. Chromatin structure will be closed and RNApol II will remain paused on c-myc promoter. Consequently, c-myc expression is shut off.

Id2 could play such a role as part of a common mechanism for transcription of E2F-driven genes. Id2 has been shown to bind to a repressor complex on c-myc promoter that affects chromatin structure (figure 4) [30]. On quiescent hepatocytes Id2, mSin3A (a co-repressor that constitutes the core of HDAC1 and HDAC2 complex), E2F4 and p130 remain bound to the c-myc promoter repressing its expression. Additionally, immunoprecipitation experiments revealed that Id2 is bound to mSin3A(HDAC), E2F4 and p130. Upon stimulation after PHx, Id2 and mSin3A(HDAC) are released from the c-myc promoter concurrently with a, at least in part c-myc transcriptional up-regulation. On the other hand, the transient c-myc up-regulation is followed by an increase of Id2 mRNA. Since c-Myc modulates Id2 transcription and Id2 modulates c-myc expression, a possible regulatory loop would finally control c-myc abundance. These observations lead to propose Id2 as part of the priming events described for liver regeneration and perhaps for some other processes [30].

This hypothesis would go further from the initial idea of Id2 as a simple effector of c-myc to bypass the repressive activity of RB. In this sense, endogenous levels of activated Id2 were shown to enhance but not to support the rate of proliferation in oligodendrocyte precursor cells at the time that slows the rate of differentiation [51]. The authors suggested that Id2 takes part of an intrinsic timing mechanism to control or limit cell proliferation in biological processes highly dependent on a sequential chain of signals that must be transiently synthesized to coordinate the process.

The significance of the mechanism proposed for the role of Id2 in the regulation of c-myc expression, might be extended to the modulation of other genes. To ask whether Id2 plays a global role on transcriptional regulation and/or if it is restricted to E2F4 target genes, we performed genome-wide ChIP-on-chip experiments with antibodies specific for mouse Id2 and E2F4 in quiescent mouse liver [manuscript in preparation]. Promoter arrays contained approximately 28,000 known mouse genes centered on the region from -6 kb to +2.5 kb relative to the transcription start site at an average resolution of 35 bp. Analysis of at least three independent experiments for each factor identified 871 target regions for Id2, and 9307 for E2F4. A comparison of Id2 and E2F4 target regions indicated a limited overlap of 550 target regions for both factors. Moreover, a genome-wide factor location analysis and region classification for E2F4 and Id2-bound regions compared to the genome revealed that although E2F4-alone showed a 100% overlap with gene promoters, positive probes for E2F4/Id2 were partially overlapping with the first exon of genes. This observation suggests that there is a common structure in those genes modulated by E2F4/Id2 that differs from those bound by E2F4 alone. Moreover, E2F4 and Id2 seem to mutually influence each other's binding position and behave like a complex on chromatin. Finally, an in silico gene expression analysis for E2F4 or Id2 positive genes showed that Id2/E2F4-bound genes were mostly repressed in liver basal conditions versus those bound by E2F4 alone.

ChIP-on-chip data confirm that although not all E2F-target genes bind Id2, a subset of these genes might be modulated by the same mechanism as c-myc. This would be a promising molecular mechanism to explain the pleiotropic activities of Id2 affecting the expression of a variety of genes. Id2 could be one of those signals shared by a plethora of biological responses to different stimuli and part of a common mechanism for transcription initiation of different genes.

Most of papers in the literature are focus on the role of Id2 in proliferating, undifferentiated or otherwise transformed cells. However, the behavior of Id2 seems to be quite different depending on the microenvironment, its expression levels, compartmentalization and/or phosphorylation. In other words, the role of Id2 in quiescent cells seems to be different from the one observed in long term proliferating cells. While "activated" Id2 seems to promote cell cycle progression after a proliferative stimulus, "inactivated" Id2 seems to limit or to control the number of cell divisions in quiescent cells

3. Signals involved in the molecular regulation of Id2 activity and function

Id2 expression levels have been classically described as a key event for Id2 function. In general, Id2 expression is high in proliferating cells and low or almost absent in non-proliferating cells such as terminally differentiated cells. However, Id2 is a pleiotropic protein involved in many other functions different from cell proliferation. TGF-β (a cytokine whose function is highly dependent on the microenvironment) represses Id2 expression in epithelial cells [34] but induces Id2 up-regulation in dendritic cells [52]. Glucocorticoids [53], starvation [54], antidiabetic agents and peroxisome proliferator-activated receptor (PPAR) gamma agonists or members of HDAC family including HDAC1-8 [9] are some of the many examples reported to inhibit Id2 expression in specific cell types. Furthermore, this signals can be connected and coordinated. For instance, it seems that HDAC is involved in the modulation of Id2 expression through the interaction with several signaling pathways such as the HDAC/Ying Yang1, the Wnt-β-catenin-TCF7L2 and the BMP pathways that can be mutually coordinated in a different way in different cell types.

On the other hand, Id2 expression can be up-regulated by many factors such as glucose [55] insulin-like growth factor, estrogen, progesterone, thyroid hormone or hypoxia-inducible factor-1α [review in ref 9]. Moreover, recently it has been published a large-scale RNAi screen to characterize genes involved in the regulation of Id2 expression [56]. To further complicate it, in addition to a growing list of up- and down-regulators of Id2 expression, the protein undergoes a rapid turnover, having a reported half-life of 20-60 min, depending on the cell type [57,58]. Thus, Id2 can be regulated at several levels, i.e. transcriptional regulation and protein stability. Although the importance of these modes of regulation cannot be denied, they do not explain the underlying mechanisms for the regulation of Id2 activity. It is important to highlight that there are reports describing an important role for Id2 in conditions in which its protein levels do not substantially change [51].

3.1. Id2 phosphorylation and cell compartmentalization

An important mechanism proposed to regulate Id2 activity is the phosphorylation of specific residues. There is a phosphorylation site for CDK-type kinases close to the amino-terminal domain of Id2 proteins. This site comprises the consensus sequence for CDK substrates (S/T-P-X-K/R) that is conserved among other members of the Id family. Id2 has been shown to be phosphorylated in Ser5 within this consensus sequence by cyclin A/E/CDK2. This phosphorylation was reported to prevent Id2 binding to some bHLH factors and to block the activity of Id2 in serum stimulated human fibroblasts. *In vitro* experiments with a mutant form of Id2 in which Ser5 was change to Ala (Id2-S5A), showed that when Id2 phosphorylation was blocked, Id2 was able to interact with the bHLH protein MyoD. In agreement with this, cyclinA/CDK2 phosphorylation of wild type Id2 prevented its binding to MyoD. The relation between cell proliferation and Id2 phosphorylation state was also established. Indeed, expression of Id2-S5A caused a 50% reduction in colony formation, suggesting that sustained unphosphorylated-Id2 is growth inhibitory [59]. Nevertheless, it seems that Id2 phosphorylation do not necessarily blocks Id2 interaction with other proteins. A latter report suggested that CDK2 phosphorylation of Ser5-Id2 is necessary for the interaction of Id2 with factors that allow nuclear transport such as E47 [60].

From these observations we should infer that Id2 phosphorylation at Ser5 does not block any of its possible interactions with other proteins. Interestingly,Id2 phosphorylated *in vitro* and *in vivo* was subject to a tryptic peptide mapping. The unique phosphopeptide found *in vitro* resulted to be phosphoSer5-Id2. However, two phosphopeptides were observed in the Id2 recovered from the experiment *in vivo*. Whereas the first phosphopeptide was also phosphoSer5-Id2, the identity of the second phosphopeptide in metabolically labeled Id2 needs to be determined. The authors suggested that it might reflect the action of a non-CDK kinase such as PKA or PKC on Id2 [59]. Although this possibility needs to be confirmed *in vivo*, these two kinases have been reported to phosphorylate Id2 *in vitro* [61]. In that case, it is reasonable to think that the different activities of Id2 or its interaction with other proteins could be dependent on the type or number of residues phosphorylated by specific kinases.

Another important consequence of Id2 phosphorylation on Ser5 has been pointed out above. This phosphorylation seems to be necessary for Id2 nuclear localization and proliferating activity. Ectopic over-expression of Id2-S5A and wild type Id2 in smooth muscle cells show a different subcellular distribution. While wild type Id2 localization was predominantly nuclear, mutant Id2-S5A was excluded from the nucleus,. Moreover, over-expression of wild type Id2 in smooth muscle cells leads to increase Id2 phosphorylation, down-regulation of p21 and enhanced cell proliferation. In contrast over-expression of unphosphorylated Id2-S5A could not promote cell proliferation [60].

The subcellular distribution is one of the major points for the regulation of Id2 activity and function. During differentiation of oligodendrocyte precursor cells (OPC) into oligodendrocytes, Id2 protein levels are similar. Interestingly, the cellular distribution of Id2 dramatically changed as OPC differentiate. Id2 was localized into the nucleus of undifferentiated OPC whereas in fully differentiated oligodendrocytes Id2 was localized in the cytoplasm [51]. Moreover, the authors show that Id2 needs to translocate from the nucleus to the cytosol prior to cell differentiation.

Id2 contains two export signals (NES1 and NES2) in the HLH domain and the C-terminal domain respectively. NES1 was found to be conserved among all members of the Id family, and NES2 was shown to be specific for Id2. Although Id2 transport between nucleus and cytosol had been proposed to be by passive diffusion, the recent data point out also to an active transport of Id2. Id2 export from the nucleus is mediated by NES2. However, Id2 does not contain a nuclear localization signal (NLS) and translocation from the cytosolic compartment into the nucleus should be mediated by its interaction with a NLS-containing protein. In this way, translocation can be mediated by interaction of Id2 with E proteins such as E47[60]. Phosphorylation of Id2 favors Id2/E47 interaction and nuclear translocation. Nevertheless, it is important to highlight that interaction with E proteins can also function sequestering Id2 in the cytosol [61]. Moreover, since Id2 can bind to non-HLH proteins, other factors up-regulated during cell differentiation can sequester Id2 preventing its transport into the nucleus. A cytoskeleton-associated protein enigma homolog (ENH) is a good example of a number of proteins described to retain Id2 in the cytosol. ENH is a member of the enigma family of PDZ-LIM domain proteins that is associated to the actin cytoskeleton by direct interaction between its PDZ domain and the α-actinin. Id2 binds to ENH through specific interaction between the ENH-LIM domain and the Id2-HLH domain. ENH, up-regulated during neural differentiation, sequesters Id2 in the cytoplasm preventing cell-cycle progression and releasing bHLH factors from the restrictive activity of Id2 [62]

3.2. Role of GSH on Id2 modulation

Id2 expression and interaction with other proteins has been shown to be modulated by GSH content [63,64]. The tripeptide glutathione is one of the most important systems against oxidative stress in the organism. Alteration of redox balance can affect cell signaling pathways through the induction of protein posttranslational modifications or, in an indirect manner, by the modulation of transcription factor binding activity and signal transduction pathways [65]. However, while the role of cell GSH content in the synthesis of DNA and protection against oxidative damage has been long established, little is known about its sub-cellular distribution and functions in specific compartments. Moreover, the nucleus of dividing cells dramatically change throughout progression into the cell-cycle. It has been recently shown that nuclear GSH content is high in proliferating cultured cells. On the contrary, quiescent cells show similar or lower GSH levels in the nucleus than in the cytosol [66]. In this sense, although most of data describe a significant increase in the hepatic GSH content at 12h after PHx [67], at earlier times, when the priming events take place, there is a 49% reduction in GSH content [68]. Finally, an increasing number of evidences establish a correlation between GSH content and gene expression. Interestingly, it has been speculated that ROS generation induced by a shift in the redox status of cells could affect gene expression by altering chromatin configuration [69,70].

3.2.1. GSH depletion and Id2 up-regulation

The nature of a rapid response triggered by a stimulus suggests pre-existing signals within the tissue that could modulate the expression of Id2 and/or its activity. Moreover, the role of GSH as part of a sensitization process has been already described. GSH depletion sensitizes cells to c-myc-induced apoptosis or proliferation in a variety of cell types, such as myoblasts, melanoma cells or hepatocytes [65,71]. Treatment of rats with l-buthionine-(S,R)-sulfoximine (BSO), the inhibitor of γ-glutamil-cysteine synthetase, induces a rapid GSH depletion in liver that in some way resembles the one observed after PHx (figure 5). Interestingly, BSO treatment also induces two marked peaks of c-myc and Id2 expression in rat liver [69]. The first peak of c-myc expression after GSH depletion shows a short up-regulation also described for other stimuli, a stereotypical transcriptional pulse that lasts for 2-3h and is followed by a shutoff [72]. The second peak of c-myc mRNA was shown to be the result of a posttranscriptional mRNA up-regulation.

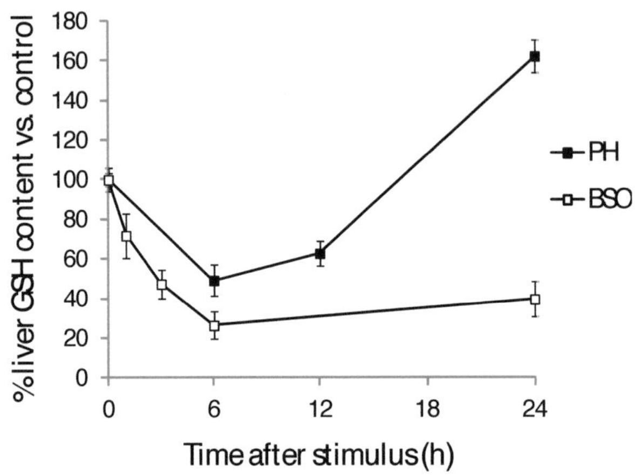

Figure 5. GSH content in rat liver after PHx or in BSO-treated animals. White squares represent GSH levels in rat liver during the time course of BSO experiment (Torres et al. refer 63) Black squares represent GSH levels in rat liver during the time course of liver regeneration after PHx (Lee *et al.* ref. 68).

GSH depletion seemed to be involved in the release of the repressor complex Id2/ mSin3A(HDAC) from the c-myc promoter as it occurred after PHx (figure 4). The proteins Id2 and mSin3A are released from the c-myc promoter as soon as the GSH content decreases 20% under basal levels. Concomitantly with the release of the repressor complex, c-myc expression is induced. When Id2 and mSin3A turns back to the c-myc promoter, the transcription of the gene is down-regulated. Nevertheless it could not be established a relationship between GSH content and the return of Id2 to the c-myc promoter. However, linking these observations to liver regeneration, it would be possible that a decrease in GSH content very early after PH could promote the release of Id2/mSin3A(HDAC) from the c-myc promoter.

Nevertheless, this event would not be enough to induce the transient transcription initiation of c-myc observed after GSH depletion with BSO. However, the release of Id2 and mSin3A(HDAC) from the c-myc promoter would induce profound changes in chromatin structure to become accessible to transcription factors. Indeed, a deeper insight into the molecular mechanisms involved in the regulation of transcription at the first peak of c-myc expression after GSH depletion, suggested an important role for STAT3 at this peak. GSH depletion induces STAT3 phosphorylation, recruitment of CBP/p300 (HAT) and binding to a region that overlaps the E2F site in the c-myc gene P2 promoter shown to be important for nucleosomal structure [73]. These observations are in agreement with the idea of GSH and Id2 as part of a general mechanism to sensitize cells to respond to a given stimulus (figure 6): Id2 release would lead to an open chromatin structure allowing transcription factors to gain access

http://dx.doi.org/10.5772/54969

to gene promoters. The specificity of the response would be achieve by the precise combination of activated-transcription factors and their binding to a particular gene promoter, like in this case occurs with STAT3 and c-myc promoter.

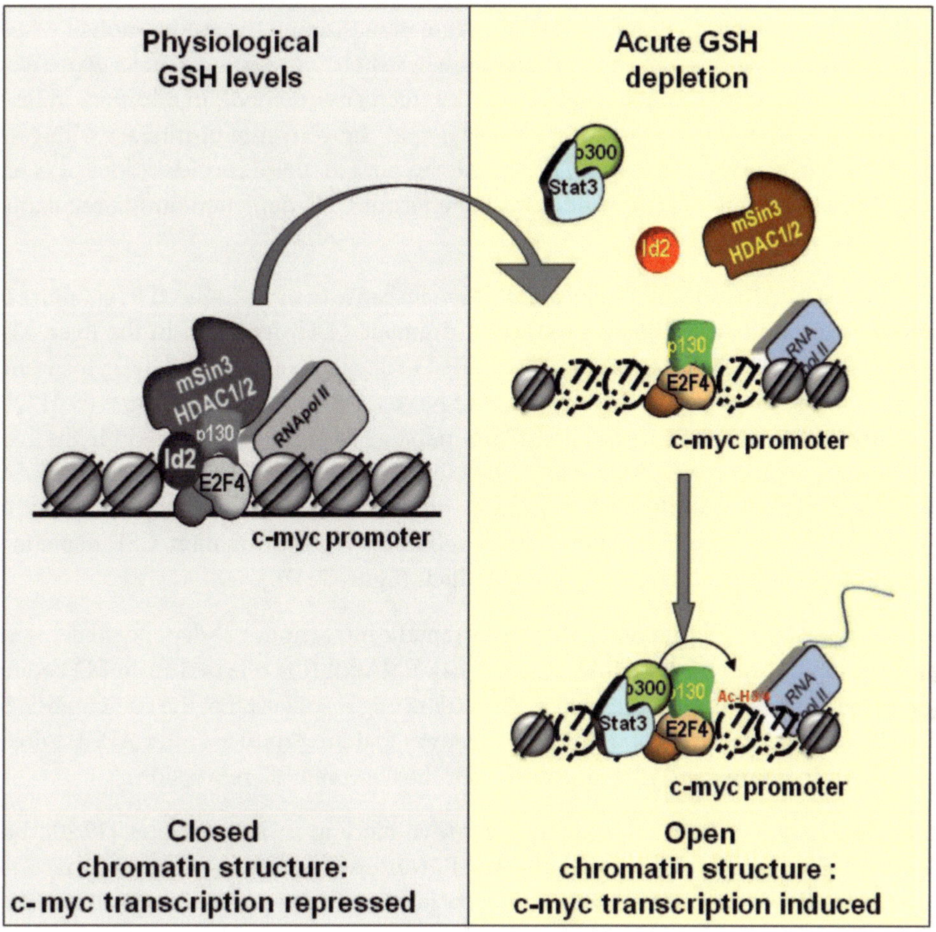

Figure 6. Model for the role of GSH on the modulation of Id2 activity. In quiescent cells, under physiological GSH content E2F4, p130, Id2 and the HDAC complex are bound on the c-myc promoter. Chromatin structure will be closed, inaccessible to transcription factors. RNApol II is paused on the c-myc promoter and unable to transcribe the gene. Early after an acute GSH depletion, Id2 and HDAC would be released from c-myc promoter. Chromatin will be now open and accessible for transcription factors like STAT3 that could now specifically induce transcription initiation. These events would enhance an open hyperacetylated chromatin structure and RNApol II progression.

3.2.2. GSH depletion and Id2 down-regulation

It has been demonstrated that drugs, infections, inflammation, or cell proliferation can alter GSH levels and cause a shift in the GSH/GSSG redox status of cells [65]. Over-expression of c-myc and GSH depletion has been described in a variety of both experimentally induced and naturally occurring liver diseases including hepatocarcinoma, HCV infection, liver cirrhosis, apoptosis and drug-induced toxicity [74]. The information about the signals mediating the induction or repression of Id2 transcription in response to different stimuli is scarce and sometimes contradictory. GSH depletion by BSO has been shown to induce Id2 expression by c-Myc [63]. Conversely, TGF-β which decreases the concentration of GSH in a variety of cell types [75], has been shown to induce Id2 down-regulation through the modulation of c-Myc [34]. Id2 is always defined as a pleiotropic protein whose behavior depends on its expression levels, cell type, stimulus and in general on the cell microenvironment. In addition, Id2 is a downstream target of multiple signaling pathways that can converge or interact with each other giving rise to a specific response. Taking into account all these considerations, it is not surprising that under pathological conditions the effect of GSH depletion on Id2 regulation could be quite different.

Acetaminophen (APAP)-induced intoxication, the main cause of drug-induced liver failure in the United States and Great Britain, produces a dramatic GSH depletion in the liver. The deleterious effect of APAP excess has been attributed to its metabolization by the cytochrome P450 system, which gives rise to the formation of N-acetyl-p-benzoquinoneimine (NAPQI). This derivative of APAP will then react with GSH, inducing its rapid depletion within the liver and generating oxidative stress. Moreover, when the formation of NAPQI exceeds the GSH content, NAPQI will covalently bind to cellular proteins. Therefore, the hepatotoxicity of APAP overdose is the consequence of the additive effect of NAPQI formation, GSH depletion, oxidative stress and the generation of protein adducts (figure 7) [76].

Concomitantly with the GSH depletion there is a dramatic transcriptional-dependent decrease of Id2 expression in response to APAP toxicity [64]. RNApol-II is released from Id2 coding region and, the promoter is hypoacetylated. These data might suggest that the combination of GSH depletion, oxidative stress and APAP derivatives that are produced after APAP intoxication (depicted in figure 7) may be responsible for the observed Id2 repression.

Id2 expression is known to be dependent on c-Myc binding to its promoter [19,20], but surprisingly GSH depletion stimulated by APAP-overdose increases c-myc transcription. However, the mRNA steady state levels do not correlate with the protein levels and consistently, c-Myc does not bind to Id2 promoter in response to APAP-overdose. Although APAP induces c-myc transcription, it also triggers the proteasome pathway leading to decreased c-Myc half life, which is in agreement with other observations showing the APAP-induced degradation of specific proteins [77,78]. On the other hand, it has been shown that c-Myc down-regulation is involved in the Id2 repression [34]. Accordingly, a decreased in c-Myc half life induced by APAP overload would lead to Id2 repression.

Data from these experiments support the idea of a regulatory loop between Id2 and c-myc: The down-regulation of Id2 would favor the release of the repressor complex mSin3A(HDAC) from c-myc promoter and would render a peak of c-myc expression.

On the other hand, although APAP-overdose induces c-myc mRNA up-regulation, it decreases c-Myc protein half life and therefore protein levels are diminished.

http://dx.doi.org/10.5772/54969

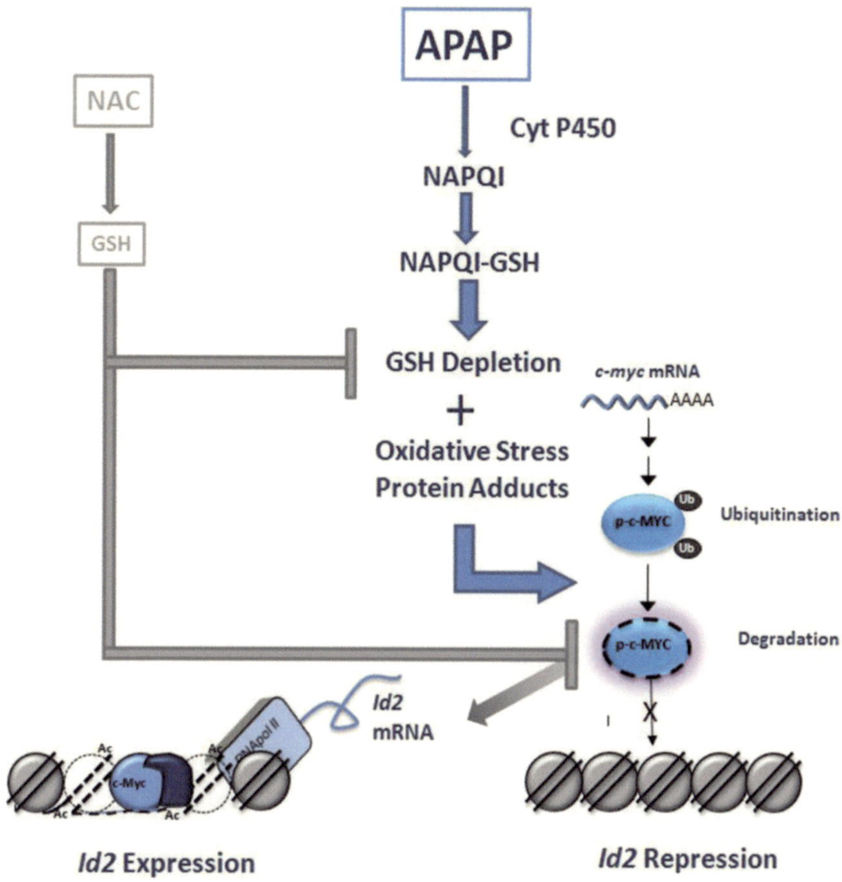

Figure 7. Model for the regulation of Id2 expression in rat liver after acetaminophen overdose and protection by N-acetylcysteine. APAP-overdose is metabolized by the cytochrome P450 system giving rise to the highly reactive derivative NAPQI. This derivative will be detoxified by covalent binding to GSH, which will be soon depleted inducing c-myc expression. When NAPQI exceeds GSH stores, oxidative stress and protein adducts formation will induce c-Myc degradation. The absence of c-Myc from Id2 promoter will block Id2 basal expression. NAC replenishes GSH stores thus preventing GSH depletion, protein adduct formation and the proteasome pathway activation. In the presence of NAC, c-Myc degradation is prevented. Therefore, c-Myc binds to Id2 promoter supporting its basal expression.

Administration of N-acetycysteine (NAC) prior to APAP-overload prevents GSH depletion. Moreover, it has been suggested that NAC interferes with the proteasome pathway induced by APAP toxicity. NAC inhibits the 26S proteasome activity in cultured cells increasing the stability of IκBα and p53 [79]. Furthermore, the proteasome has been described as a redox-sensitive system [80]. Interestingly, NAC pretreatment prevents c-Myc degradation and accordingly, RNApol-II release from Id2 coding region is also prevented. Consistently, Id2 promoter is hyperacetylated and Id2 repression prevented. It is noteworthy to mention that there is a parallelism between NAC protection and keeping Id2 expression at baseline levels.

Covalent binding of NAPQI to mitochondrial proteins has been shown to induce mitochondrial dysfunction and to enhance the formation of reactive oxygen species. The effective protection of high doses of NAC on APAP-induced liver damage has been attributed to the recovery of hepatic and mitochondrial GSH levels. Nevertheless, NAC is not only a GSH precursor, but it is also a reducing and antioxidant agent acting as a direct scavenger of free radicals. Altogether this data suggest that NAC by itself and/or GSH seem to improve the efficiency of the detoxifying system preventing, among other events, Id2 down-regulation. But more importantly, the effect of GSH and oxidative stress in the modulation of Id2 in the context of a wide spread pathology such as the intoxication by APAP seems to be the result of cumulative and converging pathways. These observations highlight the importance of establishing the correct landscape to study the role of Id2, the molecular mechanisms governing its functions, and the physiological and pathological consequences of its regulation and deregulation.

4. Conclusions and perspectives

Among the four members of Id family of proteins, Id2 is a key player in the modulation of cell proliferation. However, many questions about its function *in vivo* remain unresolved. Most of data about the role of Id2 as a proliferating factor are referred to either tumors or cultured and/or transformed cells that might reflect conditions far away from a physiological situation. This is especially relevant since it is well known and generally accepted that the modulation of Id2 activity and its many functions depend on the cell microenvironment. We already discussed the diametrically opposing effects of GSH depletion on Id2 in a pathological condition such as APAP-induced toxicity and in an experimental condition of BSO-induced GHS depletion [63,64].

In addition, the functions of Id2 are not exclusively dependent on its abundance, but also on its posttranslational modifications, sub-cellular distribution and its interaction with a number of different proteins [5,6,11-15]. Nevertheless, most studies use ectopic over-expression of Id2 as a tool to determine its functions and molecular mechanisms with independence of its microenvironment. To understand the role of Id2 during cell proliferation, we should take into account that the enzymatic activities, signaling networks and redox status of cells dramatically change throughout the different phases of the cell cycle. A static image of Id2 during cell cycle would lead to confusion. Id2 gene expression is exposed to a tight control, restrained by a precise timing and coordinated with the expression of other proteins to interact with (i.e. ENH is induced during cell differentiation to sequester Id2 within the cytoplasm).

Following this rational, we can deduce that Id2 functions will change as the cell progress through the cell cycle. Actually, Id2 shows two marked peaks of gene expression during G0-G1 and G1-S respectively that will have different effects on the regulation of the cell cycle. In quiescent cells Id2 binds to hypophosphorylated p130, E2F4 and a co-repressor complex. Id2 expression is low at this stage. The role of Id2 at this phase is most probably to limit the number of cell divisions enhancing repression of E2F-target genes.

During G0-G1 transition, at the onset of the mitogenic stimuli there is a rapid change in both, cytosolic and nuclear compartments (i.e. redox status, signaling networks, enzymatic activities) that will change the preferential Id2-p130 interaction. Initial studies suggested that HDAC complexes directly bound to RB proteins. Nevertheless, subsequent studies revealed that recruitment of HDAC complexes to RB was mediated by RBP1 [28]. As already discussed, the release of RB restrictive activity is the result of cumulative CDK-mediated phosphorylations. These phosphorylations do not have an effect exclusively on RB proteins, but also on RBP1 that bridges SAP30/mSin3(HDAC) to RB proteins. CDK-mediated phosphorylation of RBP1 induces its dissociation from RB [28]. It seems that during G1 phase the multiple and cumulative CDK-mediated phosphorylations of cell cycle-dependant proteins would set a threshold. This ensures that the G1 phase can only be overcome when CDKs reach a critical phosphorylation threshold for efficient dissociation of HDAC and RB from E2F. Therefore it is not a matter of "all or nothing", but the binding affinities between co-repressors, E2F and RB gradually change. Following the same rational, it is tempted to speculate that Id2 could remain bound to the repressor complex SAP30/mSin3/HDAC in quiescent cells and upon a stimulus, a CDK-mediated phosphorylation of Id2 or its interacting proteins would release Id2 and the repressor complex from p130. As already referred, Id2 is known to be phosphorylated during G1 phase by cyclin A/CDK2 and cyclin E/CDK2 [24,59]. This phosphorylation may target Id2 for ubiquitn-mediated proteasomal degradation and/or change its affinity for specific bHLH proteins [81,82]. Alternatively, other posttranslational modifications of Id2 or Id2-interacting proteins might condition Id2 release from E2F4/5 and p130 during G0-G1 transition. In the future it will be crucial to determine those signals that modulating Id2-binding activities can condition the transition from G0 to G1.

It is important to highlight that independently of the molecular mechanism that trigger Id2 release, this event seems to have a profound effect on chromatin structure changing its accessibility to specific transcription factors that on their behalf could recruit HATs (as depicted in figure 6). This mechanism seems to operate not only in a small subset of genes, but on the contrary it can be extended to a larger group of genes (we have observed almost 400 Id2/E2F4-bound genes in our ChIP-on-chip experiments). We propose here the suggestive hypothesis that Id2 could take part of a common mechanism for cell sensitization or priming to fully respond to a mitogenic stimulus inducing an open chromatin structure. The resultant expression of a particular gene will depend on the activation and DNA-binding of the precise combination of transcription factors for the specific gene. Nevertheless, this hypothesis remains as a challenge to cover and understand the molecular mechanisms of Id2 regulation and more importantly to unveil Id2 role during G0-G1 transition.

Acknowledgements

This work was supported in part by grants from Ministerio de Ciencia e Innovación (FIS PS09-02360) to E.R.G-T and Plan Nacional I+D+I (BFU2010-18253) and Generalitat Valenciana (PROMETEO 2010-075) to J.R.V.

Author details

Elena R. García-Trevijano, Luis Torres, Rosa Zaragozá and Juan R. Viña

*Address all correspondence to: elena.ruiz@uv.es

Department of Biochemistry and Molecular Biology, University of Valencia, Valencia, Spain

References

[1] Michalopoulos GK Liver regenerationJ. Cell Physiol.(2007)., 213, 286-300.

[2] Leist, M, Gantner, F, Bohlinger, I, Germann, P. G, Tiegs, G, & Wendel, A. Murine hepatocyte apoptosis induced in vitro and in vivo by TNF-alpha requires transcriptional arrest. J Immunol.(1994)., 153, 1778-1788.

[3] Benezra, R, Davis, R. L, Lockshon, D, Turner, D. L, & Weintraub, H. The protein Id: a negative regulator of helix-loop-helix DNA binding proteins. Cell. (1990). , 61(1), 49-59.

[4] Murre, C, Mccaw, P. S, Vaessin, H, Caudy, M, Jan, L. Y, Jan, Y. N, Cabrera, C. V, Buskin, J. N, Hauschka, S. D, Lassar, A. B, et al. Interactions between heterologous helix-loop-helix proteins generate complexes that bind specifically to a common DNA sequence. Cell. (1989)., 58(3), 537-44.

[5] Massari, M. E, & Murre, C. Helix-loop-helix proteins: regulators of transcription in eucaryotic organisms. Mol Cell Biol. (2000)., 20, 429-440.

[6] Uzinova, M. B, & Benezra, R. Id proteins in development, cell cycle and cancer. Trends Cell Biol. (2003)., 13(8), 410-8.

[7] Kim, H. J, Hong, J. M, Yoon, K. A, Kim, N, Cho, D. W, Choi, J. Y, Lee, I. K, & Kim, S. Y. Early growth response 2 negatively modulates osteoclast differentiation through upregulation of Id helix-loop-helix proteins. Bone. (2012)., 51(4), 643-50.

[8] Yokota, Y, Mansouri, A, Mori, S, Sugawara, S, Adachi, S, Nishikawa, S, & Gruss, P. Development of peripheral lymphoid organs and natural killer cells depends on the helix-loop-helix inhibitor Id2. Nature. (1999)., 397(6721), 702-6.

[9] Chen, X. S, Zhang, Y. H, Cai, Q. Y, & Yao, Z. X. ID2: A negative transcription factor regulating oligodendroglia differentiation. J Neurosci Res. (2012)., 90(5), 925-32.

[10] Iavarone, A, King, E. R, Dai, X. M, Leone, G, Stanley, E. R, & Lasorella, A. Retinoblastoma promotes definitive erythropoiesis by repressing Id2 in fetal liver macrophages. Nature. (2004)., 432(7020), 1040-5.

[11] Norton, J. D, & Helix-loop, I. D. helix proteins in cell growth, differentiation and tumorigenesis J. Cell Sci. (2000). , 113, 3897-3905.

[12] Lasorella, A, Uo, T, & Iavarone, A. Id proteins at the cross-road of development and cancer. Oncogene. (2001). , 20, 8326-8333.

[13] Zebedee, Z, & Hara, E. Id proteins in cell cycle control and cellular senescence Oncogene. (2001). , 20, 8317-8325.

[14] Yokota, Y, & Mori, S. Role of Id family proteins in growth control J. Cell. Physiol. (2002). , 190, 21-28.

[15] Fong, S, Debs, R. J, & Desprez, P. Y. Id genes and proteins as promising targets in cancer therapy.Trends Mol Med. (2004). , 10(8), 387-92.

[16] Coma, S, Amin, D. N, Shimizu, A, Lasorella, A, Iavarone, A, & Klagsbrun, M. Id2 promotes tumor cell migration and invasion through transcriptional repression of semaphorin 3F. Cancer Res. (2010). , 70(9), 3823-32.

[17] Iavarone, A, Garg, P, Lasorella, A, Hsu, J, & Israel, M. A. The helix-loop-helix protein Id-2 enhances cell proliferation and binds to the retinoblastoma protein. Genes Dev. (1994). , 8(11), 1270-84.

[18] Norton, J. D, & Atherton, G. T. Coupling of cell growth control and apoptosis functions of Id proteins. Mol Cell Biol. (1998). , 18(4), 2371-81.

[19] Lasorella, A, Boldrini, R, Dominici, C, Donfrancesco, A, Yokota, Y, Inserra, A, & Iavarone, A. Id2 is critical for cellular proliferation and is the oncogenic effector of N-myc in human neuroblastoma. Cancer Res. (2002). , 62(1), 301-6.

[20] Lasorella, A, Noseda, M, Beyna, M, & Iavarone, A. Id2 is a retinoblastoma protein target and mediates signalling by Myc oncoproteins. Nature. (2000). , 407(6804), 592-8.

[21] Maruyama, H, Kleeff, J, Wildi, S, Friess, H, Büchler, M. W, Israel, M. A, & Korc, M. Id-1 and Id-2 are overexpressed in pancreatic cancer and in dysplastic lesions in chronic pancreatitis. Am J Pathol. (1999). , 155(3), 815-22.

[22] Gray, M. J, Dallas, N. A, Van Buren, G, Xia, L, Yang, A. D, Somcio, R. J, Gaur, P, Mangala, L. S, Vivas-mejia, P. E, Fan, F, Sanguino, A. M, Gallick, G. E, Lopez-berestein, G, Sood, A. K, & Ellis, L. M. Therapeutic targeting of Id2 reduces growth of human colorectal carcinoma in the murine liver. Oncogene. (2008). , 27(57), 7192-200.

[23] Hasskarl, J, & Münger, K. Id proteins--tumor markers or oncogenes? Cancer Biol Ther. (2002). , 1(2), 91-6.

[24] Matsumura, M. E, Lobe, D. R, & Mcnamara, C. A. Contribution of the helix-loop-helix factor Id2 to regulation of vascular smooth muscle cell proliferation. J Biol Chem. (2002). , 277(9), 7293-7.

[25] Rothschild, G, Zhao, X, Iavarone, A, & Lasorella, A. E Proteins and Id2 converge on to regulate cell cycle in neural cells. Mol Cell Biol. (2006). , 57Kip2.

[26] Lasorella, A, Iavarone, A, & Israel, M. A. Id2 specifically alters regulation of the cell cycle by tumor suppressor proteins. Mol Cell Biol. (1996). , 16(6), 2570-8.

[27] Chen, H. Z, Tsai, S. Y, & Leone, G. Emerging roles of E2Fs in cancer: an exit from cell cycle control. Nat Rev Cancer. (2009). , 9(11), 785-97.

[28] Suryadinata, R, Sadowski, M, Steel, R, & Sarcevic, B. Cyclin-dependent kinase-mediated phosphorylation of RBP1 and pRb promotes their dissociation to mediate release of the SAP30 mSin3 HDAC transcriptional repressor complex.J Biol Chem. (2011). , 286(7), 5108-18.

[29] Fan, L. X, Li, X, Magenheimer, B, & Calvet, J. P. Li X Inhibition of histone deacetylases targets the transcription regulator Id2 to attenuate cystic epithelial cell proliferation. Kidney Int. (2012). , 81(1), 76-85.

[30] Rodríguez, J. L, Sandoval, J, Serviddio, G, Sastre, J, Morante, M, Perrelli, M. G, Martínez-chantar, M. L, Viña, J, Viña, J. R, Mato, J. M, Avila, M. A, Franco, L, López-rodas, G, & Torres, L. Id2 leaves the chromatin of the E2F4-c-myc promoter during hepatocyte priming for liver regeneration. Biochem J. (2006). , 130.

[31] Zhang, J. M, Zhao, X, Wei, Q, & Paterson, B. M. Direct inhibition of G(1) cdk kinase activity by MyoD promotes myoblast cell cycle withdrawal and terminal differentiation. EMBO J. (1999). , 18(24), 6983-93.

[32] Roberts, E. C, Deed, R. W, Inoue, T, & Norton, J. D. Sharrocks AD Id helix-loop-helix proteins antagonize pax transcription factor activity by inhibiting DNA binding. Mol Cell Biol. (2001). , 21(2), 524-33.

[33] Stinson, J, Inoue, T, Yates, P, Clancy, A, Norton, J. D, & Sharrocks, A. D. Regulation of TCF ETS-domain transcription factors by helix-loop-helix motifs. Nucleic Acids Res. (2003). , 31(16), 4717-28.

[34] Siegel, P. M, Shu, W, & Massagué, J. Mad upregulation and Id2 repression accompany transforming growth factor (TGF)-beta-mediated epithelial cell growth suppression. J Biol Chem. (2003). , 278(37), 35444-50.

[35] Morrow, M. A, Mayer, E. W, Perez, C. A, Adlam, M, & Siu, G. Overexpression of the Helix-Loop-Helix protein Id2 blocks T cell development at multiple stages. Mol Immunol. (1999). , 36(8), 491-503.

[36] Vandeputte, D. A, Troost, D, Leenstra, S, Ijlst-keizers, H, Ramkema, M, Bosch, D. A, Baas, F, Das, N. K, & Aronica, E. Expression and distribution of id helix-loop-helix proteins in human astrocytic tumors. Glia. (2002). , 38(4), 329-38.

[37] Cao, Y, Liu, X, Zhang, W, Deng, X, Zhang, H, Liu, Y, Chen, L, & Thompson, E. A. Townsend CM Jr, Ko TC. TGF-beta repression of Id2 induces apoptosis in gut epithelial cells. Oncogene. (2009). , 28, 1089-1098.

[38] Kim, N. S, Kim, H. T, Kwon, M. C, Choi, S. W, Kim, Y. Y, Yoon, K. J, Koo, B. K, Kong, M. P, Shin, J, & Cho, Y. Kong YY Survival and differentiation of mammary epithelial cells in mammary gland development require nuclear retention of Id2 due to RANK signaling. Mol Cell Biol. (2011). , 31(23), 4775-88.

[39] Prisco, M, Peruzzi, F, Belletti, B, & Baserga, R. Regulation of Id gene expression by type I insulin-like growth factor: roles of Stat3 and the tyrosine 950 residue of the receptor. Mo.l Cell. Biol. (2001). , 21, 5447-5458.

[40] Oster, S. K, Ho, C. S, Soucie, E. L, & Penn, L. Z. The myc oncogene: MarvelouslY Complex. Adv Cancer Res. (2002). , 84, 81-154.

[41] Vervoorts, J, Lüscher-firzlaff, J, & Lüscher, B. The ins and outs of MYC regulation by posttranslational mechanisms. J Biol Chem. (2006). , 281, 34725-3479.

[42] Langa, F, Lafon, I, Vandormael-pournin, S, Vidaud, M, Babinet, C, & Morello, D. Healthy mice with an altered c-myc gene: role of the 3' untranslated region revisited..Oncogene. (2001). , 20, 4344-4353.

[43] Levens, L. D. Making Myc. Curr. Top. Microbiol. Immunol., (2006). , 302, 1-32.

[44] Thomas, L. R, & Tansey, W. P. Proteolytic control of the oncoprotein transcription factor Myc. Adv. Cancer Res. (2011). , 110, 77-106.

[45] Albert, T, Wells, J, Funk, J. O, Pullner, A, Raschke, E. E, Stelzer, G, Meisterernst, M, Farnham, P. J, & Eick, D. The chromatin structure of the dual c-myc promoter P2 is regulated by separate elements. J Biol Chem. (2001). , 1.

[46] Bentley, D. L, & Groudine, M. A block to elongation is largely responsible for decreased transcription of c-myc in differentiated HL60 cells. Nature. (1986). , 321, 702-6.

[47] Hamel, P. A, Gill, R. M, Phillips, R. A, & Gallie, B. L. Transcriptional repression of the E2-containing promoters EIIaE, c-myc, and RB1 by the product of the RB1 gene. Mol Cell Biol. (1992). , 12, 3431-3438.

[48] Iavarone, A, & Massagué, J. E. F and histone deacetylase mediate transforming growth factor beta repression of cdc25A during keratinocyte cell cycle arrest. Mol. Cell. Biol. (1999). , 19, 916-922.

[49] Morello, D, Fitzgerald, M. J, Babinet, C, & Fausto, N. c-m. y. c. c-fos, and c-jun regulation in the regenerating livers of normal and H-2K/c-myc transgenic mice. Mol Cell Biol. (1990). , 10(6), 3185-93.

[50] Eick, D, & Bornkamm, G W. Transcriptional arrest within the first exon is a fast control mechanism in c-myc gene expression. Nucleic Acids Res.(1986). , 14, 8331-8346.

[51] Wang, S, Sdrulla, A, Johnson, J. E, Yokota, Y, & Barres, B. A. A role for the helix-loop-helix protein Id2 in the control of oligodendrocyte development. Neuron. (2001). , 29(3), 603-14.

[52] Hacker, C, Kirsch, R. D, Ju, X. S, Hieronymus, T, Gust, T. C, Kuhl, C, Jorgas, T, Kurz, S. M, Rose-john, S, Yokota, Y, & Zenke, M. Transcriptional profiling identifies Id2 function in dendritic cell development.Nat Immunol. (2003). , 4(4), 380-6.

[53] Zilberfarb, V, Siquier, K, Strosberg, A. D, & Issad, T. Effect of dexamethasone on adipocyte differentiation markers and tumour necrosis factor-alpha expression in human PAZ6 cells. Diabetologia. (2001). , 44(3), 377-86.

[54] González Mdel CCorton JC, Acero N, Muñoz-Mingarro D, Quirós Y, Alvarez-Millán JJ, Herrera E, Bocos C Peroxisome proliferator-activated receptorα agonists differentially regulate inhibitor of DNA binding expression in rodents and human cells. PPAR Res. (2012).

[55] Grønning, L. M, Tingsabadh, R, Hardy, K, Dalen, K. T, Jat, P. S, Gnudi, L, & Shepherd, P. R. Glucose induces increases in levels of the transcriptional repressor Id2 via the hexosamine pathway.Am J Physiol Endocrinol Metab. (2006). E, 599-606.

[56] Wu, N, Castel, D, Debily, M. A, Vigano, M. A, Alibert, O, Mantovani, R, Iljin, K, Romeo, P. H, & Gidrol, X. Large scale RNAi screen reveals that the inhibitor of DNA binding 2 (ID2) protein is repressed by family member p63 and functions in human keratinocyte differentiation. J Biol Chem. (2011). , 53.

[57] Deed, R. W, Armitage, S, Brown, M, & Norton, J. D. Regulation of Id-HLH transcription factor function in third messenger signalling. Biochem Soc Trans. (1996). S.

[58] Bounpheng, M. A, Dimas, J. J, Dodds, S. G, & Christy, B. A. Degradation of Id proteins by the ubiquitin-proteasome pathway.FASEB J. (1999). , 13(15), 2257-64.

[59] Hara, E, Hall, M, & Peters, G. Cdk2-dependent phosphorylation of Id2 modulates activity of E2A-related transcription factors. EMBO J. (1997). , 16(2), 332-42.

[60] Matsumura, M. E, Lobe, D. R, & Mcnamara, C. A. Contribution of the helix-loop-helix factor Id2 to regulation of vascular smooth muscle cell proliferation. J Biol Chem. (2002). , 277(9), 7293-7.

[61] Samanta, J, & Kessler, J. A. Interactions between ID and OLIG proteins mediate the inhibitory effects of BMP4 on oligodendroglial differentiation Development. (2004). , 131(17), 4131-42.

[62] Lasorella, A. Iavarone A The protein ENH is a cytoplasmic sequestration factor for Id2 in normal and tumor cells from the nervous system Proc Natl Acad Sci U S A. (2006). , 103(13), 4976-81.

[63] Torres, L, Sandoval, J, Penella, E, Zaragozá, R, García, C, Rodríguez, J. L, Viña, J. R, & García-trevijano, E. R. In vivo GSH depletion induces c-myc expression by modulation of chromatin protein complexes.Free Radic Biol Med. (2009). , 46(11), 1534-42.

[64] Penella, E, Sandoval, J, Zaragozá, R, García, C, Viña, J. R, Torres, L, & García-trevijano, E. R. Molecular mechanisms of Id2 down-regulation in rat liver after acetaminophen overdose. Protection by N-acetyl-L-cysteine. Free Radic Res. (2010). , 44(9), 1044-53.

[65] Han, D, Hanawa, N, Saberi, B, & Kaplowitz, N. Mechanisms of liver injury. III. Role of glutathione redox status in liver injury. Am. J. Physiol. Gastrointest. Liver Physiol. (2006). G, 1-7.

[66] Diaz Vivancos PWolff T, Markovic J, Pallardó FV, Foyer CH.A nuclear glutathione cycle within the cell cycle. Biochem J. (2010). , 431(2), 169-78.

[67] Huang, Z. Z, Li, H, Cai, J, Kuhlenkamp, J, Kaplowitz, N, & Lu, S. C. Changes in glutathione homeostasis during liver regeneration in the rat. Hepatology. (1998). , 27, 147-53.

[68] Lee, S. J, & Boyer, T. D. The effect of hepatic regeneration on the expression of the glutathione S-transferases. Biochem. J. (1993). , 293, 137-142.

[69] Hitchler, M. J, & Domann, F. E. An epigenetic perspective on the free radical theory of development. Free Radic Biol Med. (2007). , 43, 1023-36.

[70] Hitchler, M. J, & Domann, F. E. Redox regulation of the epigenetic landscape in Cancer: A role for metabolic reprogramming in remodeling the epigenome. Free Radic Biol Med. (2012).

[71] Biroccio, A, Benassi, B, Filomeni, G, Amodei, S, Marchini, S, Chiorino, G, Rotilio, G, Zupi, G, & Ciriolo, M. R. Glutathione influences c-Myc-induced apoptosis in M14 human melanoma cells. J Biol Chem.(2002). , 277, 43763-43770.

[72] Levens, D. How the c-myc promoter works and why it sometimes does not. J Natl Cancer Inst Monogr. (2008). , 39, 41-43.

[73] Kiuchi, N, Nakajima, K, Ichiba, M, Fukada, T, Narimatsu, M, Mizuno, K, Hibi, M, & Hirano, T. STAT3 is required for the gp130-mediated full activation of the c-myc gene. J Exp Med. (1999). , 189, 63-73.

[74] Chan, K. L, Guan, X. Y, & Ng, I. O. High-throughput tissue microarray analysis of c-myc activation in chronic liver diseases and hepatocellular carcinoma. Hum Pathol. (2004). , 35, 1324-1331.

[75] Liu, R. M. Gaston Pravia KA.Oxidative stress and glutathione in TGF-beta-mediated fibrogenesis. Free Radic Biol Med. (2010). , 48(1), 1-15.

[76] Jaeschke, H, Mcgill, M. R, & Ramachandran, A. Oxidant stress, mitochondria, and cell death mechanisms in drug-induced liver injury: lessons learned from acetaminophen hepatotoxicity. Drug Metab Rev. (2012). , 44(1), 88-106.

[77] Lee, Y-S, Wan, J, Kim, B. J, Bae, M-A, & Song, B. J. Ubiquitin-dependent degradation of protein despite phosphorylation at its N terminus by acetaminophen. J Pharm Exp Ther (2006). , 53.

[78] Abdelmegeed, M. A, Moon, K-H, Chen, C, Gonzalez, F. J, & Song, B-J. Role of cytochrome E1 in protein nitration and ubiquitin-mediated degradation during acetaminophen toxicity. Biochem Pharmacol. (2010). , 450.

[79] Pajonk, F, Riess, K, & Sommer, A. McBride W.H. N-acetyl-L-cysteine inhibits 26S proteasome function: implications for effects on NF-kappaB activation. Free Rad Biol Med. (2002). , 32, 536-543.

[80] Breusing, N, & Grune, T. Regulation of proteasome-mediated protein degradation during oxidative stress and aging. Biol Chem. (2008). , 389, 203-209.

[81] Lasorella, A, Stegmüller, J, Guardavaccaro, D, Liu, G, Carro, M. S, Rothschild, G, De La Torre-ubieta, L, Pagano, M, Bonni, A, & Iavarone, A. Degradation of Id2 by the anaphase-promoting complex couples cell cycle exit and axonal growth. Nature. (2006). , 442, 471-474.

[82] Williams, S. A, Maecker, H. L, French, D. M, Liu, J, Gregg, A, Silverstein, L. B, Cao, T. C, Carano, R. A, & Dixit, V. M. USP1 deubiquitinates ID proteins to preserve a mesenchymal stem cell program in osteosarcoma. Cell. (2011). , 146(6), 918-30.

Section 3

Chromatin Remodeling in DNA Damage, Development and Human Disease

Chapter 6

Role of Enhancer of Zeste Homolog 2 Polycomb Protein and Its Significance in Tumor Progression and Cell Differentiation

Irene Marchesi and Luigi Bagella

Additional information is available at the end of the chapter

http://dx.doi.org/10.5772/55370

1. Introduction

Epigenetics is a branch of genetics that focuses on the heritable changes of DNA or associated proteins, other than DNA sequence variations, which carry information content during cell division [1,2]. These heritable changes are ascribed to chromatin, which constitutes the ultrastructure of DNA and whose modifications affect the genetic material functionality. Differences in chromatin structure have been associated to transcription regulation [3-5] and chromosome stability [6,7], affecting both gene's information, expression and heritability. Noteworthy, these epigenetic modifications are involved in both transcriptional activation and repression, indicating their widespread role as modulators of gene expression in numerous biological processes [8,9].

Chromatin is subjected to numerous modifications roughly classified in two groups: DNA and histone post-translational modifications (histone-PTMs).

DNA methylation is the most studied epigenetic modification of DNA and corresponds to the covalent addition of a methyl (CH_3) group to the nucleotide cytosine within CG dinucleotides or CNG trinucleotides where N can be C, A, G or T. Usually, DNA methylation induces decreased protein-DNA binding of transcription factors and leads to the repression of gene expression [10].

DNA "methylable" sequences are not uniform across the human genome but restricted in CpG rich DNA regions termed CpG islands (CGI). CGI are localized at repetitive sequences, heavy methylated, to prevent the reactivation of endoparasitic sequences such as transposons, and at gene promoter sequences, which are normally refractory to methylation in normal somatic cells [8,11].

DNA methylation is specifically established by DNA methyltransferases proteins (DNMTs), which can be recruited by numerous DNA-binding molecular complexes. These enzymes were classically classified in two categories: de novo DNMTs, as mammalian DNMT3a and DNMT3b, in charge of the addition of the methyl group on a previously unmethylated DNA, and maintenance DNMTs, whose only known member is DNMT1, responsible for methylation renewal in the newly synthesized DNA copy. However, this classification does not entirely explain methylation establishment and maintenance in various molecular processes [10]. For instance, a number of studies demonstrated that all DNMTs are important in the maintenance of methylation during DNA replication, therefore indicating that it is not possible to distinguish classes of DNMTs based on their functional role [12-15]. Another important functional role in DNA methylation dynamics is constituted by the removal of methyl group, which is required to activate methylated genes. However, demethylation is a process not fully understood, in fact, until recently, it was current opinion that only a passive demethylation could occur, as a consequence of a lack of methylation maintenance during DNA replication. The discovery of several putative demethylases, as thymine DNA glycosylase (TDG), methyl-binding domain 2 (MBD2), and GADD45 [16-18], strongly suggested that an active mechanism of demethylation can occur in specific contexts, such as germ line reprogramming [19-22].

The second group of epigenetic changes is represented by histone post-translational modifications (PTM), which consist in the addition of chemical groups to amino acid residues of both canonical histones (H2A, H2B, H3 and H4) and variant histones (such as H3.1, H3.3 and HTZ.1).

Differently from DNA modifications, there are at least eight distinct types of histone post-translational modifications: acetylation, methylation, phosphorylation, ubiquitylation, sumoylation, ADP ribosylation, deimination, and proline isomerization. Each chemical group can be established at multiple amino acid residues of nucleosomes in multiple levels of substrate modification by specific classes of enzymes. For example, lysine methylation can be established at numerous aminoacidic residues of N-terminus tails of histones H3 and H4, such as K4, K9, K20 and K27, in mono-, di- or tri-methylated forms. This variety of histone PTMs and its timing of appearance depends on the particular cell conditions giving the cells different functional responses [23]. Differently from DNA methylation, histone PTMs feature numerous functional roles. For instance, histone acetylation regulates DNA replication, repair and condensation; methylation, phosphorylation and ubiquitylation are involved in DNA repair or condensation. Moreover, all PTMs regulate transcription processes; acetylation is generally a marker of transcriptionally active genes, and methylation can be a marker of repressed or active genes depending on the amino-acid residues involved. For example, methylation of histone H3 lysine 4 (H3K4me) is considered a mark of transcriptionally active genes, while methylation of histone H3 lysine 9 and 27 (H3K9me; H3K27) are considered a mark of transcriptionally repressed genes [8,11,23].

Almost all cellular processes that require transcription dynamics and genetic stability can be considered epigenetic processes. Cellular differentiation is a good example of biological process, which is strictly connected to epigenetics. The genome sequence is static and it is the same for each cell of an organism (with some exceptions); however, cells are able to differentiate into many different types, with different morphology and physiological functions. During organism

http://dx.doi.org/10.5772/55370

development, the zygote, derived form a single fertilized egg cell, originates totipotent cells, able to potentially differentiate in all cell types of adult organisms. After several divisions, totipotent cells originate pluripotent cells, which are partially differentiated and able to differentiate in several cell types. Finally, pluripotent cells complete differentiation becoming adult somatic cells. The differentiation processes are characterized by transcriptional activation and repression of specific genes and, once completed, the cells maintain their characteristic gene-expression pattern, strictly dependent on the epigenetic modifications previously established [24]. Therefore, cell differentiation is rigorously related to the establishment of the correct epigenetic status and to the proper epigenetic maintenance. Epigenetic abnormalities alter gene expression, counteracting regular differentiation and cell physiology [25]. In support of this theory, cancer cells feature an aberrant epigenetic landscape, indicating the causal relationship between epigenome dynamics and cellular processes as proliferation, cellular identity maintenance and genomic instability. [26-28]. Frequently, CGIs in the proximity of tumor suppressor genes (TSG) are methylated in various cancers, inducing TSGs transcriptional repression and promoting cancer progression [29]. Furthermore, specific patterns of histones H3 and H4 acetylation and methylation are associated with numerous cancer types, and it has been shown that several epigenetic patterns enable to distinguish disease subtypes [30,31].

This chapter explores the role of the Enhancer of Zeste Homolog 2 (EZH2). EZH2, the catalytic subunit of Polycomb repressive complex 2, catalyzes the addition of methyl groups to lysine 27 of the N-tail of histone H3 (H3K27me). The importance to specifically focus on EZH2 raises from the evidence that it is involved in several differentiation processes and is often overexpressed in a wide variety of cancer types [32].

2. PcG proteins and PRC-mediated silencing

Polycomb group proteins (PcG) were discovered in *Drosophila melanogaster* as responsible of homeotic gene silencing, also referred as Hox clusters. Hox proteins are a group of transcription factors that determine cell identity along the anteroposterior axis of the body plan by the transcriptional regulation of hundreds of genes [33-42]. After the initial discovery in fruit flies, PcG proteins were detected in plants and in mammals, where they are involved in development, stem cell biology and cancer [43-48]. Polycomb-mediated gene silencing is required in many processes like mammalian X-chromosome inactivation and imprinting [49,50]. Furthermore, PcG proteins are required to maintain stem cell identity [51]. Indeed, their numerous target genes encode for transcription factors and signaling components involved in cell fate decision, therefore in differentiation processes [32].

Principal PcG proteins are conserved from Drosophila to human indicating that PcG-mediated gene silencing is conserved among eukaryotes [42,52,53]. In mammals, each of the fly proteins has two or more homologs [54]. PcG proteins form two main complexes: Polycomb-repressive complex 1 and 2 (PRC1, PRC2) [55-59].

In mammals PRC1 is formed by BMI1, RING1A/B, CBX, and PHC subunits [60]. RING1A/B are ubiquitin E3 ligases that catalyze the monoubiquitylation of histone H2A at lysine 119 (H2AK119ub1), a histone PTM associated with transcriptional silencing [48,53].

As previously explained, PRC2 has a histone methyltransferase activity on lysine-27 of histone H3 [56-59]. EZH2 is the catalytic subunit of the complex and is activated by other PRC2 subunits like EED, SUZ1 and RbAp46 [61,62]. Recent studies have identified an EZH2 homolog, EZH1 that originates an alternative PRC2 complex and, as EZH2, is able to methylate H3K27. EZH1 and EZH2 can occupy similar target genes, and in some cases have been proposed to play redundant roles. However, during development, it has been demonstrated that the two proteins, can also have distinct and context-dependent roles [63-65].

PRC1 and PRC2 are able to induce gene silencing independently by each other [66,67] or by a synergistic mechanism. In fact, establishment of H3K27me3 by PRC2 complex can induce the recruitment of PRC1 by binding the chromodomain of the PHC subunits [39,58]. Once recruited, PRC1 induces transcriptional repression of target gene by catalyzing the ubiquitilation of lysine 119 of histone H2 or by an H2Aub-independent mechanism [68-70]. Therefore, in gene promoters of PRC1 and PRC2 common target genes, H3K27me3, can be reckoned as the hallmark of PcG mediated repression, whereas PRC1 carries out the gene silencing (Figure 1) [48,71].

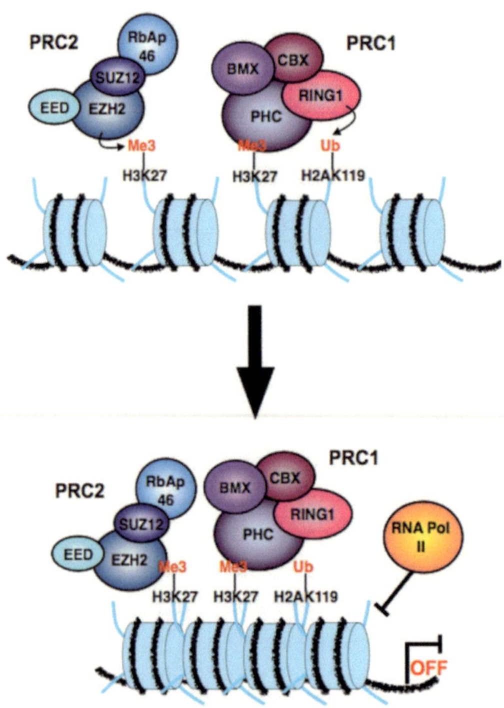

Figure 1. Epigenetic gene silencing PcG-mediated. PRC2 induces EZH2-mediated H3K27me3. H3K27me3 recruits PRC1 that ubiquitylates H2AK119 promoting chromatin compaction and gene silencing.

http://dx.doi.org/10.5772/55370

For what concerns PRC1-independent target genes, it has been shown that PRC2 is able to catalyze *in vitro* the methylation of lysine 26 of histone H1, which in turn recruits heterochromatin binding protein 1 (HP1) to chromatin, influencing its structure [72,73].

PRC2 is also able to cooperate with other epigenetic silencing enzymes. Recent studies demonstrated that it acts upstream of DNMTs in order to silence target genes [74]. The mechanism is not yet clear, but a hypothesis is that target genes are initially repressed through histone H3K27 methylation. Afterwards, PRC2 induces a more stable transcriptional silencing by recruiting DNMTs and establishing CGI methylation [75-77]. Moreover, PRC2 associates with histone deacetylases, reinforcing transcriptional repression and providing functional synergy to stable silencing of target genes (Figure 2) [32,56-59,61,78,79].

The functional link between PcG proteins, HDACs and DMTs demonstrated a synergic control of gene silencing involved in both physiological and pathological processes.

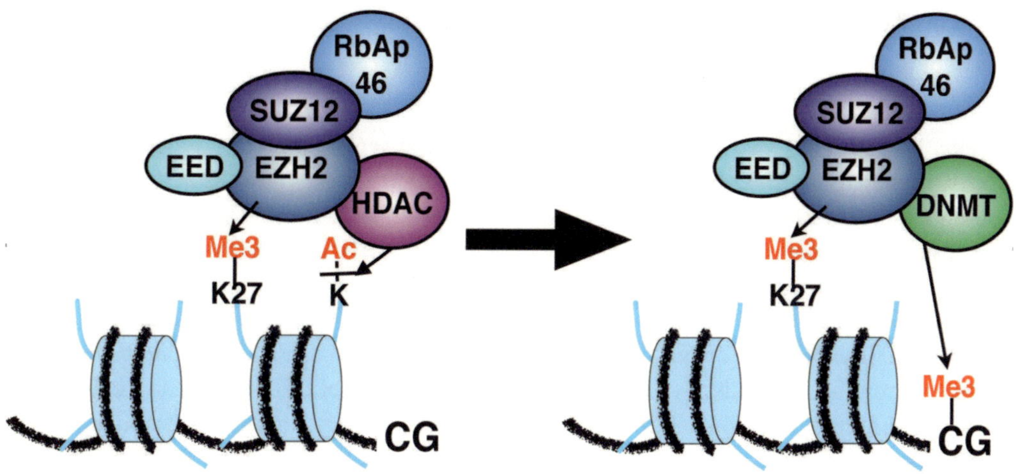

Figure 2. Functional link between PRC2 HDACs and DNMTs. Target genes are initially deacetylated by a histone deacetylase. PRC2 silences target genes by H3K27me3. PRC2 may also recruit DNMTs that methylate DNA promoting a more strongly silenced chromatin state.

3. Regulation of PRC2 activity

Polycomb group proteins are epigenetic regulators of embryonic development and stem cell maintenance [48,51,80] and their deregulation contributes to cancer [28,81]. The crucial role of Polycomb-repressive complexes in the regulation of these biological processes strongly supports the presence of multiple molecular mechanisms involved in PRC activity modulation, such as regulation of expression, post-translational modification and recruitment of other molecular complexes to target genes.

3.1. Regulation of PRC2 components expression

As already explained, PRC2 functions are strictly tissue-specific. Therefore, it should not surprise that the expression of PRC2 subunits has been reported to be context- and tissue-specific, despite the activity of PRC2 promoters has not yet fully understood. Recently, it has been proposed a general rule by which PRC2 expression is maintained by molecular factors that control cell proliferation and self-renewal, such as E2F factors and c-myc, whereas its transcriptional repression is induced by differentiation-promoting factors, such as pRb and p16INK4b [65,82-85].

For what concerns the transcriptional regulation by the pRb/E2F pathway, it has been demonstrated that E2F factors are required for the transcriptional activity of EZH2 and EED in mouse embryonic fibroblasts (MEF). Ectopic expression of pRb and p16INK4b, both involved in E2F target gene repression, induces PRC2 subunits transcriptional repression, whereas pRb silencing increases their transcript levels [82-84].

Furthermore, it has been recently reported that c-myc, a key regulator of ES cells pluripotency maintenance, is directly involved in transcriptional upregulation of all components of PRC2; c-myc binds PRC2 subunits promoters and induces the acetylation of histones H3 and H4, an epigenetic modification involved in transcriptional activation [85].

Finally, it has been demonstrated that EZH2 is post-transcriptionally regulated by a micro-RNAs-mediated translation-inhibition mechanism. MicroRNAs (miRNAs) are small non-coding RNA ~22 nt long (ncRNA), involved in various biological processes, which exert gene expression regulation. Several studies showed a role of miRNA in chromatin structure, they are indeed able to regulate transcriptional levels of epigenetic enzymes as for example PcG proteins [86,87]. Initially, it has been shown that miRNA-101 and miRNA-26a negatively regulate EZH2 expression by binding to its 3′-UTR. However, recent studies have reported an increasing number of miRNAs, able to inhibit the translation of PRC2 subunits (reviewed in [87]). For example, miR-214 regulates EZH2 expression during muscle differentiation [88]. Furthermore, downregulation of several miRNAs promotes EZH2 overexpression in cancer; for instance, miR-25 and miR30d in thyroid carcinoma [89], let-7 in prostate cancer [90], miR-98 and miR-214 in esophageal squamous cell carcinoma.

3.2. Post-translational modification of EZH2

Several studies demonstrated that post-translational modifications of PRC2 subunits can regulate their recruitment to target genes and molecular activity [91-93].

The first post-translational modification that will be analyzed is EZH2 phosphorylation, which has been extensively studied. In order to bind to PRC2 complex and exert its molecular function, EZH2 must be phosphorylated in several specific sites. EZH2 phosphorylation can be classified in two groups: dependent by cell-cycle-dependent signals and dependent by extracellular-regulated kinases [94]. In the first mechanism, EZH2 is phosphorylated by Cdk1 and Cdk2 during cell cycle progression [92,93,95]. In murine model, phosphorylation of threonine 345 (Thr345) increases the binding of EZH2 to specific regulatory ncRNAs as HOTAIR that induces the recruitment of PRC2 to HOX gene promoters, and Xist RepA that

http://dx.doi.org/10.5772/55370

induces the inactivation of X chromosome [93]. In humans, phosphorylation of threonine 350 (Thr350) corresponds to murine Thr345. Recently, Chen *and collaborators* demonstrated a crucial role for the phosphorylation of Thr350 by Cdk1 and Cdk2 in both EZH2-dependent gene silencing and EZH2-mediated cell proliferation and migration [92].

Moreover, Cdk1 is able to phosphorylate EZH2 at Thr487. This modification is associated with the disruption of EZH2 binding with other PRC2 components with subsequent methyltransferase activity inhibition [95]. Surprisingly, these data are in contrast with studies of Kaneco *and coworkers*, which demonstrated that EZH2 phosphorylated at Thr487 is able to bind other subunits of PRC2 complex and to maintain its activity. In addition, another recent work showed that inhibition of Cdk1 suppresses hoxA gene expression in contrast to the findings of Chen *and colleagues*. [92,93,95]. Bearing in mind that these three findings use different models to analyze EZH2 phosphorylation, becomes noticeable that the apparent discrepancies could be explained with different mechanisms of tissue-specific regulation. Further studies are needed to resolve these specific incongruities. Mechanisms of EZH2 regulation during cell cycle are summarized in figure 3.

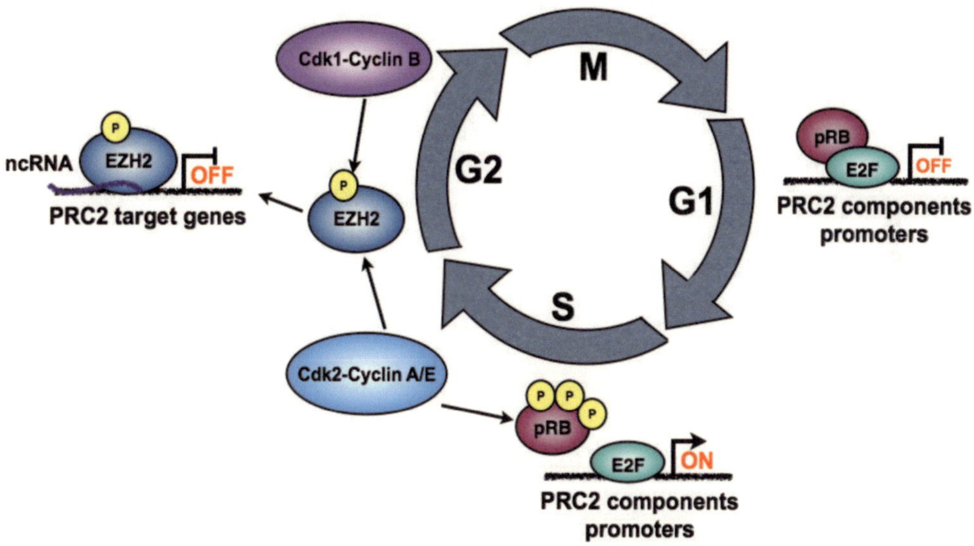

Figure 3. Model for regulation of EZH2 activity during cell cycle. PRC2 subunits are E2Fs target genes. E2Fs activity is inhibited by hypo-phosphorylated pRb during G1 phase of cell cycle. Activity of Cdk/cyclin complexes triggers the transition from G1 to S phase through phoshorylation of pRb and consequent activation of E2F target genes. Moreover Cdk2 and Cdk1 are able to phosphorylate EZH2 promoting the binding of ncRNA, a crucial step for the recruitment of PRC2 to its target genes.

Phosphorylation of EZH2 is also modulated by environmental signals. Extracellular signals induce Akt activation that in turn is able to phosphorylate EZH2 at Serine 21 (Ser21), which results in a suppression of the PRC2 activity. Differently by previous phosphorylation mechanisms, Akt-dependent phosphorylation does not affect the binding with other PRC2 components but it reduces the affinity of EZH2 with histone H3, which results in a decrease of the H3K27 methylation and consequent de-repression of the EZH2-silenced genes [96].

Furthermore, recent studies reported that EZH2 can be phosphorylated at threonine 372 (Thr372) by p38α kinase in muscle stem (satellite) cells in response to tumor necrosis factor (TNF), an inflammatory cytokine highly expressed in muscle regeneration process [97]. The phosphorylation of EZH2 at Thr372 promotes the repression of Pax7, a marker of stem cells, by inducing the interaction between PRC2, YY1 and PRC1. This leads to the transcriptional activation of genes involved in muscle regeneration and to transcriptional repression of genes involved in cell proliferation. This data are in apparent conflict with the fully studied role of EZH2 in the cell proliferation promotion, but it is possible that in response to specific signals and in particular cell types, PRC2 can silence genes involved in cell cycle regulation, resulting in an antiproliferative activity [97]. Other studies are needed to confirm this hypothesis.

Finally EZH2 and SUZ12 can be sumoylated *in vitro* and *in vivo* but the role of this modification is still not yet clear [91].

3.3. PRC2 recruitment to target genes

PRC2 core subunits bind to the DNA sequences with low affinity, this, therefore, suggests the existence of recruiting mechanisms that direct PRC2 to target genes [98].

In *Drosophila melanogaster*, PcGs are recruited by Polycomb response elements (PREs), DNA sequences of several hundred base pairs [42,48,99] located both in proximal region of gene promoters and in long-range enhancer elements. PREs contain consensus sequences for various transcription factors [100]. For instance, Drosophila's pleiohomeotic (PHO) and pleiohomeotic-like (PHO-like) are PcG proteins conserved in mammalian cells and involved in the recruitment of PRC complexes.

It is important to stress that PREs are element and not short stretches of nucleotides and contain numerous TF binding sites, therefore, although several Drosophila transcription factors are essential for the recruitment of PRC complexes to specific promoters, a single TF is not sufficient alone. Moreover, "universal" factors able to bind all PcG target genes have not been found yet, and it is strongly suggested that the PcG protein recruitment is a cell type-specific mechanism dependent by various combinations of TFs [52,53]. Mammalian PREs have been just recently discovered [101]. The mammalian orthologue of *Drosophila* DNA-binding protein PHO is YY1, however, studies in mouse stem cells showed a little overlap between sequences bound by YY1 and PRC2 suggesting a cell-type specific role rather than a general one [47].

Similar to YY1, the embryonic stem (ES) cell-related transcription factors OCT4, SOX2 and NANOG co-occupy a subset of PcG target genes in human and mouse ES cells [45,46]. Interestingly, recent studies demonstrated that the serine/threonine protein phosphatase-1 (PP1), together with its regulatory partner NPP1, is capable of complexing PRC2 at its target genes, modulating the DNA occupancy of EZH2 and therefore its activity [102].

Current data suggest that, similarly to flies, various transcription factors may be involved in the recruitment of mammalian PRC2, varying in different cell types and context. Recent studies showed that Twist-1 recruits EZH2 at ARF-INK4a locus in Mesenchymal Stem Cells (MSCs), inducing transcriptional repression of both p14ARF and p16INK4a, and suppression of senescence initiation [103].

Moreover, PRC2 can also be associated with another PcG protein, called PHF1. PHF1 is not a core subunit of PRC2 but its association with the complex influences the recruitment of PRC2 to target genes and stimulates the enzymatic activity [104,105].

Furthermore, several reports have identified in mouse and human ES cells, a novel DNA-binding component of PRC2 complex, Jarid2, which is a member of the Jumonji C (JmjC) family that binds GC and GA-rich motifs [106-109]. Despite this, it has been demonstrated that Jarid2 promotes PRC2 recruitment to target genes, but its precise role in PRC2 activity has not yet been defined. Knockdown of Jarid2 causes an increase of H3K27me3 levels on some PRC2-target genes [106,107] and a decrease on others [108,109]. Different effects of Jarid2 on PRC2 activity could depend from additional factors, and it has been suggested that it acts as a "molecular rheostat" that finely calibrates PRC2 functions at developmental genes [106].

Finally, long ncRNAs have been implicated in the recruitment of PRC2 [48,53,80,81,110]. For example, in primary human fibroblasts the ncRNA HOTAIR recruits PRC2 complex to HOXD locus for regulating gene silencing in *trans* [111]. Several long ncRNA have been discovered and its tissue-specific expression allows assuming PRC2-dependent roles in organogenesis [112].

4. Role of PRC2 in differentiation and cell fate commitment

In past decades, several studies demonstrated that PcG proteins play a key role during invertebrate differentiation but, only recently, the involvement of these proteins during vertebrate organogenesis as regulators of developmental gene expression has been confirmed. Various tissues are regulated by PRC2 during development (Table 1).

Embryonic stem cells (ESC) are able to differentiate into all derivatives of the three primary germ layers and their pluripotency is preserved by the inhibition of differentiation and the promotion of proliferation [71]. Therefore, ESC can be an extremely valuable model to study cell fate transition mechanisms involved in mammalian development. As previously explained, during development, epigenetic changes regulate the activation determining cell fate.

Genome wide analysis revealed that epigenetic changes regulate the activation or the inhibition of lineage-specific transcription factors in cell fate transition, suggesting their role in the maintenance of ESC pluripotency. For what concerns the polycomb repressive complexes, they occupy gene promoter sequences of the main developmental genes, impeding their transcriptional activation through repressive marks [44-46].

Major targets of PRC2 are tumor suppressor genes, such as Ink4b/Arf/Ink4a locus and their inhibition promotes cell proliferation [44,132,136-141].

In ESC, numerous differentiation-related genes feature a bivalent epigenetic regulation in preparation of lineage commitment [65]. This bivalent epigenetic regulation consists in the

Tissue	Specie	Role/Stage	References
Brain	human mouse	Neuronal stem cell maintenance; oligodendrocytes differentiation	[113-118]
Spinal Cord	chicken	Dorsoventral patterning	[119]
Skin	human mouse	Epidermal stem cell maintenance; hair follicle homeostasis	[120-122]
Cardiac Muscle	mouse	Endocardial cushion formation and cardiomyocyte proliferation	[123-125]
Skeletal Muscle	mouse	Skeletal muscle stem cells maintenance; somites developing and myoblasts proliferation	[88,126-129]
Liver	mouse	Hepatic stem/progenitor cells proliferation and self-renewal	[130,131]
Pancreas	mouse	β-cell proliferation	[132,133]
Adipose Tissue	mouse	Adipogenesis promotion	[134]
Mammary Gland	mouse	Alveolar progenitors maintenance	[135]

Table 1. Tissues under PRC2 regulation

presence of both H3K27me3 and H3K4me3, which respectively are a repressing and an activating mark of transcription [142]. Upon differentiation, PRC2 complex dissociates from these gene promoters, inducing H3K27me3 removal and gene expression [45,46].

Similarly to ESC, PRC2 is involved in organ development through tissue-dependent mechanisms. As a general rule, EZH2 prevents differentiation by inhibiting genes involved in its completion. For instance, EZH2 negatively regulates skin development by repressing premature differentiation of skin progenitors. Specifically, it has been shown that in this specific differentiation model, EZH2 prevents epidermal differentiation by inhibiting the recruitment of AP1, a transcriptional activator, to Ink4/ARF locus, thus maintaining proliferative potential of epidermal progenitors [120]. Likewise, it has been reported that silencing of EZH2 in hepatic stem/progenitor cells promotes the differentiation into hepatocytes and further enhances the maturation of hepatocytes through Ink4a-Ink4b dependent and independent mechanisms [130].

EZH2 also contributes to pancreatic regeneration, by the suppression of Arf/Ink4a locus and the promotion of pancreatic β-cells proliferation, [132] and to terminal differentiation inhibition of mammary gland alveolar cells during pregnancy, in order to prevent milk production and secretion until parturition [135].

In opposition to PRC2-dependent mechanisms mentioned above, there are some tissues and organs, which require PRC2 activity for differentiation completion. For instance, recent studies showed a promoting role of EZH2 methyltransferase activity in adipogenesis. EZH2 is required, indeed, for silencing of Wnt1, -6, -10a, and -10b genes, which are inhibitors of adipogenesis [134]. Moreover, EZH2 contributes to the correct development by preventing the inappropriate gene expression, typical of different cell types. The cardiac differentiation is an example of this PRC2-dependent regulatory function; indeed, EZH2 is involved in transcriptional repression of genes as Six1, responsible of skeletal muscle genes activation in cardiomyocytes. EZH2-knockout mice feature postnatal myocardial pathologies and altered cardiac gene expression [123,125]. EZH2 promotes evenly, by indirect mechanism, liver differentiation by the inhibition of Pdx1 gene, which is involved in pancreatic differentiation promotion [133].

The complexity of PRC2-dependent molecular pathways in organogenesis has been specifically demonstrated by extensive studies in neurogenesis and myogenesis.

4.1. Role of EZH2 in neurogenesis

Neurons and astrocytes derive from common neural precursors (neuronal stem cells: NSC), which sequentially pass through phases of expansion, neurogenesis and astrogenesis. The timing of the switch from neurogenic to astrocyte differentiation is crucial for the determination of neuron numbers.

Analysis of EZH2 expression in neurogenesis showed that EZH2 decreases when NSCs differentiate into neurons and is completely suppressed in astrocyte differentiation. In contrast, EZH2 expression remains high in oligodendrocyte differentiation, from precursor cells to the immature stage [113]. EZH2 silencing and overexpression in NSCs confirmed these results, indeed forced expression of EZH2 increases the number of oligodendrocytes and reduces the number of astrocytes [113]. Furthermore, forced expression of EZH2 in astrocytes induces a partially dedifferentiation to NSCs [117], supporting a key role for EZH2 towards oligodendrocyte commitment. For what concerns EZH2 silencing, it has been reported that inhibition of EZH2 or EED in neural precursor cells extends neurogenic phase, inducing an increased production of neurons and a delay in gliogenesis [114]. However, Pereira and colleagues found that loss of EZH2 results in a shift from self-renewal towards differentiation, accelerating the timing for both cortical neurogenesis and gliogenesis [115]. These differences could be accounted to differential EZH2 inhibition timing before or after neurogenesis onset; further studies are required to clarify this pathway, but all data confirm an essential role for PRC2 in the regulation of developmental transitions timing.

4.2. Role of EZH2 in skeletal myogenesis

Proliferation and differentiation of skeletal muscle cells are controlled by a family of myogenic transcription factors, known as bHLH proteins. MyoD is one of the most important bHLH factors, which is crucial for complete muscle differentiation [143]. In ESC, PRC2 binds and represses numerous MyoD target genes [46]. In skeletal myoblasts, despite MyoD expression, PRC2 is recruited by YY1 to muscle-specific genes, inhibiting their expression and preventing premature differentiation. After the commitment of myogenesis, EZH2 expression decreases and H3K27me3 at MyoD-target loci is removed. Consequently, muscle-specific genes are transcriptionally active [126]. This process is finely regulated by miR-214, a miRNA expressed after myogenic commitment of MyoD. In myoblasts, PRC complexes occupy and repress transcription of the intronic region containing miR-214. During myogenesis decreased levels of EZH2 allow derepression of the miR-214 locus. miR-214, on the other hand, targets EZH2 3′UTR reducing its mRNA translation, thus inhibiting EZH2 mRNA translation [88].

It has been shown that UTX, a specific demethylase that accomplish the muscle specific genes activation, is specifically involved in removal of H3K27me3 and in establishment of H3K4me3, an epigenetic marker of active genes [127].

Interestingly, EZH1 expression increases during myogenesis and its levels remain elevated in differentiated myoblasts [144]. It has been demonstrated that PRC2-EZH1 complex has a crucial role in the correct timing of transcriptional activation of muscle specific genes, as myogenin, allowing proper recruitment of MyoD on its target promoters. This mechanism involves another epigenetic modification, the phosphorylation of serine 28 of the histone H3 (H3S28ph), which is fundamental for the displacement of the PRC2-EZH2 complex [129].

This example proves the complexity of PRC2 dependent mechanism during development and demonstrates how distinctive complexes can regulates various stages of differentiation.

Despite the numerous roles of PRC2 in differentiation and organogenesis are attributable to a tissue-specific behavior, further studies are required to clarify each time its role in any process of differentiation.

It is certainly clear that both PRC2 and its catalytic subunit EZH2 can be defined as key factors in the regulation of development and in preserving cell identity.

5. EZH2 and cancer

Epigenetic abnormalities lead to altered gene expression and cellular physiology and occur in several pathologies such as cancer [145,146]. Cancer epigenetics is a branch of cancer biology that focuses on the epigenetic malfunctions involved in cancer initiation and progression [11]. EZH2 is differentially expressed in many tumors with abnormally elevated levels in cancer tissues versus the corresponding normal ones. Of interest is that EZH2 expression is generally correlated with metastatic cancer cells and poor prognosis [32].

Microarray studies in breast and prostate cancers were the first reports addressing the implication of EZH2 in tumor progression [79,147]. Currently, a wide number of human cancers associated with the deregulation of EZH2 have been discovered (Table 2).

The role of PcG proteins in cancer epigenetics is partially attributed to their contribution in transcriptional repression of INK4b-ARF-INK4a locus, which encode p15INK4b, p16INK4a and p14ARF proteins. These proteins constitute a homeostatic mechanism that protect organism from inappropriate growth signals, which would eventually lead to uncontrolled proliferation, promoting in contrast senescence or apoptosis [139]. Various tumors are characterized by mutations or transcriptional repression at INF4b-ARF-INKa locus, which is frequently a consequence of an aberrant epigenetic landscape established by factors as EZH2.

p15INK4b and p16INK4a are cyclin-dependent kinase inhibitors (CdkI) that function upstream in the retinoblastoma protein (pRb) pathway. pRb can be found in two isoforms: hypophosphorylated pRb is the biologically active form, while hyper-phosphorylated pRb is inactive. Hypo-phosphorylated pRb binds and inhibits E2F transcriptional factor activity. Cdks, through phosphorylation of pRb, render E2F an active transcriptional activator on the E2F target genes. INK4 proteins bind Cdk4 and Cdk6, blocking the assembly of catalytically active Cyclin–Cdk complexes.

The result of an elevated transcription of INK4 proteins is a pRb-dependent cell-cycle arrest in G1-phase [44,132,136-141,188,189]. Differently from INK4 proteins, p14ARF activates p53 pathway by inhibiting MDM2 functions. Indeed, MDM2 modulates p53 activity by inducing its transcriptional repression and by promoting its proteasome-mediated degradation. p14ARF induction generally causes cell-cycle arrest in G1 and G2 phases and apoptosis [139,190,191]. Interestingly, EZH2 activity on p16INK4a promoter is Rb family-dependent. Indeed, EZH2 is not able to bind INK4a locus in Rb proteins-deficient cells. A model has been proposed where pRb recruits PRC2 to the p16INK4a promoter, which in turn promotes its transcriptional repression [192].

EZH2 has shown a functional role evenly on pRb2/p130. pRb2/p130 is a member of Rb family that binds and recruits HDAC1 at Cyclin A promoter, inducing gene silencing. Cyclin A is a protein with a crucial role in cell cycle advancement. EZH2 competes with HDAC1 for its binding with pRb2/p130, disrupting both proteins occupancy on cyclin A promoter, inducing cyclin A activation and cell cycle progression [193,194].

As well as Rb family members, EZH2 inhibits tumor suppressor genes as p21 and phosphatase and tensin homolog (PTEN) [170,195]. For example, oncogenic stimuli in melanocytes provoke an oncogene-induced senescence, termed melanocytic nevus, which is a benign precursor of melanoma. EZH2 overexpressing cells escape senescence through the inhibition of p21. EZH2 depletion indeed, results in p21 activation and senescence induction in human melanoma cells [195]. A similar functional role has been reported in B-cell acute lymphoblastic leukemia (B-ALL) cells, where EZH2 overexpression induces p21, p53 and PTEN silencing whereas its knockdown induces cell cycle arrest and apoptosis [170].

As already stated, EZH2 is involved in apoptosis regulation [196,197]. High levels of EZH2 induce silencing of DAB2IP, a Ras GTPase-activating protein that promotes apoptosis through the tumor necrosis factor-mediated JNK signaling pathway [196], and Bim, a protein that promotes E2F1-dependent apoptosis [197].

DAB2IP is downregulated by epigenetic modifications in multiple aggressive cancers such as lung, breast and prostate. In medulloblastoma, EZH2-dependent-DAB2IP repression correlates significantly with a poor prognosis, independent by the metastatic stage [187].

Recent reports, using genome-wide technologies, reported that a large number of differentiation-related factors are PRC2-target genes [43-47]. Consequently, numerous differentiation-related factors as Gata, Sox, Fox, Pou, Pax, components of Wnt, TGF-β, Notch, FGF and retinoic acid pathways are silenced by EZH2 [32,44-46]. It has been proposed that similarly to ESC, the role of EZH2 in cancer is linked to its activity in self-renewal promotion and in the maintenance of undifferentiated state of cells; EZH2 deregulation indeed, strongly contributes to the transcriptional silencing of tumor suppressor and differentiation genes, promoting therefore uncontrolled cell proliferation and cancer progression [32]. For instance, EZH2 is upregulated in Rhabdomyosarcoma (RMS) cell lines and primary tumors [180]. RMS is a tumor that arises from muscle precursor cells, characterized by a partial myogenic differentiation. RMS cells do not form functional muscle units and feature a strong proliferative ability. Specifically, as shown in a recent study, EZH2 binds and silences several muscle gene promoters evenly under differentiated conditions. The silencing of EZH2 promotes the reduction of H3K27me3 establishment, the recruitment of elongating RNA Polymerase II at these loci and the activation of muscle specific genes, with a partial recovery of skeletal muscle phenotype [182].

Finally, PRC2 complex inhibits the expression of several tumor suppressor miRNA. For instance, downregulation of miR-31, a common event of various melanomas, is caused by epigenetic silencing of EZH2-mediated histone methylation [177].

Moreover, in metastatic liver cancers, up-regulation of EZH2 inhibits miR-139-5p, miR-125b, miR-101, let-7c, and miR-200b, promoting cell motility and metastasis-related pathways [163].

Cancer	Histological Origin	References
Breast	Epithelial	[84,147-151]
Prostate	Epithelial	[79,149,152-157]
Lung	Epithelial	[158-160]
Colon	Epithelial	[161]
Liver	Epithelial	[162,163]
Gastric	Epithelial	[164]
Lymphoma	Mesenchymal	[165-171]
Myeloma	Mesenchymal	[172-174]
Ovarian	Epithelial	[175]
Skin	Epithelial	[149,176,177]
Bladder	Epithelial	[178]
Endometrial	Epithelial	[149,179]
Sarcoma	Mesenchymal	[180-182]
Pancreas	Epithelial	[156,183,184]
Kidney	Epithelial	[185]
Brain	Nervous Tissue	[186,187]

Table 2. Human cancers associated with overexpression of EZH2

5.1. Extra-nuclear function of EZH2

The role of EZH2 as chromatin regulator has been extensively analyzed in a number of normal and pathological models. Recent studies demonstrated a localization of EZH2 and other PRC2 components in the cytoplasm of murine and human cells [198]. Cytoplasmic EZH2 maintains its methyltransferase activity and interacts with Vav1, a GDP-GTP exchange factor (GEF) for members of the Rho-family of GTPases. EZH2-Vav1 complex is necessary for actin reorganization and cellular proliferation in T-lymphocytes and fibroblasts, promoting cytoskeletal dynamics and cell migration as well as proliferation [198]. An example of this specific cytoplasmic function could be found in prostate cancer cells, characterized by increased levels of both nuclear and cytoplasmic EZH2. Cytoplasmic EZH2 might influence cell adhesion and migration, contributing to invasiveness and metastatic ability of tumors [199,200]. The nuclear and cytoplasmic functions of PRC2 thereby could co-operate to promote tumorigenesis.

5.2. Tumor suppressor roles of EZH2

Up to few years ago, EZH2 and PRC2 upregulation were assumed to hypermethylate H3K27, repressing the transcription of tumor suppressor genes. In 2010, Morin and colleagues identified a somatic mutation (Tyr641), which affects the EZH2 catalytic domain activity in diffuse large B-cell lymphoma but not in mantle cell or T-cell lymphoma. Specifically, mutations in lymphoma were heterozygous but haploinsufficient for the enzymatic activity, resulting in global deficit of H3K27 methylation and derepression of gene expression [168]. It has been supposed that the loss of EZH2 in lymphoma may lead to derepression of genes, promoting cell growth [201]. Other reports demonstrated that specific mutations in the EZH2 enzyme display limited capacity to carry out H3K27 monomethylation but have high efficiency for driving di- and tri-methylation. In B-cell lymphomas, mutant and wild type EZH2 co-operate increasing the trimethylated form [202].

Although the data analyzed as of now allow us to classify EZH2 as an oncogene, it must be stated that in particular cellular environments the picture becomes less clear, like for example in malignant myeloid diseases. Three different reports showed the inactivation of EZH2 in myelodysplastic syndromes (MDSs) and in myeloproliferative disorder (MPD) [203-205]. Point mutations of EZH2 gene in MDSs, MPD, and primary myelofibrosis (PMF) are predictors of poor overall survival, independently by risk factors [206,207]. Similarly, three studies conducted in T-acute lymphoblastic leukemia (T-ALL) demonstrated that PRC2 displays a tumor suppressor role in this pathology [171,208,209]. Particularly, Simon and colleagues demonstrated that in mouse, loss of EZH2 in hematopoietic stem cells induces aggressive T-ALL. Similar studies in human showed a comparable decrease of EZH2 levels in T-ALL [171]. Moreover, Ntziachristos and coworkers found that EZH2 and other PRC2 core components are frequently mutated in T-ALL samples [209]. Of interest is that the frequency of PRC2 mutations is higher in pediatric subtype of leukemia [208].

Despite mutations of EZH2 seem specific for a few type of cancers, latest reports suggest a fine balance of H3K27 methylation, necessary for normal cell growth. Recent studies showed an indirect EZH2-dependent mechanism involved in pancreatic cancer inhibition. Jon Mallen-St. and co-authors investigated the role of EZH2 in pancreatic regeneration and in cancer progression using a mouse model characterized by KRas activation, frequently mutated in pancreatic tumors. In particular, they show that KRas mutated mice developed preneoplastic lesions but rarely progressed into invasive adenocarcinoma. The loss of EZH2 function in this experimental model increases by 6 times the development of pancreatic intraepithelial neoplasia, suggesting a protective role of EZH2 in pancreatic carcinogenesis. Since EZH2 is transiently upregulated after injury and returns to basal levels after tissue recovery, it has been proposed that, in injured tissue, surviving acinar cells de-differentiate into metaplastic epithelial intermediates are able to proliferate and restore pancreatic injury. Proliferation is induced by EZH2 activation through P16INK4a inhibition. Subsequently, acinar cell mass and function is finally restored through re-differentiation, which corresponds to restored basal levels of EZH2. EZH2 is involved therefore in homeostatic mechanisms that controls pancreatic regeneration, decreasing the risk of pancreatic cancer in patient with chronic pancreatic injury [156,184].

6. Conclusions

Epigenetic alterations in cancer cells represent an important aspect of tumor biology. Differently from genetic modifications, epigenetic alterations can be reversed by specific drugs inducing the restoration of "normal" cellular pathways, which in turn promote cellular senescence or apoptosis. Therefore, epigenetic changes are excellent target candidates for chemotherapeutic intervention in cancer.

Several HDAC and DNMT inhibitors are already available as putative anticancer drugs, and several clinical trials are underway [210,211].

A pharmacological therapy, which specifically targets EZH2, may constitute a novel approach to the treatment of cancer, assuming its role in inhibition of several tumor suppressor or differentiation genes.

Recently, an S-adenosyl-L-homocysteine (AdoHcy) hydrolase inhibitor, 3-Deazaneplanocin A (DZNep), has been demonstrated to deplete EZH2 and remove H3K27me3 at PRC2 target genes. The inhibition of AdoHcy hydrolase fosters accumulation of AdoHcy, which in turn stops S-adenosyl-L-methionine (SAH)-dependent methyltransferases.

DZNep promotes apoptosis in cancer cell lines as breast and colorectal cancer cells, but not in normal cells. DZNep reduces cellular levels of PRC2 subunits, inhibits H3K27 methylation and promotes the reactivation of PRC2 silenced genes and apoptosis [212]

Of interest is that, in several non-small cell lung cancer (NSCLC) cell lines, DZNep treatment results in p27 accumulation, G1 cell cycle arrest and apoptosis, whereas immortalized bronchial epithelial and fibroblast cell lines are less sensitive and show apoptosis with lesser extent, which render it a potential candidate in anti-cancer therapy [160].

Studies in various gastric cancer cell lines and in primary human gastric cancer cells showed that the DZNep responsiveness is attenuated in p53-depleted cells. p53 genomic status is therefore a potential predictive marker of DZNep response in this specific cell type [213].

Despite its potential usefulness in cancer therapy, further studies need to address its target specificity. Indeed, it has been reported that DZNep inhibits H4K20 methylation, another epigenetic modification, which is involved with chromosome stability [212]. The effect of DZNep on several methyl transferases activity is a strong limiting factor for its use as anticancer drug.

New PRC2 targets have been recently developed. GSK126 is a small molecule, competitor of S-adenosyl-L-methionine. Unlike DZNep, that reduce levels of EZH2 indirectly, GSK126 specifically inhibits EZH2 methyltransferase activity with no alterations in EZH2 expression. In lymphoma cells, GSK126 treatment decreases global H3K27me3 levels and reactivates PRC2 target genes. [169]. Finally, it has been discovered a natural compound, 16-hydroxyclero-da-3,13-dien-15,16-olide (PL3), which is able to promote apoptosis in leukemia K562 cells by the modulation of various histone-modifying enzymes among which EZH2 and SUZ12 [214].

Other studies are needed to design inhibitors specific for PRC2 and to develop new strategies for epigenetic therapy in cancer.

Acknowledgements

We are grateful to Dr. Francesco Paolo Fiorentino for his helpful comments on this manuscript.

This work was supported by a grant from POR FSE 2007–2013 "Regione Autonoma della Sardegna, Programma Master and Back" and a grant from "Fondazione Banco di Sardegna" (Rif. Vs Prot. 469/2011.271).

Author details

Irene Marchesi[1] and Luigi Bagella[1,2]

1 Department of Biomedical Sciences, Division of Biochemistry and National Institute of Biostructures and Biosystems, University of Sassari, Sassari, Italy

2 Sbarro Institute for Cancer Research and Molecular Medicine, Center for Biotechnology, College of Science and Technology, Temple University, Philadelphia, USA

References

[1] Van Speybroeck L. From epigenesis to epigenetics: the case of C. H. Waddington. Annals New York Academy of Sciences 2002;981: 61–81.

[2] Feinberg AP, Tycko B. The history of cancer epigenetics. Nature Review Cancer 2004;4(2): 143–53.

[3] Grunstein M. Yeast heterochromatin: regulation of its assembly and inheritance by histones. Cell 1998;93(3): 325–8.

[4] Turner BM. Histone acetylation as an epigenetic determinant of long-term transcriptional competence. Cellular and Molecular Life Sciences 1998;54(1): 21–31.

[5] Strahl BD, Allis CD. The language of covalent histone modifications. Nature 2000;403(6765): 41–5.

[6] Karpen GH, Allshire RC. The case for epigenetic effects on centromere identity and function. Trends in Genetics 1997;13(12): 489–96.

[7] Wei Y, Yu L, Bowen J, Gorovsky MA, Allis CD. Phosphorylation of histone H3 is required for proper chromosome condensation and segregation. Cell 1999;97(1): 99–109.

[8] Berger SL. The complex language of chromatin regulation during transcription. Nature 2007;447(7143): 407–12.

[9] Probst AV, Dunleavy E, Almouzni G. Epigenetic inheritance during the cell cycle. Nature Reviews Molecular and Cellular Biology 2009;10(3): 192–206.

[10] Bird A. DNA methylation patterns and epigenetic memory. Genes & Development 2002;16(1): 6–21.

[11] Fiorentino FP, Marchesi I, Giordano A. On the role of Retinoblastoma family proteins in the establishment and maintenance of the epigenetic landscape. Journal of Cellular Physiology 2013;228(2): 276-84.

[12] Liang G, Chan MF, Tomigahara Y, Tsai YC, Gonzales FA, Li E, et al. Cooperativity between DNA methyltransferases in the maintenance methylation of repetitive elements. Molecular and Cellular Biology 2002;22(2): 480–91.

[13] Chen T, Ueda Y, Dodge JE, Wang Z, Li E. Establishment and maintenance of genomic methylation patterns in mouse embryonic stem cells by Dnmt3a and Dnmt3b. Molecular and Cellular Biology 2003;23(16): 5594–605.

[14] Riggs AD, Xiong Z. Methylation and epigenetic fidelity. Proceedings of the National Academy of Sciences 2004;101(1): 4–5.

[15] Jeong S, Liang G, Sharma S, Lin JC, Choi SH, Han H, et al. Selective Anchoring of DNA Methyltransferases 3A and 3B to Nucleosomes Containing Methylated DNA. Molecular and Cellular Biology 2009;29(19): 5366–76.

[16] Ooi SKT, Bestor TH. The Colorful History of Active DNA Demethylation. Cell 2008;133(7): 1145–8.

[17] Rai K, Huggins IJ, James SR, Karpf AR, Jones DA, Cairns BR. DNA demethylation in zebrafish involves the coupling of a deaminase, a glycosylase, and gadd45. Cell 2008;135(7): 1201–12.

[18] Cortellino S, Xu J, Sannai M, Moore R, Caretti E, Cigliano A, et al. Thymine DNA Glycosylase Is Essential for Active DNA Demethylation by Linked Deamination-Base Excision Repair. Cell 2011;146(1): 67–79.

[19] Métivier R, Gallais R, Tiffoche C, Le Péron C, Jurkowska RZ, Carmouche RP, et al. Cyclical DNA methylation of a transcriptionally active promoter. Nature 2008;452(7183): 45–50.

[20] Kangaspeska S, Stride B, Métivier R, Polycarpou-Schwarz M, Ibberson D, Carmouche RP, et al. Transient cyclical methylation of promoter DNA. Nature 2008;452(7183): 112–5.

[21] Kim M-S, Kondo T, Takada I, Youn M-Y, Yamamoto Y, Takahashi S, et al. DNA demethylation in hormone-induced transcriptional derepression. Nature 2009;461(7266): 1007–12.

[22] Cohen NM, Dighe V, Landan G, Reynisdottir S, Palsson A, Mitalipov S, et al. DNA methylation programming and reprogramming in primate embryonic stem cells. Genome Research 2009;19(12): 2193–201.

[23] Kouzarides T. Chromatin Modifications and Their Function. Cell 2007;128(4): 693–705.

[24] Reik W. Stability and flexibility of epigenetic gene regulation in mammalian development. Nature 2007;447(7143): 425–32.

[25] Feinberg AP, Ohlsson R, Henikoff S. The epigenetic progenitor origin of human cancer. Nature Review Genetics 2006;7(1): 21–33.

[26] Jones PA, Baylin SB. The fundamental role of epigenetic events in cancer. Nature Review Genetics 2002;3(6): 415–28.

[27] Ting AH, McGarvey KM, Baylin SB. The cancer epigenome--components and functional correlates. Genes & Development 2006;20(23): 3215–31.

[28] Sparmann A, van Lohuizen M. Polycomb silencers control cell fate, development and cancer. Nature Review Cancer 2006;6(11): 846–56.

[29] Esteller M. Cancer epigenomics: DNA methylomes and histone-modification maps. Nature Review Genetics 2007;8(4): 286–98.

[30] Fraga MF, Ballestar E, Villar-Garea A, Boix-Chornet M, Espada J, Schotta G, et al. Loss of acetylation at Lys16 and trimethylation at Lys20 of histone H4 is a common hallmark of human cancer. Nature Genetics 2005;37(4): 391–400.

[31] Seligson DB, Horvath S, Shi T, Yu H, Tze S, Grunstein M, et al. Global histone modification patterns predict risk of prostate cancer recurrence. Nature Cell Biology 2005;435(7046): 1262–6.

[32] Simon JA, Lange CA. Roles of the EZH2 histone methyltransferase in cancer epigenetics. Mutation Research 2008;647(1-2): 21–9.

[33] Lewis EB. A gene complex controlling segmentation in Drosophila. Nature 1978;276(5688): 565–70.

[34] Struhl G. A gene product required for correct initiation of segmental determination in Drosophila. Nature 1981;293(5827): 36–41.

[35] Duncan IM. Polycomblike: a gene that appears to be required for the normal expression of the bithorax and antennapedia gene complexes of Drosophila melanogaster. Genetics 1982;102(1): 49–70.

[36] Jurgens G. A Group of Genes-Controlling the Spatial Expression of the Bithorax Complex in Drosophila. Nature 1985;316(6024): 153–5.

[37] Schwartz YB, Kahn TG, Nix DA, Li X-Y, Bourgon R, Biggin M, et al. Genome-wide analysis of Polycomb targets in Drosophila melanogaster. Nature Genetics 2006;38(6): 700–5.

[38] Nègre N, Hennetin J, Sun LV, Lavrov S, Bellis M, White KP, et al. Chromosomal Distribution of PcG Proteins during Drosophila Development. Plos Biology 2006;4(6): e170.

[39] Tolhuis B, Muijrers I, de Wit E, Teunissen H, Talhout W, van Steensel B, et al. Genome-wide profiling of PRC1 and PRC2 Polycomb chromatin binding in Drosophila melanogaster. Nature Genetics 2006;38(6): 694–9.

[40] Oktaba K, Gutiérrez L, Gagneur J, Girardot C, Sengupta AK, Furlong EEM, et al. Dynamic Regulation by Polycomb Group Protein Complexes Controls Pattern Formation and the Cell Cycle in Drosophila. Developmental Cell 2008;15(6): 877–89.

[41] Kwong C, Adryan B, Bell I, Meadows L, Russell S, Manak JR, et al. Stability and Dynamics of Polycomb Target Sites in Drosophila Development. PLoS Genetics 2008;4(9): e1000178.

[42] Schuettengruber B, Cavalli G. Recruitment of Polycomb group complexes and their role in the dynamic regulation of cell fate choice. Development 2009;136(21): 3531–42.

[43] Kirmizis A, Bartley SM, Kuzmichev A, Margueron R, Reinberg D, Green R, et al. Silencing of human polycomb target genes is associated with methylation of histone H3 Lys 27. Genes & Development 2004;18(13): 1592–605.

[44] Bracken AP. Genome-wide mapping of Polycomb target genes unravels their roles in cell fate transitions. Genes & Development 2006;20(9): 1123–36.

[45] Boyer LA, Plath K, Zeitlinger J, Brambrink T, Medeiros LA, Lee TI, et al. Polycomb complexes repress developmental regulators in murine embryonic stem cells. Nature Cell Biology 2006;441(7091): 349–53.

[46] Lee TI, Jenner RG, Boyer LA, Guenther MG, Levine SS, Kumar RM, et al. Control of Developmental Regulators by Polycomb in Human Embryonic Stem Cells. Cell 2006;125(2): 301–13.

[47] Squazzo SL. Suz12 binds to silenced regions of the genome in a cell-type-specific manner. Genome Research 2006;16(7): 890–900.

[48] Simon JA, Kingston RE. Mechanisms of Polycomb gene silencing: knowns and unknowns. Nature Review Molecular Cell Biology 2009;10(10): 697-708.

[49] Plath K, Fang J, Mlynarczyk-Evans SK, Cao R, Worringer KA, Wang H, et al. Role of histone H3 lysine 27 methylation in X inactivation. Science 2003;300(5616): 131–5.

[50] Umlauf D, Goto Y, Cao R, Cerqueira F, Wagschal A, Zhang Y, et al. Imprinting along the Kcnq1 domain on mouse chromosome 7 involves repressive histone methylation and recruitment of Polycomb group complexes. Nature Genetics 2004;36(12): 1296–300.

[51] Pietersen AM, van Lohuizen M. Stem cell regulation by polycomb repressors: postponing commitment. Current Opinion in Cell Biology 2008;20(2): 201–7.

[52] Morey L, Helin K. Polycomb group protein-mediated repression of transcription. Trends in Biochemical Sciences 2010;35(6): 323–32.

[53] Margueron R, Reinberg D. The Polycomb complex PRC2 and its mark in life. Nature 2011;469(7330): 343–9.

[54] Levine SS, Weiss A, Erdjument-Bromage H, Shao Z, Tempst P, Kingston RE. The core of the polycomb repressive complex is compositionally and functionally conserved in flies and humans. Molecular and Cellular Biology 2002;22(17): 6070–8.

[55] Shao Z, Raible F, Mollaaghababa R, Guyon J, Wu C, Bender W, et al. Stabilization of Chromatin Structure by PRC1, a Polycomb Complex. Cell 1999;98(1): 37–46.

[56] Cao R. Role of Histone H3 Lysine 27 Methylation in Polycomb-Group Silencing. Science 2002;298(5595): 1039–43.

[57] Czermin B, Melfi R, McCabe D, Seitz V, Imhof A, Pirrotta V. Drosophila enhancer of Zeste/ESC complexes have a histone H3 methyltransferase activity that marks chromosomal Polycomb sites. Cell 2002;111(2): 185–96.

[58] Kuzmichev A. Histone methyltransferase activity associated with a human multiprotein complex containing the Enhancer of Zeste protein. Genes & Development 2002;16(22): 2893–905.

[59] Müller J, Hart CM, Francis NJ, Vargas ML, Sengupta A, Wild B, et al. Histone methyltransferase activity of a Drosophila Polycomb group repressor complex. Cell 2002;111(2): 197–208.

[60] Surface LE, Thornton SR, Boyer LA. Polycomb Group Proteins Set the Stage for Early Lineage Commitment. Cell Stem Cell 2010;7(3): 288–98.

[61] Cao R, Zhang Y. SUZ12 Is Required for Both the Histone Methyltransferase Activity and the Silencing Function of the EED-EZH2 Complex. Molecular Cell 2004;15(1): 57–67.

[62] Pasini D, Bracken AP, Helin K. Polycomb group proteins in cell cycle progression and cancer. Cell Cycle 2004;3(4): 396–400.

[63] Margueron R, Li G, Sarma K, Blais A, Zavadil J, Woodcock CL, et al. Ezh1 and Ezh2 maintain repressive chromatin through different mechanisms. Molecular Cell 2008;32(4): 503–18.

[64] Shen X, Liu Y, Hsu Y-J, Fujiwara Y, Kim J, Mao X, et al. EZH1 mediates methylation on histone H3 lysine 27 and complements EZH2 in maintaining stem cell identity and executing pluripotency. Molecular Cell 2008;32(4): 491–502.

[65] Aldiri I, Vetter ML. PRC2 during vertebrate organogenesis: A complex in transition. Develomental Biology 2012;367(2): 91–9.

[66] Leeb M, Pasini D, Novatchkova M, Jaritz M, Helin K, Wutz A. Polycomb complexes act redundantly to repress genomic repeats and genes. Genes & Development 2010;24(3): 265–76.

[67] Ku M, Koche RP, Rheinbay E, Mendenhall EM, Endoh M, Mikkelsen TS, et al. Genomewide Analysis of PRC1 and PRC2 Occupancy Identifies Two Classes of Bivalent Domains. van Steensel B, editor. PLoS Genetics 2008;4(10): e1000242.

[68] Wang L, Brown JL, Cao R, Zhang Y, Kassis JA, Jones RS. Hierarchical Recruitment of Polycomb Group Silencing Complexes. Molecular Cell 2004;14(5): 637–46.

[69] Cao R, Tsukada Y-I, Zhang Y. Role of Bmi-1 and Ring1A in H2A Ubiquitylation and Hox Gene Silencing. Molecular Cell 2005;20(6): 845–54.

[70] Eskeland R, Leeb M, Grimes GR, Kress C, Boyle S, Sproul D, et al. Ring1B Compacts Chromatin Structure and Represses Gene Expression Independent of Histone Ubiquitination. Molecular Cell 2010;38(3): 452–64.

[71] Richly H, Aloia L, Di Croce L. Roles of the Polycomb group proteins in stem cells and cancer. Cell Death and Disease 2012;2(9): e204–7.

[72] Kuzmichev A, Jenuwein T, Tempst P, Reinberg D. Different EZH2-containing complexes target methylation of histone H1 or nucleosomal histone H3. Molecular Cell 2004;14(2): 183–93.

[73] Daujat S. HP1 Binds Specifically to Lys26-methylated Histone H1.4, whereas Simultaneous Ser27 Phosphorylation Blocks HP1 Binding. Journal of Biological Chemistry 2005;280(45): 38090–5.

[74] Viré E, Brenner C, Deplus R, Blanchon L, Fraga M, Didelot C, et al. The Polycomb group protein EZH2 directly controls DNA methylation. Nature Cell Biology 2005;439(7078): 871–4.

[75] Ohm JE, McGarvey KM, Yu X, Cheng L, Schuebel KE, Cope L, et al. A stem cell–like chromatin pattern may predispose tumor suppressor genes to DNA hypermethylation and heritable silencing. Nature Genetics 2007;39(2): 237–42.

[76] Schlesinger Y, Straussman R, Keshet I, Farkash S, Hecht M, Zimmerman J, et al. Polycomb-mediated methylation on Lys27 of histone H3 pre-marks genes for de novo methylation in cancer. Nature Genetics 2006;39(2): 232–6.

[77] Widschwendter M, Fiegl H, Egle D, Mueller-Holzner E, Spizzo G, Marth C, et al. Epigenetic stem cell signature in cancer. Nature Genetics 2006;39(2): 157–8.

[78] van der Vlag J, Otte AP. Transcriptional repression mediated by the human polycomb-group protein EED involves histone deacetylation. Nature Genetics 1999;23(4): 474–8.

[79] Varambally S, Dhanasekaran SM, Zhou M, Barrette TR, Kumar-Sinha C, Sanda MG, et al. The polycomb group protein EZH2 is involved in progression of prostate cancer. Nature 2002;419(6907): 624–9.

[80] Kerppola TK. Polycomb group complexes – many combinations, many functions. Trends in Cell Biology 200919(12): 692–704.

[81] Bracken AP, Helin K. Epigenetics and genetics: Polycomb group proteins: navigators of lineage pathways led astray in cancer. Nature Review Cancer 2009;9(11): 773-84

[82] Weinmann AS, Bartley SM, Zhang T, Zhang MQ, Farnham PJ. Use of chromatin immunoprecipitation to clone novel E2F target promoters. Molecular and Cellular Biology 2001;21(20): 6820–32.

[83] Müller HH, Bracken APA, Vernell RR, Moroni MCM, Christians FF, Grassilli EE, et al. E2Fs regulate the expression of genes involved in differentiation, development, proliferation, and apoptosis. Genes & Development 2001;15(3): 267–85.

[84] Bracken AP, Pasini D, Capra M, Prosperini E, Colli E, Helin K. EZH2 is downstream of the pRB-E2F pathway, essential for proliferation and amplified in cancer. EMBO Journal 2003;22(20): 5323–35.

[85] Neri F, Zippo A, Krepelova A, Cherubini A, Rocchigiani M, Oliviero S. Myc Regulates the Transcription of the PRC2 Gene To Control the Expression of Developmental Genes in Embryonic Stem Cells. Molecular and Cellular Biology 2012;32(4): 840–51.

[86] Guil S, Esteller M. DNA methylomes, histone codes and miRNAs: Tying it all together. The International Journal of Biochemistry & Cell Biology 2009;41(1): 87–95.

[87] Benetatos L, Voulgaris E, Vartholomatos G, Hatzimichael E. Non coding RNAs and EZH2 interactions in cancer: Long and short tales from the transcriptome. International Journal of Cancer 2012; doi: 10.1002/ijc.27859.

[88] Juan AH, Kumar RM, Marx JG, Young RA, Sartorelli V. Mir-214-Dependent Regulation of the Polycomb Protein Ezh2 in Skeletal Muscle and Embryonic Stem Cells. Molecular Cell 2009;36(1): 61–74.

[89] Esposito F, Tornincasa M, Pallante P, Federico A, Borbone E, Pierantoni GM, et al. Down-Regulation of the miR-25 and miR-30d Contributes to the Development of Anaplastic Thyroid Carcinoma Targeting the Polycomb Protein EZH2. Journal of Clinical Endocrinology & Metabolism 2012;97(5): e710–8.

[90] Kong D, Heath E, Chen W, Cher ML, Powell I, Heilbrun L, et al. Loss of Let-7 Up-Regulates EZH2 in Prostate Cancer Consistent with the Acquisition of Cancer Stem Cell Signatures That Are Attenuated by BR-DIM. PLoS ONE 2012;7(3): e33729.

[91] Riising EM, Boggio R, Chiocca S, Helin K, Pasini D. The Polycomb Repressive Complex 2 Is a Potential Target of SUMO Modifications. PLoS ONE 2008;3(7): e2704.

[92] Chen S, Bohrer LR, Rai AN, Pan Y, Gan L, Zhou X, et al. Cyclin-dependent kinases regulate epigenetic gene silencing through phosphorylation of EZH2. Nature Cell Biology 2010;12(11): 1108-14.

[93] Kaneko S, Li G, Son J, Xu CF, Margueron R, Neubert TA, et al. Phosphorylation of the PRC2 component Ezh2 is cell cycle-regulated and up-regulates its binding to ncRNA. Genes & Development 2010;24(23): 2615–20.

[94] Caretti G, Palacios D, Sartorelli V, Puri PL. Phosphoryl-EZH-ion. Cell Stem Cell 2011;8(3): 262–5.

[95] Wei Y, Chen Y-H, Li L-Y, Lang J, Yeh S-P, Bin Shi, et al. CDK1-dependent phosphorylation of EZH2 suppresses methylation of H3K27 and promotes osteogenic differentiation of human mesenchymal stem cells. Nature Cell Biology 2010;13(1): 87–94.

[96] Cha T-LT, Zhou BPB, Xia WW, Wu YY, Yang C-CC, Chen C-TC, et al. Akt-mediated phosphorylation of EZH2 suppresses methylation of lysine 27 in histone H3. Science 2005;310(5746): 306–10.

[97] Palacios D, Mozzetta C, Consalvi S, Caretti G, Saccone V, Proserpio V, et al. TNF/p38α/Polycomb Signaling to Pax7 Locus in Satellite Cells Links Inflammation to the Epigenetic Control of Muscle Regeneration. Stem Cell 2010;7(4): 455–69.

[98] Margueron R, Justin N, Ohno K, Sharpe ML, Son J, Drury WJ III, et al. Role of the polycomb protein EED in the propagation of repressive histone marks. Nature 2009;461(7265): 762–7.

[99] Ringrose L, Paro R. Polycomb/Trithorax response elements and epigenetic memory of cell identity. Development 2007;134(2): 223–32.

[100] Müller J, Kassis JA. Polycomb response elements and targeting of Polycomb group proteins in Drosophila. Current Opinion in Genetics & Development 2006;16(5): 476–84.

[101] Sing A, Pannell D, Karaiskakis A, Sturgeon K, Djabali M, Ellis J, et al. A Vertebrate Polycomb Response Element Governs Segmentation of the Posterior Hindbrain. Cell 2009;138(5): 885–97.

[102] Van Dessel N, Beke L, Gornemann J, Minnebo N, Beullens M, Tanuma N, et al. The phosphatase interactor NIPP1 regulates the occupancy of the histone methyltransferase EZH2 at Polycomb targets. Nucleic Acids Research 2010;38(21): 7500–12.

[103] Cakouros D, Isenmann S, Cooper L, Zannettino A, Anderson P, Glackin C, et al. Twist-1 Induces Ezh2 Recruitment Regulating Histone Methylation along the Ink4A/Arf Locus in Mesenchymal Stem Cells. Molecular and Cellular Biology 2012;32(8): 1433–41.

[104] Sarma K, Margueron R, Ivanov A, Pirrotta V, Reinberg D. Ezh2 Requires PHF1 To Efficiently Catalyze H3 Lysine 27 Trimethylation In Vivo. Molecular and Cellular Biology 2008;28(8): 2718–31.

[105] Cao R, Wang H, He J, Erdjument-Bromage H, Tempst P, Zhang Y. Role of hPHF1 in H3K27 Methylation and Hox Gene Silencing. Molecular and Cellular Biology 2008;28(5): 1862–72.

[106] Peng JC, Valouev A, Swigut T, Zhang J, Zhao Y, Sidow A, et al. Jarid2/Jumonji Coordinates Control of PRC2 Enzymatic Activity and Target Gene Occupancy in Pluripotent Cells. Cell 2009;139(7): 1290–302.

[107] Shen X, Kim W, Fujiwara Y, Simon MD, Liu Y, Mysliwiec MR, et al. Jumonji Modulates Polycomb Activity and Self-Renewal versus Differentiation of Stem Cells. Cell 2009;139(7): 1303–14.

[108] Li G, Margueron R, Ku M, Chambon P, Bernstein BE, Reinberg D. Jarid2 and PRC2, partners in regulating gene expression. Genes & Development 2010;24(4): 368–80.

[109] Pasini D, Cloos PAC, Walfridsson J, Olsson L, Bukowski J-P, Johansen JV, et al. JARID2 regulates binding of the Polycomb repressive complex 2 to target genes in ES cells.Nature 2010;464(7286): 306–10.

[110] Khalil AM, Guttman M, Huarte M, Garber M, Raj A, Rivea Morales D, et al. Many human large intergenic noncoding RNAs associate with chromatin-modifying complexes and affect gene expression. Proceedings of the National Academy of Sciences 2009;106(28): 11667–72.

[111] Rinn JL, Kertesz M, Wang JK, Squazzo SL, Xu X, Brugmann SA, et al. Functional demarcation of active and silent chromatin domains in human HOX loci by noncoding RNAs. Cell 2007;129(7): 1311–23.

[112] Pauli A, Rinn JL, Schier AF. Non-coding RNAs as regulators of embryogenesis. Nature Review Genetics 2011;12(2): 136–49.

[113] Sher F, Rössler R, Brouwer N, Balasubramaniyan V, Boddeke E, Copray S. Differentiation of neural stem cells into oligodendrocytes: involvement of the polycomb group protein Ezh2. Stem Cells 2008;26(11): 2875–83.

[114] Hirabayashi Y, Suzki N, Tsuboi M, Endo TA, Toyoda T, Shinga J, et al. Polycomb Limits the Neurogenic Competence of Neural Precursor Cells to Promote Astrogenic Fate Transition. Neuron 2009;63(5): 600–13.

[115] Pereira JD, Sansom SN, Smith J, Dobenecker M-W, Tarakhovsky A, Livesey FJ. Ezh2, the histone methyltransferase of PRC2, regulates the balance between self-renewal and differentiation in the cerebral cortex. Proceedings of the National Academy of Sciences 2010;107(36): 15957–62.

[116] Yu YL, Chou RH, Chen LT, Shyu WC, Hsieh SC, Wu CS, et al. EZH2 Regulates Neuronal Differentiation of Mesenchymal Stem Cells through PIP5K1C-dependent Calcium Signaling. Journal of Biological Chemistry 2011;286(11): 9657–67.

[117] Sher F, Boddeke E, Copray S. Ezh2 Expression in Astrocytes Induces Their Dedifferentiation Toward Neural Stem Cells. Cellular Reprogramming 2011;13(1): 1–6.

[118] Sher F, Boddeke E, Olah M, Copray S. Dynamic Changes in Ezh2 Gene Occupancy Underlie Its Involvement in Neural Stem Cell Self-Renewal and Differentiation towards Oligodendrocytes. PLoS ONE 2012;7(7): e40399.

[119] Akizu N, Estaras C, Guerrero L, Marti E, Martinez-Balbas MA. H3K27me3 regulates BMP activity in developing spinal cord. Development 2010;137(17): 2915–25.

[120] Ezhkova E, Pasolli HA, Parker JS, Stokes N, Su I-H, Hannon G, et al. Ezh2 Orchestrates Gene Expression for the Stepwise Differentiation of Tissue-Specific Stem Cells. Cell 2009;136(6): 1122–35.

[121] Ezhkova E, Lien WH, Stokes N, Pasolli HA, Silva JM, Fuchs E. EZH1 and EZH2 cogovern histone H3K27 trimethylation and are essential for hair follicle homeostasis and wound repair. Genes & Development 2011;25(5): 485–98.

[122] Mulder KW, Wang X, Escriu C, Ito Y, Schwarz RF, Gillis J, et al. Diverse epigenetic strategies interact to control epidermal differentiation. Nature Cell Biology 2012;14(7): 753–63.

[123] Delgado-Olguín P, Huang Y, Li X, Christodoulou D, Seidman CE, Seidman JG, et al. Epigenetic repression of cardiac progenitor gene expression by Ezh2 is required for postnatal cardiac homeostasis. Nature Genetics 2012;44(3): 343-7.

[124] He M, Zhang W, Bakken T, Schutten M, Toth Z, Jung JU, et al. Cancer angiogenesis induced by Kaposi's sarcoma-associated herpesvirus is mediated by EZH2. Cancer Research 2012;72(14): 3582-92.

[125] Chen L, Ma Y, Kim EY, Yu W, Schwartz RJ, Qian L, et al. Conditional Ablation of Ezh2 in Murine Hearts Reveals Its Essential Roles in Endocardial Cushion Formation, Cardiomyocyte Proliferation and Survival. PLoS ONE 2012;7(2): e31005.

[126] Caretti G. The Polycomb Ezh2 methyltransferase regulates muscle gene expression and skeletal muscle differentiation. Genes & Development 2004;18(21): 2627–38.

[127] Seenundun S, Rampalli S, Liu Q-C, Aziz A, Palii C, Hong S, et al. UTX mediates demethylation of H3K27me3 at muscle-specific genes during myogenesis. EMBO Journal 2010;29(8): 1401–11.

[128] Juan AH, Derfoul A, Feng X, Ryall JG, Dell'Orso S, Pasut A, et al. Polycomb EZH2 controls self-renewal and safeguards the transcriptional identity of skeletal muscle stem cells. Genes & Development 2011;25(8): 789–94.

[129] Stojic L, Jasencakova Z, Prezioso C, Stützer A, Bodega B, Pasini D, et al. Chromatin regulated interchange between polycomb repressive complex 2 (PRC2)-Ezh2 and PRC2-Ezh1 complexes controls myogenin activation in skeletal muscle cells. Epigenetics & Chromatin 2011;4(1): 16.

[130] Aoki R, Chiba T, Miyagi S, Negishi M, Konuma T, Taniguchi H, et al. The polycomb group gene product Ezh2 regulates proliferation and differentiation of murine hepatic stem/progenitor cells. Journal of Hepatology 2010;52(6): 854–63.

[131] Xu C, Bian C, Yang W, Galka M, Ouyang H, Chen C, et al. Binding of different histone marks differentially regulates the activity and specificity of polycomb repressive complex 2 (PRC2). Proceedings of the National Academy of Sciences 2010;107(45): 19266–71.

[132] Chen H, Gu X, Su I-H, Bottino R, Contreras JL, Tarakhovsky A, et al. Polycomb protein Ezh2 regulates pancreatic -cell Ink4a/Arf expression and regeneration in diabetes mellitus. Genes & Development 2009;23(8): 975–85.

[133] Xu CR, Cole PA, Meyers DJ, Kormish J, Dent S, Zaret KS. Chromatin "Prepattern" and Histone Modifiers in a Fate Choice for Liver and Pancreas. Science 2011;332(6032): 963–6.

[134] Wang L, Jin Q, Lee JE, Su I-H, Ge K. Histone H3K27 methyltransferase Ezh2 represses Wnt genes to facilitate adipogenesis. Proceedings of the National Academy of Sciences 2010;107(16): 7317–22.

[135] Shore AN, Kabotyanski EB, Roarty K, Smith MA, Zhang Y, Creighton CJ, et al. Pregnancy-Induced Noncoding RNA (PINC) Associates with Polycomb Repressive Complex 2 and Regulates Mammary Epithelial Differentiation. PLoS Genetics 2012;8(7): e1002840.

[136] Gil J, Bernard D, Martínez D, Beach D. Polycomb CBX7 has a unifying role in cellular lifespan. Nature Cell Biology 2003;6(1): 67–72.

[137] Leung C, Lingbeek M, Shakhova O, Liu J, Tanger E, Saremaslani P, et al. Bmi1 is essential for cerebellar development and is overexpressed in human medulloblastomas. Nature 2004;428(6980): 337–41.

[138] Bruggeman SWM. Ink4a and Arf differentially affect cell proliferation and neural stem cell self-renewal in Bmi1-deficient mice. Genes & Development 2005;19(12): 1438–43.

[139] Gil J, Peters G. Regulation of the INK4b–ARF–INK4a tumour suppressor locus: all for one or one for all. Nature Review Molecular Cell Biology 2006;7(9): 667–77.

[140] Dietrich N, Bracken AP, Trinh E, Schjerling CK, Koseki H, Rappsilber J, et al. Bypass of senescence by the polycomb group protein CBX8 through direct binding to the INK4A-ARF locus. EMBO Journal 2007;26(6): 1637–48.

[141] Dhawan S, Tschen SI, Bhushan A. Bmi-1 regulates the Ink4a/Arf locus to control pancreatic -cell proliferation. Genes & Development 2009;23(8): 906–11.

[142] Bernstein BE, Mikkelsen TS, Xie X, Kamal M, Huebert DJ, Cuff J, et al. A Bivalent Chromatin Structure Marks Key Developmental Genes in Embryonic Stem Cells. Cell 2006;125(2): 315–26.

[143] Puri PL, Sartorelli V. Regulation of muscle regulatory factors by DNA-binding, interacting proteins, and post-transcriptional modifications. Journal of Cellular Physiology 2000;185(2): 155–73.

[144] Mousavi K, Zare H, Wang AH, Sartorelli V. Polycomb Protein Ezh1 Promotes RNA Polymerase II Elongation. Molecular Cell 2012;45(2): 255–62.

[145] Gaudet F. Induction of Tumors in Mice by Genomic Hypomethylation. Science 2003;300(5618): 489–92.

[146] Feinberg AP. Epigenetics at the epicenter of modern medicine. JAMA: The journal of the American Medical Association 2008;299(11): 1345–50.

[147] Kleer CG, Cao Q, Varambally S, Shen R, Ota I, Tomlins SA, et al. EZH2 is a marker of aggressive breast cancer and promotes neoplastic transformation of breast epithelial cells. Proceedings of the National Academy of Sciences 2003;100(20): 11606–11.

[148] Raaphorst FMF, Meijer CJLMC, Fieret EE, Blokzijl TT, Mommers EE, Buerger HH, et al. Poorly differentiated breast carcinoma is associated with increased expression of the human polycomb group EZH2 gene. Neoplasia 2003;5(6): 481–8.

[149] Bachmann IM. EZH2 Expression Is Associated With High Proliferation Rate and Aggressive Tumor Subgroups in Cutaneous Melanoma and Cancers of the Endometrium, Prostate, and Breast. Journal of Clinical Oncology 2005;24(2): 268–73.

[150] Collett K. Expression of Enhancer of Zeste Homologue 2 Is Significantly Associated with Increased Tumor Cell Proliferation and Is a Marker of Aggressive Breast Cancer. Clinical Cancer Research 2006;12(4): 1168–74.

[151] Ding L. Identification of EZH2 as a Molecular Marker for a Precancerous State in Morphologically Normal Breast Tissues. Cancer Research 2006;66(8): 4095–9.

[152] Rhodes DRD, Sanda MGM, Otte APA, Chinnaiyan AMA, Rubin MAM. Multiplex biomarker approach for determining risk of prostate-specific antigen-defined recurrence of prostate cancer. Journal of the National Cancer Institute 2003;95(9): 661–8.

[153] Saramäki OR, Tammela TLJ, Martikainen PM, Vessella RL, Visakorpi T. The gene for polycomb group protein enhancer of zeste homolog 2 (EZH2) is amplified in late-stage prostate cancer. Genes Chromosomes and Cancer 2006;45(7): 639–45.

[154] Berezovska OPO, Glinskii ABA, Yang ZZ, Li X-MX, Hoffman RMR, Glinsky GVG. Essential role for activation of the Polycomb group (PcG) protein chromatin silencing pathway in metastatic prostate cancer. Cell Cycle 2006;5(16): 1886–901.

[155] van Leenders GJLH, Dukers D, Hessels D, van den Kieboom SWM, Hulsbergen CA, Witjes JA, et al. Polycomb-Group Oncogenes EZH2, BMI1, and RING1 Are Overexpressed in Prostate Cancer With Adverse Pathologic and Clinical Features. European Urology 2007;52(2): 455–63.

[156] Mallen-St Clair J, Soydaner-Azeloglu R, Lee KE, Taylor L, Livanos A, Pylayeva-Gupta Y, et al. EZH2 couples pancreatic regeneration to neoplastic progression. Genes & Development 2012;26(5): 439–44.

[157] Duan Z, Zou JX, Yang P, Wang Y, Borowsky AD, Gao AC, et al. Developmental and androgenic regulation of chromatin regulators EZH2 and ANCCA/ATAD2 in the prostate Via MLL histone methylase complex. Prostate 2012; doi: 10.1002/pros.22587.

[158] Breuer RHJ, Snijders PJF, Smit EF, Sutedja TG, Sewalt RGAB, Otte AP, et al. Increased Expression of the EZH2 Polycomb Group Gene in BMI-1–Positive Neoplastic Cells During Bronchial Carcinogenesis. Neoplasia 2004;6(6): 736–43.

[159] McCabe MT, Brandes JC, Vertino PM. Cancer DNA Methylation: Molecular Mechanisms and Clinical Implications. Clinical Cancer Research 2009;15(12): 3927–37.

[160] Kikuchi J, Takashina T, Kinoshita I, Kikuchi E, Shimizu Y, Sakakibara-Konishi J, et al. Epigenetic therapy with 3-deazaneplanocin A, an inhibitor of the histone methyltransferase EZH2, inhibits growth of non-small cell lung cancer cells. Lung Cancer 2012;78(2): 138–43.

[161] Mimori K, Ogawa K, Okamoto M, Sudo T, Inoue H, Mori M. Clinical significance of enhancer of zeste homolog 2 expression in colorectal cancer cases. European Journal of Surgical Oncology 2005;31(4): 376–80.

[162] Sudo T, Utsunomiya T, Mimori K, Nagahara H, Ogawa K, Inoue H, et al. Clinicopathological significance of EZH2 mRNA expression in patients with hepatocellular carcinoma. British Journal of Cancer 2005;92(9): 1754–8.

[163] Au SL-K, Wong CC-L, Lee JM-F, Fan DN-Y, Tsang FH, Ng IO-L, et al. Enhancer of zeste homolog 2 epigenetically silences multiple tumor suppressor microRNAs to promote liver cancer metastasis. Hepatology 2012;56(2): 622-31.

[164] Matsukawa Y, Semba S, Kato H, Ito A, Yanagihara K, Yokozaki H. Expression of the enhancer of zeste homolog 2 is correlated with poor prognosis in human gastric cancer. Cancer Science 2006;97(6): 484–91.

[165] van Kemenade FJ, Raaphorst FM, Blokzijl T, Fieret E, Hamer KM, Satijn DP, et al. Coexpression of BMI-1 and EZH2 polycomb-group proteins is associated with cycling cells and degree of malignancy in B-cell non-Hodgkin lymphoma. Blood 2001;97(12): 3896–901.

[166] Visser HPJ, Gunster MJ, Kluin Nelemans HC, Manders EMM, Raaphorst FM, Meijer CJLM, et al. The Polycomb group protein EZH2 is upregulated in proliferating, cultured human mantle cell lymphoma. British journal of haematology 2001;112(4): 950–8.

[167] Park SW, Chung NG, Eom HS, Yoo NJ, Lee SH. Mutational analysis of EZH2 codon 641 in non-Hodgkin lymphomas and leukemias. Leukemia Research 2010;35(1): e6-7.

[168] Morin RD, Johnson NA, Severson TM, Mungall AJ, An J, Goya R, et al. Somatic mutations altering EZH2 (Tyr641) in follicular and diffuse large B-cell lymphomas of germinal-center origin. Nature Genetics 2010;42(2): 181–5.

[169] McCabe MT, Ott HM, Ganji G, Korenchuk S, Thompson C, Van Aller GS, et al. EZH2 inhibition as a therapeutic strategy for lymphoma with EZH2-activating mutations. Nature 2012; doi: 10.1038/nature11606.

[170] Chen J, Li J, Han Q, Sun Z, Wang J, WANG S, et al. Enhancer of zeste homolog 2 is overexpressed and contributes to epigenetic inactivation of p21 and phosphatase and tensin homolog in B-cell acute lymphoblastic leukemia. Experimental Biology and Medicine 2012;237(9): 1110–6.

[171] Simon C, Chagraoui J, Krosl J, Gendron P, Wilhelm B, Lemieux S, et al. A key role for EZH2 and associated genes in mouse and human adult T-cell acute leukemia. Genes & Development 2012;26(7): 651–6.

[172] Croonquist PA, Van Ness B. The polycomb group protein enhancer of zeste homolog 2 (EZH2) is an oncogene that influences myeloma cell growth and the mutant ras phenotype. Oncogene 2005;24(41): 6269–80.

[173] Tanaka S, Miyagi S, Sashida G, Chiba T, Yuan J, Mochizuki-Kashio M, et al. Ezh2 augments leukemogenecity by reinforcing differentiation blockage in acute myeloid leukemia. Blood 2012;120(5): 1107-17.

[174] Neff T, Sinha AU, Kluk MJ, Zhu N, Khattab MH, Stein L, et al. Polycomb repressive complex 2 is required for MLL-AF9 leukemia. Proceedings of the National Academy of Sciences 2012;109(13): 5028–33.

[175] Rizzo S, Hersey JM, Mellor P, Dai W, Santos-Silva A, Liber D, et al. Ovarian Cancer Stem Cell-Like Side Populations Are Enriched Following Chemotherapy and Overexpress EZH2. Molecular Cancer Therapeutics 2011;10(2): 325–35.

[176] McHugh JB, Fullen DR, Ma L, Kleer CG, Su LD. Expression of polycomb group protein EZH2 in nevi and melanoma. Journal of Cutaneous Pathology 2007;34(8): 597–600.

[177] Asangani IA, Harms PW, Dodson L, Pandhi M, Kunju LP, Maher CA, et al. Genetic and epigenetic loss of microRNA-31 leads to feed-forward expression of EZH2 in melanoma. Oncotarget 2012 3(9): 1011-25.

[178] Raman JD. Increased Expression of the Polycomb Group Gene, EZH2, in Transitional Cell Carcinoma of the Bladder. Clinical Cancer Research 2005;11(24): 8570–6.

[179] Zhou J, Roh J-W, Bandyopadhyay S, Chen Z, Munkarah A, Hussein Y, et al. Overexpression of enhancer of zeste homolog 2 (EZH2) and focal adhesion kinase (FAK) in high grade endometrial carcinoma. Gynecologic Oncology 2012; http://dx.doi.org/10.1016/j.ygyno.2012.07.128.

[180] Ciarapica R, Russo G, Verginelli F, Raimondi L, Donfrancesco A, Rota R, et al. Deregulated expression of miR-26a and Ezh2 in rhabdomyosarcoma. Cell Cycle 2009;8(1): 172–5.

[181] Venneti S, Le P, Martinez D, Xie SX, Sullivan LM, Rorke-Adams LB, et al. Malignant rhabdoid tumors express stem cell factors, which relate to the expression of EZH2 and Id proteins. The American Journal of Surgical Pathology 2011;35(10): 1463–72.

[182] Marchesi I, Fiorentino FP, Rizzolio F, Giordano A, Bagella L. The ablation of EZH2 uncovers its crucial role in rhabdomyosarcoma formation. Cell Cycle 2012;11(20): 3828–36.

[183] Avan A, Crea F, Paolicchi E, Funel N, Galvani E, Marquez VE, et al. Molecular mechanisms involved in the synergistic interaction of the EZH2 inhibitor 3-deazaneplanocin A (DZNeP) with gemcitabine in pancreatic cancer cells. Molecular Cancer Therapeutics 2012;11(8): 1735-46.

[184] Lasfargues C, Pyronnet S. EZH2 links pancreatitis to tissue regeneration and pancreatic cancer. Clinics and Research in Hepatology and Gastroenterology 2012;36(4): 323-4

[185] Shen Y, Guo X, Wang Y, Qiu W, Chang Y, Zhang A, et al. Expression and significance of histone H3K27 demethylases in renal cell carcinoma. BMC Cancer 2012;12(1):470.

[186] Suva ML, Riggi N, Janiszewska M, Radovanovic I, Provero P, Stehle JC, et al. EZH2 Is Essential for Glioblastoma Cancer Stem Cell Maintenance. Cancer Research;69(24): 9211–8.

[187] Smits M, van Rijn S, Hulleman E, Biesmans D, van Vuurden DG, Kool M, et al. EZH2-Regulated DAB2IP Is a Medulloblastoma Tumor Suppressor and a Positive Marker for Survival. Clinical Cancer Research 2012;18(15): 4048-58.

[188] Molofsky AV. Bmi-1 promotes neural stem cell self-renewal and neural development but not mouse growth and survival by repressing the p16Ink4a and p19Arf senescence pathways. Genes & Development 2005;19(12): 1432–7.

[189] Fiorentino FP, Symonds CE, Macaluso M, Giordano A. Senescence and p130/Rbl2: a new beginning to the end. Cell Research 2009;19(9): 1044–51.

[190] Sherr CJ. The INK4a/ARF network in tumour suppression. Nature Review Molecular Cell Biology 2001;2(10): 731–7.

[191] Lowe SW, Sherr CJ. Tumor suppression by Ink4a–Arf: progress and puzzles. Current Opinion in Genetics & Development 2003;13(1): 77–83.

[192] Kotake Y, Cao R, Viatour P, Sage J, Zhang Y, Xiong Y. pRB family proteins are required for H3K27 trimethylation and Polycomb repression complexes binding to and silencing p16INK4a tumor suppressor gene. Genes & Development 2007;21(1): 49–54.

[193] Tonini T, Bagella L, D'andrilli G, Claudio PP, Giordano A. Ezh2 reduces the ability of HDAC1-dependent pRb2/p130 transcriptional repression of cyclin A. Oncogene 2004;23(28): 4930–7.

[194] Tonini T, D'andrilli G, Fucito A, Gaspa L, Bagella L. Importance of Ezh2 polycomb protein in tumorigenesis process interfering with the pathway of growth suppressive key elements. Journal of Cellular Physiology 2007;214(2): 295–300.

[195] Fan T, Jiang S, Chung N, Alikhan A, Ni C, Lee CCR, et al. EZH2-Dependent Suppression of a Cellular Senescence Phenotype in Melanoma Cells by Inhibition of p21/ CDKN1A Expression. Molecular Cancer Research 2011;9(4): 418–29.

[196] Chen H. Down-regulation of Human DAB2IP Gene Expression Mediated by Polycomb Ezh2 Complex and Histone Deacetylase in Prostate Cancer. Journal of Biological Chemistry 2005;280(23): 22437–44.

[197] Wu ZL, Zheng SS, Li ZM, Qiao YY, Aau MY, Yu Q. Polycomb protein EZH2 regulates E2F1-dependent apoptosis through epigenetically modulating Bim expression. Cell Death and Differentiation 2009;17(5): 801–10.

[198] Su I-H, Dobenecker M-W, Dickinson E, Oser M, Basavaraj A, Marqueron R, et al. Polycomb Group Protein Ezh2 Controls Actin Polymerization and Cell Signaling. Cell 2005;121(3): 425–36.

[199] Bryant RJ, Cross NA, Eaton CL, Hamdy FC, Cunliffe VT. EZH2 promotes proliferation and invasiveness of prostate cancer cells. Prostate 2007;67(5): 547–56.

[200] Bryant RJ, Winder SJ, Cross SS, Hamdy FC, Cunliffe VT. The polycomb group protein EZH2 regulates actin polymerization in human prostate cancer cells. Prostate 2008;68(3): 255–63.

[201] Martinez-Garcia E, Licht JD. Deregulation of H3K27 methylation in cancer. Nature Genetics 2010;42(2): 100–1.

[202] Sneeringer CJ, Scott MP, Kuntz KW, Knutson SK, Pollock RM, Richon VM, et al. Coordinated activities of wild-type plus mutant EZH2 drive tumor-associated hypertrimethylation of lysine 27 on histone H3 (H3K27) in human B-cell lymphomas. Proceedings of the National Academy of Sciences 2010;107(49): 20980–5.

[203] Ernst T, Chase AJ, Score J, Hidalgo-Curtis CE, Bryant C, Jones AV, et al. Inactivating mutations of the histone methyltransferase gene EZH2 in myeloid disorders. Nature Genetics 2010;42(8): 722–6.

[204] Nikoloski G, Langemeijer SMC, Kuiper RP, Knops R, Massop M, Tönnissen ERLTM, et al. Somatic mutations of the histone methyltransferase gene EZH2 in myelodysplastic syndromes. Nature Genetics 2010;42(8): 665–7.

[205] Makishima H, Jankowska AM, Tiu RV, Szpurka H, Sugimoto Y, Hu Z, et al. Novel homo- and hemizygous mutations in EZH2 in myeloid malignancies. Leukemia 2010;24(10): 1799–804.

[206] Bejar R, Stevenson K, Abdel-Wahab O, Galili N, Nilsson B, Garcia-Manero G, et al. Clinical Effect of Point Mutations in Myelodysplastic Syndromes.The New England Journal of Medicine 2011;364(26): 2496–506.

[207] Guglielmelli P, Biamonte F, Score J, Hidalgo-Curtis C, Cervantes F, Maffioli M, et al. EZH2 mutational status predicts poor survival in myelofibrosis. Blood 2011;118(19): 5227–34.

[208] Zhang J, Ding L, Holmfeldt L, Wu G, Heatley SL, Payne-Turner D, et al. The genetic basis of early T-cell precursor acute lymphoblastic leukaemia. Nature 2012;481(7380): 157–63.

[209] Ntziachristos P, Tsirigos A, Vlierberghe PV, Nedjic J, Trimarchi T, Flaherty MS, et al. Genetic inactivation of the polycomb repressive complex 2 in T cell acute lymphoblastic leukemia. Nature Medicine 2012;18(2): 298–303.

[210] Lyko F, Brown R. DNA Methyltransferase Inhibitors and the Development of Epigenetic Cancer Therapies. Journal of the National Cancer Institute 2005;97(20): 1498–506.

[211] Federico M, Bagella L. Histone Deacetylase Inhibitors in the Treatment of Hematological Malignancies and Solid Tumors. Journal of Biomedicine and Biotechnology 2011; doi:10.1155/2011/475641

[212] Tan J, Yang X, Zhuang L, Jiang X, Chen W, Lee PL, et al. Pharmacologic disruption of Polycomb-repressive complex 2-mediated gene repression selectively induces apoptosis in cancer cells. Genes & Development 2007;21(9): 1050–63.

[213] Cheng LL, Itahana Y, Lei ZD, Chia NY, Wu Y, Yu Y, et al. TP53 Genomic Status Regulates Sensitivity of Gastric Cancer Cells to the Histone Methylation Inhibitor 3-Deazaneplanocin A (DZNep). Clinical Cancer Research 2012;18(15): 4201-12.

[214] Lin Y-H, Lee C-C, Chang F-R, Chang W-H, Wu Y-C, Chang J-G. 16-Hydroxycleroda-3,13-dien-15,16-olide regulates the expression of histone-modifying enzymes PRC2 complex and induces apoptosis in CML K562 cells. Life Sciences 2011;89(23-24): 886-95.

Chapter 7

Chromatin Remodeling in DNA Damage Response and Human Aging

Lili Gong, Edward Wang and Shiaw-Yih Lin

Additional information is available at the end of the chapter

http://dx.doi.org/10.5772/55272

1. Introduction

Chromatin consists of the DNA and all proteins involved in organizing and regulating DNA structure. The building block of chromatin is the nucleosome, which is composed of 146 base pairs of DNA and a core histone octamer. The core histone oactomer is composed of two heterodimers of histone H2A and histone H2B and a tetramer of histone H3 and histone H4 [1]. The overall chromatin structure is very dynamic in response to diverse biological events. Regulation of chromatin structure is achieved by two major mechanisms. The first is post-translational modification (PTM) of histones and other chromatin proteins via phosphorylation, methylation, acetylation, ubiquitination and sumoylation [2, 3]. The second is through ATP-dependent nucleosome structure alteration. Cooperation between histone PTMs and chromatin remodelers allows chromatin remodeling to regulate diverse biological events including transcription, chromosome segregation, DNA replication, and DNA repair. In this chapter, we summarize how chromatin structure is regulated during DNA damage response (DDR), focusing particularly on three PTMs: phosphorylation, Poly(ADP-ribosyl)ation (PARylation) and sumoylation. We discuss the DDR in a highly compacted chromatic structure, heterochromatin, as well as the interplay between chromatin remodeling, DNA damage and human aging.

2. DNA damage response

2.1. Sources leading to DNA damage

In order to maintain DNA fidelity, cells must overcome multiple challenges that threaten genome stability. Cues cause DNA damages can be divided into spontaneous and environment-induced. Spontaneous DNA damages are usually caused by intracellular metabolism stress, or formed during genetically programmed processes such as V (variable), D (diversity), and J (joining) (V(D)J) recombination in developing vertebrate lymphocytes or meiotic recombination in germ cells [4, 5]. The major types of damage include aberrant conformations of DNA, chemical instability of DNA, free radicals of oxygen, endogenous mutagens and errors in DNA replications [6]. Environmental DNA damages generally refer to exposure of cells to various genotoxic agents. These agents contain both physical factors, such as ultraviolet (UV), visible light and ionizing radiation; as well as chemical factors, such as alkylating agents, benzopyrene, aflatoxins and cis-Platinum. These DNA damages can lead to single base mutation or more deleterious chromosomal lesion.

2.2. DDR pathway

To maintain genome stability, cells have developed a global signaling network, known as the DNA damage response (DDR), to sense different types of genotoxic stress, to modulate cell cycle transitions and transcriptional process, and to stimulate DNA repair. Mechanistically, proteins involved in the DDR signaling network can be grouped into three major classes: 1) Sensors, acting at the upstream of DDR by recognizing the DNA damage and initiating DDR; 2) Transducers, proteins that pass and amplify DNA damage signals to downstream effectors. Notably, among diverse transducers, ATM (Ataxia Telangiectasia Mutated) and ATR (ATM and Rad3 Related) are central to the entire DDR; 3) Effector, proteins determine the physiological outcome of DNA damage response. Depending on the context of DNA damage, effectors can regulate cell cycle, transcription or cell apoptosis. Nevertheless, we need to point out that although DDR is often referred to as a signaling pathway, it is more accurately described as a network of interacting pathways that coordinate the damage response.

2.3. DNA damage repair

The various types of DNA damage include aberrant base or nucleotide modifications, single strand DNA (ssDNA) breaks, and chromosomal lesions caused by double strand breaks (DSBs). Among these, DSBs are regarded as the most cytotoxic. If left unrepaired, DSBs will affect genome integrity by causing mutations, chromosome deletions or translocations, because there is no intact complimentary template to repair the damaged strand. In this chapter, we will use DSBs as a model lesion.

DSBs can be repaired by two principle mechanisms, the non-homologous end joining (NHEJ) and homologous recombination (HR) [7]. These two pathways differ in their functional enzymes, the repair efficiency and also the cell cycle phases where they are active (Figure 1).

Molecular Basis of NHEJ. In the process of NHEJ, DSBs are repaired by direct ligation of the exposed ends regardless of their DNA sequences. Enzymes involved specifically in NHEJ capture both ends of the broken DNA molecule, bringing them together to form a DNA-protein complex to repair the break. Therefore NHEJ is a very efficient but error-prone way to repair damaged DNA, and it occurs in all phases of the cell cycle [8]. In NHEJ pathway, the Ku70/80 heterodimer initiates NHEJ by binding to both ends of the broken DNA molecule, which

http://dx.doi.org/10.5772/55272

creates a scaffold for the assembly of other NHEJ enzymes. After association of Ku70/80, the DNA-dependent protein kinase catalytic subunit (DNA-PKcs) is recruited to the DSB, forming a synaptic complex that brings the broken DNA ends together. Once the DNA ends have been captured and tethered, non-ligatable DNA termini must be processed (single strand fill in) or removed by nucleases and polymerases. Lastly, the processed DNA ends are joint by ligase IV/XRCC4 complex [9]. It was demonstrated that in higher eukaryotes, and especially in mammals, NHEJ is the preferred pathway for DNA DSB repair [10].

Molecular Basis of HR. HR is an error-free, template-dependent strategy to repair DNA DSBs. It occurs during the S and G2 phases, when the sister chromatids are more easily available [11]. The key reactions in HR are homology search and DNA strand invasion, which are catalyzed by the RecA homolog Rad51 [12]. Principally, HR can be divided into three steps: 1) Presynapsis. During this process, DSB ends are recognized and processed to a single-stranded tail with a 3′-OH ending. This ssDNA is then bound by the eukaryotic ssDNA binding protein RPA (replication protein A). 2) Synapsis. With aid of cofactors, such as Rad 52 and Rad 55-57 complexes [13, 14], Rad51 binds to RPA-coated ssDNA, forming Rad51-DNA filament. After this, DNA strand invasion by the Rad51-ssDNA filament generates a D-loop intermediate. 3) Postsynapsis. In DSBs repair, both ends of the DSB are engaged, leading to double Holliday junction formation. Finally, following the actions of polymerases, nucleases and helicases, DNA ligation and substrate resolution occur.

How cells choose between NHEJ or HR to repair the DSBs is unclear. As mentioned above, HR is initiated by ssDNA resection and requires sequence homology, but NHEJ requires neither resection at initiation nor a homologous template. Thus, resection appears to be a pivotal step in DSB repair initiation that determines whether HR or NHEJ occurs. However, an alternative end-joining (A-EJ) pathway, which is also initiated by ssDNA resection but does not require a homologous partner, was recently identified. It is proposed that the presence of ssDNA resection will determine the selection among canonical NHEJ, A-EJ or HR; the size of the resection, which is associated with the cell cycle phase, will then direct the DSB repair to either HR or A-EJ [15].

3. Chromatin remodeling during DNA damage

In 1998, functions of phosphorylation at the Serine139 residue of a histone variant, H2AX, were first discovered in DDR [16]. Since then, extensive studies regarding how chromatin alters its structures in response of DNA damage were made. It is now recognized that small DNA lesion can lead to global chromatin remodeling, with changes including histone modifications, nucleosome positioning and higher-order folding of the chromatin fiber. Furthermore, if the DDR-induced chromatin remodeling is not properly restored, then the epigenetic changes can be heritable and contribute to terminal cell fate, such as transformation, cell senescence and cell apoptosis [17, 18]. In this part, we will discuss recent progress made about chromatin structures regulations in the detecting and repairing process of DNA damage. Specifically, we will focus on H2AX phosphorylation regulation, Poly (ADP-ribosyl)ation, and sumoylation in DDR.

3.1. H2AX phosphorylation

One of the key events that initiates DDR is phosphorylation at the Ser139 of histone H2AX, a chromatin-bound histone variant compromising up to 25% of the H2A [16]. This phosphorylation process is catalyzed by the master regulator of DDR, ATM and ATR. Phosphorylation of H2AX at Ser139 is very rapid and this phosphorylated H2AX (γH2AX) serves as a platform, directly recruiting Mdc1 (mediator of DNA-damage checkpoint 1), and additional factors such as 53BP1, RNF8, and the BRCA1A complex to affected sites [19].

Although γH2AX is a well-recognized marker for DNA damage, its precise role in chromatin remodeling is only just becoming clear. It was recently found that phosphorylation at a tyrosine site, Tyr142, plays a pivotal role in regulating H2AX functions in DDR [20]. Basal phosphorylation of H2AX at Tyr142 was carried out by WSTF (Williams syndrome transcription factor), a component of the WICH ATP-dependent chromatin remodeling complex [20]. At the early stage of DDR (<1hr), inhibition of phosphorylation at Tyr142 by knocking down WICH did not affect γH2AX foci formation, but during the later recovery stages, γH2AX foci was greatly reduced[20]. So it seems that in the absence of Tyr142 phosphorylation, the kinetics of the phosphorylation/dephosphorylation cycle of γ-H2AX may be altered. Following this finding, the phosphatase EYA (eye absent) responsible for dephosphorylating H2AX at Tyr142 was identified [21]. Dephosphorylation of Tyr142 was suggested to be a prerequisite for γH2AX to be recognized by damage repair proteins. When persistent phosphorylation at Tyr142 happens during DNA damage, MDC1-dependent binding of DNA repair factors is inhibited, but recruitment of pro-apoptotic factors, such as JNK1, is promoted [21]. A more recent study demonstrated that the doubly phosphorylated H2AX interact with Microcephalin (MCPH1), an early DNA damage response protein [22]. Although the exact functions of such interaction is still unknown, we speculate that the precise regulation of γH2AX will be an area of great potential for future DNA damage studies.

3.2. Poly(ADP-ribosyl)ation

In addition to H2AX-dependent recruitment, several additional pathways have also been shown to direct the recruitment of various proteins to DNA lesion. Poly(ADP-ribosyl)ation (PARylation) is one of the early events in DDR [2]. Poly(ADP-ribose) polymerases-1 (PARP-1), the founding member of PARP family, sense DNA break through its zinc-finger domain. Structural studies also showed that engaging into the damaged DNA causes PARP-1 conformation change and increases the dynamics of its catalytic domain [23]. In this way, the occurrence of a DNA break is immediately translated into a posttranslational modification of histones H1 and H2B leading to chromatin structure change [24]. Two waves of accumulation of PARP-1 were observed in living cells. The initial recruitment of PARP-1 activates and locates poly(ADP-ribose) synthesis, which in turn generates binding sites for a second wave of PARP-1 recruitment and other DDR proteins [25]. Recently, it was found that polycomb group (PcG) members and nucleosome remodeling and deacetylase (NuRD) complex are recruited by PARP-1 and -2 to DNA lesions [26]. Both PcG and NuRD are negative regulators of gene transcription, and indeed, rapid loss of nascent RNA and elongating RNA polymerase were observed at DNA damage sites. This finding suggests that part of PARP's regulatory role in DDR involves repression of transcription.

3.3. Sumoylation

Sumoylation, the covalent attachment of the small proteins known as SUMO (small ubiquitin modifier) to protein substrate, is a very dynamic and reversible PTM [27]. Compared to ubiquitination, knowledge about sumoylation in DDR is relative rudimentary. In 2009, two papers demonstrated the importance of this ubiquitin-like protein modification in DDR [28, 29]. A series of immunofluorescence and live-cell image experiments showed that components in the sumoylation pathway, including enzymes E1 (SAE1), E2 (Ubc9), two of the diverse E3 enzymes (PIAS1 and PIAS4) and the conjugates SUMO1, 2 and 3, are rapidly recruited to DNA damage sites. Functionally, sumoylation of BRCA1 is necessary for its ubiquitin ligase activity. While association of 53BP1, BRCA1 and RNF168 with the DNA damage sites requires accumulation of PIAS1 and PIAS4 to the damaged sites [29].

Several more studies have further revealed that sumoylation and ubiquitination signaling pathways are integrated in the cellular response to DNA damage. For example, two groups showed that the human RNF4, a SUMO-targeted ubiquitin E3 ligase, was recruited to DSBs depending on its SUMO interacting motifs [30, 31] Depletion of RNF4 impairs ubiquitin adduct formation at DSB sites, causes persistent histone H2AX phosphorylation [30] and affects the clearance of 53BP1, RNF8, and RNF168 from DNA damage foci [31]. It is proposed that through physical interaction with the SUMO moiety, RNF4 promotes DNA repair by mediating ubiquitylation of sumoylated DDR components at sites of DNA damage.

The role of sumoylation in DNA repair is emphasized by modification of the RPA (replication protein A) complex [32]. RPA was found to physically associate with a SUMO specific protease, SENP6, to maintain its desumoylation status in normal conditions [32]. Under DNA damage, such as those caused by campothecin or IR, the 70 kD subunit of RPA is sumoylated, which in turn recruits Rad51 to DNA lesions, initiating DNA repair through HR. In addition to the specific study of RPA, a recent study in yeast identified a large group of proteins participating in DNA repair and undergoing sumoylation. They showed that defective sumoylation results in failure to complete replication of a damaged genome and impaired DNA end processing, highlighting the importance of sumoylation in maintaining genome stability [33].

4. DNA damage processed in heterochromatin

4.1. The heterochromatin feature

Chromatin can be divided into euchromatin and heterochromatin, on the basis of differential compaction at interphase. Euchromatin is loosely compacted, more accessible to transcriptional machinery and thus usually actively transcribed. Heterochromatin is typically densely packed, and was previously thought to be inaccessible to the transcription components [34]. Molecularly, heterochromatin is featured with specific histone modifications, such as di- or tri-methylation of histone H3 at lysine 9, and the subsequent recruitment of chromatin association protein such as heterochromatin protein1 (Hp1) [35]. Heterochromatin can be further divided into two groups. First is the constitutive heterochromatin, which contains a high density of repetitive DNA elements, such as satellite sequences and transposable elements. They remain condensed throughout the cell cycle. A second group is facultative heterochromatin, which is dynamic chromosomal loci, condensation of which is regulated by cellular and environmental signals [36].

4.2. The functions of heterochromatin

The major function of heterochromatin is to repress transcription and recombination of the embedded repetitive DNA sequences. Disruption of heterochromatin increases the occurrence of spontaneous DSBs, leads to the expansion of DNA repeat arrays, and is correlated with chromosomal defects, such as translocations and loss of heterozygosity [37]. Mechanistically, methylated H3 at Lysine9 (H3K9me) and the chromatin-bound Hp1 serve as a platform, recruiting various proteins to maintain the highly compact feature of heterochromatin. For example, the HDAC Clr3 is recruited to heterochromatic domains by the yeast Hp1 homolog Swi6. Deacytylation by Clr3 stabilizes H3 tri-methylation, increase chromatin condensation and precludes access of Polymerase II [38]. In addition to physically preventing the access of transcription machinery, heterochromatin structure also promotes the post-transcriptional silencing of repetitive sequences. This function is achieved by preferentially targeting the RNA interference components, such as RITS (RNA-induced transcriptional gene silencing) and RDRC (RNA-directed RNA polymerase complex) through H3K9me and Hp1 [39] [40, 41]. On the other side, the recruited RNAi machinery can also contribute to the heterochromatic architecture. In mammalian and drosophila cells, Hp1 shows RNA binding activity, which is required for assembling of condensed chromatin [42, 43]. It is proposed that the RNA derived from repetitive DNA sequence might function as a glue to promote folding or clustering of dispersed heterochromatic loci [36, 41].

4.3. Detection of DSBs in heterochromatin: focusing on γH2A foci

With the realization of heterochromatin structure and functions, the question is how DNA damages in heterochromatin are detected and repaired. In the following sections, we will discuss the recent understanding about these issues.

Abundant reports suggest that heterochromatin is refractory to γH2A foci formation upon ionizing radiation [44-46]. However, it remains to be determined whether this phenomenon is due to inaccessible to phosphorylation of H2AX, or heterochromatin is more resistant to DNA damage. Particularly, following DNA damage, chromatin in the vicinity of damaged sites are rapidly de-condensed, which makes the idea that γH2A foci is absent in highly packed chromatin a topic of debate [46-48]. On the other side, a recent study utilizing fluorescence in situ hybridization found that the high amount of proteins bound to heterochromatin, including Hp1, acts as a protective layer that prevents access to the DNA. Therefore, it seems that heterochromatin may internally act as an isolator to inhibit DNA damage [49].

However, those thoughts were revisited by a recent study conducted in drosophila cells. In 2011, Chiolo *et al.* demonstrated that γH2A foci can be formed in heterochromatin upon DSBs [50]. Through a serious of live-cell images and immunofluorescence studies, they found that DSBs and γH2A foci were absent at later time points of IR-induced DSBs (>60 mins post IR), which is consistent with previous studies. However, at earlier time points of IR treatment (<10 min), both γH2Ax and ATRIP foci can be observed in heterochromatin, with a level equal to that of non-heterochromatic sites. This study suggests that a complete DDR can occur within heterochromatin (Figure 2A).

4.4. DSBs repair in heterochromatin

The next question is how cell repairs the DSBs in heterochromatin. Two issues are raised when considering repair of DNA lesions in heterochromatin. The first is that chromatin compaction in heterochromatin might restrict the access of DDR proteins to damaged sites. Indeed, it was found that DSB repair occurs with slower kinetics and is less effective in heterochromatin [51]. Furthermore, a delay in repair of heterochromatic DSBs was observed in human cells [52]. To overcome the challenge given by tightly compacted chromatin, it was found that the cell can employ the ATM signaling pathway to relax chromatin [51]. Goodarzi *et al.* found that ATM signaling was specifically required for DSBs repair within heterochromatin, by phosphorylating a transcription repressor, KAP1 (KRAB-associated protein1). KAP1 induces transcriptional repression and chromatin condensation through recruitment of Hp1 [53] and Mi2α [54]. In the absence of ATM, association of KAP1 to chromatin was increased, suggesting phosphorylation by ATM decreases the affinity of KAP1 for chromatin, which in turn reduces chromatin condensation [51].

The second issue regarding repair of DSBs in heterochromatin is whether NHEJ or HR pathway occurs. In the presence of the closely clustered repeats, HR might produce dicentric and acentric chromosomes, which are known to contribute to human diseases such as cancer and infertility [55]. In this sense, it would be very risky for cells to choose HR to repair the DSBs, since this may lead to abnormal genome rearrangements. In other words, NHEJ repair seems less problematic because small deletions or mutations generally do not affect the function of tandem repeats as severely as genes. However, reports form Chiolo *et al.* demonstrated that DSBs occuring in heterochromatin are repaired by HR, but the underlying mechanism is distinct from euchromatin [50] (Figure 2A). The most prominent difference is the exclusion of Rad51, which mediates strand invasion, from the DSBs in the heterochromatic domain. Exclusion of Rad51 is achieved by protrusion of heterochromatin, which facilitates DSBs relocalization to the Hp1α periphery. The movement of the DSBs from inside to outside of heterochromatin depends on checkpoint proteins, such as ATR and resection proteins. Furthermore, relocalization of heterochromatic DSBs is blocked by the Smc5/6 SUMO ligase complex, the yeast homolog of which is required to prevent recombinational repair within the repetitive rDNA locus [56]. It is proposed that Smc5/6 could catalyze sumoylation of one or more components of the recombination machinery and block further assembly of the HR machinery [57].

Together, multiple mechanisms exist to guarantee proper DDR in heterochromatin to repair the damaged DNA without compromising genome stability. With improvements in live-cell imaging, we speculate that more details, like the process of DNA damage-induced heterochromatin expansion and reunion of the repaired heterochromatic region, will be revealed.

5. Human aging and chromatin remodeling

Aging is a complex process that has been long thought to be a consequence of unprogrammed deleterious events and accumulation of random gene mutation. However, with extensive studies in yeast, worm and mouse, and with the research in premature human aging disease, novel insights have been gained into the molecular mechanisms underlying aging. In this section, we will focus on recent understanding about the contributions that chromatin defects and DNA damage have on human aging.

5.1. Heterochromatin defects in human aging

Through studying the premature aging disorder Hutchinson–Gilford Progeria Syndrome (HGPS), the molecular mechanisms leading to chromatin defects in aging are being uncovered. HGPS is an extremely rare genetic disease caused by a point mutation in the *LMNA* gene, which encodes the major structural protein Lamin A in the nuclear envelope [58]. *LMNA* mutation leads to abnormal splicing defects and consequent production of a truncated form of lamin A protein, referred to as progerin [59, 60]. Notably, in healthy individuals, the same splice site in lamin A was used to cause age-related nuclear defects [61], suggesting conserved mechanism might be shared by both premature and physical human aging process.

One hallmark of human aging, and also in the aging process of other species, is global change in chromatin structure [62, 63].Particularly, loss of heterochromatin structure, loss of heterochromatin proteins and altered patterns of histone modifications, such as decreased H3K9me3, are found in both physiological and premature aging [61, 64-67]. Furthermore, more open chromatin structure, as indicated by tri-methylation at histone3 lysine4, is implicated in shorter lifespan in worm [68, 69].

5.2. Molecular mechanisms underlying heterochromatin loss and aging

The above evidence suggests that heterochromatin maintenance is critical for longevity. Now the question is how such densely compacted chromatin structure regulates human aging. Unfortunately, due to the complex nature of the aging process and hence experimentally intractability, it is hard to find a direct causal-effect relationship. But recent studies do shed light on the heterochromatic sequence transcription and human aging. Shumaker *et al* found that associated with the down-regulation of H3K9me3, the satellite III repeat transcripts, which is locating in the pericentric heterochromatin, were up-regulated. This up-regulation seems to be sequence-specific since transcription of other group of pericentric repeat, such as α satellite, was not altered [66]. Interestingly, Larson *et al*. reported that during *Drosophila* aging, loss of heterochromatin leads to an increased transcription of ribosomal DNA [67]. This rDNA locus contains exceeded ribosomal genes and usually only 10% of them are transcribed [70]. How abnormal transcription of heterochromatic sequences regulate aging is currently unknown. But it is proposed that loss of heterochromatic repeat silencing may affect gene expression patterns and hence affect the integrity of the transcriptome. It is also intriguing to link the heterochromatin status, ribosomal RNA synthesis and aging by taking energy metabolism into account. That is, ribosomal RNA transcription is a rate-limiting step in protein synthesis, increased RNA transcription would promote growth and accelerate aging [71, 72]

5.3. DNA damage and human aging

Persistent DNA damage is another hallmark in human aging. Most human premature aging syndromes are caused by various types of DNA damage, and in particular, DSBs [73, 74]. There is no doubt that chromatin defects and DNA damage are major contributors to human aging. The question is which one comes first? Do the DNA damage and the DDR lead to chromatin defects and thus human aging? Or it is that loss of chromatin structure makes the cell more susceptible to DNA damage, increases genome instability, and therefore promotes human aging? Observations made by Pegoraro *et al.* support that chromatin defects occur prior to DNA damage [75]. They identified that NURD, a protein complex involved in establishment of heterochromatin [76], is a key modulator in aging-associated chromatin defects. Knocking down a subunit of NURD complex lead to aberrant chromatin structure (indicated by loss of H3K9me3 foci) about 50 h earlier than DNA damage (indicated by existence of γH2AX foci). This observation suggests that epigenetic and chromatin structure changes are in the upstream of DNA damage events.

How could aberrant chromatin structure cause DNA damage and thus human aging? There might be two mechanisms. 1) The heterochromatic sequences are highly repetitive. Loss of chromatin condensation can leads to abnormal recombination of such sequence and thus genome rearrangement; 2) Heterochromatin confirmation can protect DNA from various insults and repair the damaged lesion with specific mechanisms, as mentioned above.

The next question is how DNA damage leads to human aging? Numerous studies showed that DNA damage and mutations accumulate in human aging. In aged human cells, cytogenetically visible lesions such as translocations, insertions, dicentrics, and acentric fragments are frequently detected [77]. Several signaling pathways linking DNA damage and aging are also proposed, such as the ATM-p53 axis [77] and the BRCA1 dependent aging process [78].However, in addition to being a driver in the accumulation of mutation, recent reports imply that DNA damage-induced RNA transcription change might be a novel mechanism leading human aging. The involvement of RNA processing components in DNA repair strengthens the role of DNA damage in global gene expression changes. For example, a proteomic screen for mediators of DDR showed that enrichment for RNA processing factors, such as splicing-regulator phosphatase PPM1G [79]. Furthermore, the deregulation of gene expression induced by DNA damage resembles increased transcription heterogeneity seen in aged heart tissue [80]. Specifically, Francia *et al.* found that small RNA produced by DICER and DROSHA, two RNases type III enzymes that process non-coding RNA [81], are required to activate DDR and efficiently repair DNA at the damaged sites [82]. The DICER- and

DROSHA-dependent small RNA products have the sequence of the damaged locus, and can restore DDR in RNase-treated cells [82]. Intriguingly, these DNA damage-induced RNA can regulate cellular senescence in cultured human and mouse cells, and in living zebrafish larvae [82]. Genetic ablation of DICER has been reported to cause premature senescence in both developing and adult mice [83]. Do the DICER- and DROSHA-dependent, DNA damaged-induced RNAs affect heterochromatin structure and thus regulating cell senescence and human aging? Although the methylation status of H3K9 did not alter with DICER or DROSHA knockdown [82], it is still interesting to check if other heterochromatic proteins, such as Hp1, which has RNA binding activity, could be affected (Figure 2). Furthermore, does the site-specific RNA production have any role in the dynamic movement of heterochromatic domain during DNA damage, for example, the protrusion of heterochromatin? Answering these questions will be important to gain a comprehensive understanding of the interplay between chromatin structure and RNA transcription during DDR.

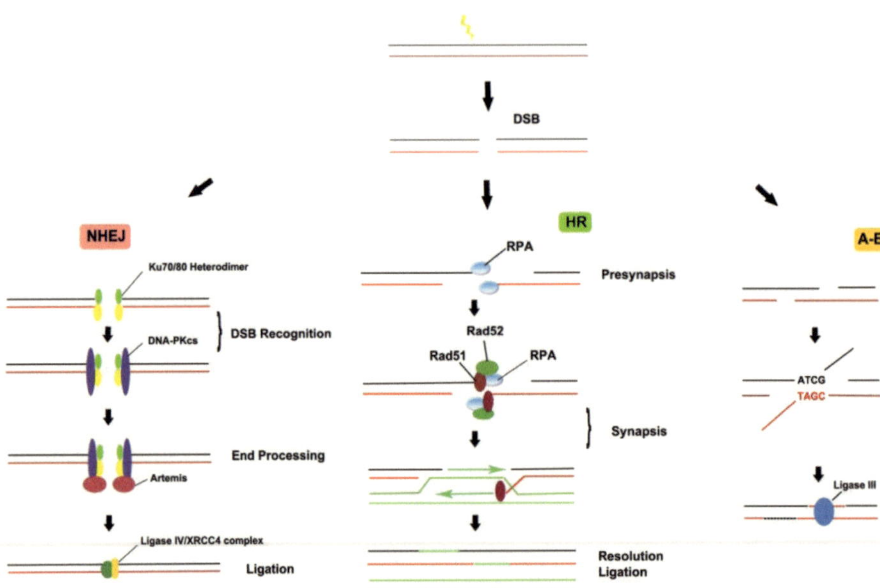

Figure 1. In **NHEJ**, the heterodimer Ku70/80 interacts with the end of damaged DNA and recruits DNA-PKcs. Artemis, which processes the ends of DNA and makes them compatible for ligation, is also recruited. Finally, the DNA breaks were joined by XRCC4/Ligase IV. In **HR**, a homologous stretch on a sister chromatid is utilized to accurately repair the DSB. DNA ends are first processed in order to create single strand overhangs. RPA is then coated to these overhangs, which recruits Rad51 and other co-factors such as Rad52. The Rad51 coated DNA filament then invade the undamaged strands, and a joint molecule is formed by the damaged and undamaged strands. Finally, template guides DNA synthesis and resolution of the two strands. **A-EJ** shares the initial resection step with HR but it requires neither extended resection nor extended sequence homology. DNA ends that are not bound by Ku70/80 are degraded. Single strand DNA resection reveals 2-4 (indicated by ATCG in the figure) or more nucleotides which can anneal, creating branched intermediate structures. The resolution of this intermediate structure results in deletions at the repair junctions. A-EJ is independent of Ku70/80 but dependent on Ligase III to join the DNA ends.

http://dx.doi.org/10.5772/55272

6. Conclusions

Since discovery of the function of γH2AX in DDR, dynamic regulation of chromatin in response to DNA damage has received great attention during these past decades. In this chapter, we have discussed the contribution of three posttranslational modifications: phosphorylation, PPAR and sumoylation in DDR. We also discussed the current understanding about heterochromatin changes during DDR and how it regulates human aging. We emphasize the function of heterochromatin in DDR because this condensed chromatin structure is particularly involved in human aging. Emerging evidence suggests that heterochromatin is not refractory to DNA damage, but utilize a different downstream mechanism to repair the damaged sites and thus prevent unwanted genome recombination. DNA damage may change the heterochromatin structure by abnormal generation of non-coding RNA at the damaged locus, which could titrate the RNA-binding heterochromatin proteins (such as Hp1) and lead to subsequent abnormal heterochromatin structure. The integrity of the transcriptome can also be affected by DNA damage and regulate human aging. We speculate that the pathways regarding DNA damage repair in heterochromatin and the interplay between heterochromatic sequence transcription and human aging will be a hot area for future research (Figure 3).

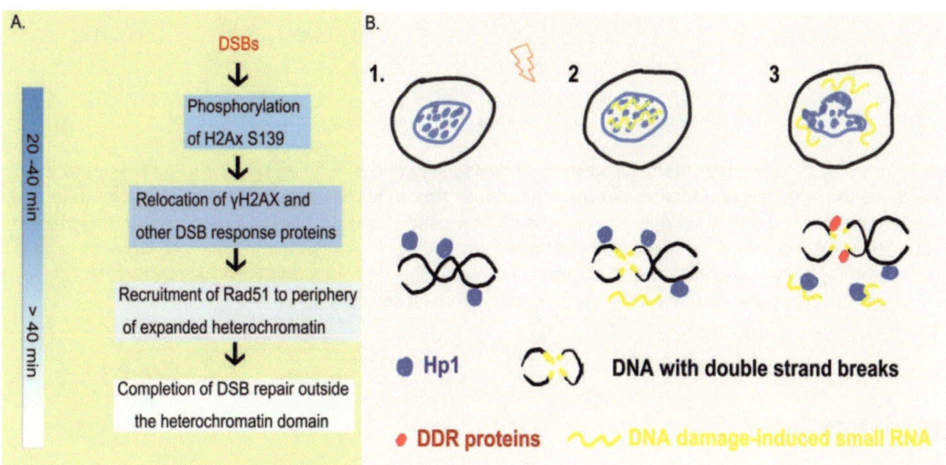

Figure 2. A. Schematic diagram shows DNA damage response in heterochromatin. Initial DSB recognition is very rapid in heterochromatin. Rapid phosphorylation and relocalization of H2Ax S139 and other DSB proteins (such as ATRIP) occur in heterochromatic region. Rad51 recombinase recruitment is inhibited in Hp1-rich heterochromatin, which allows DSB processing to induce heterochromatin expansion and DSB repaired in euchromatic site. In this way, unwanted homologous recombination is prevented in heterochromatin. **B**. A potential model for DNA damage response in heterochromatin. A typical heterochromatic domain is indicated by the enrichment of Hp1 protein (step 1). Under DNA damage, double strand breaks occur, which might result in production of site-specific small RNA with sequence of the damaged site (step 2). Hp1 might bind to the DNA damage-induced small RNA, which leads to its relocalization and consequent dynamic movement of the heterochromatic domain during DNA damage. Binding of Hp1 to the small RNA might also facilitate recruiting of other DDR proteins to the damaged heterochromatic sequences, and thus promoting damage repair. Notably, it still needs to be determined whether the damage-induced RNA is generated in heterochromatin (step [2]). If this is the case, the role of this RNA in the dynamic movement of heterochromatin during DNA damage also awaits investigation (step 3).

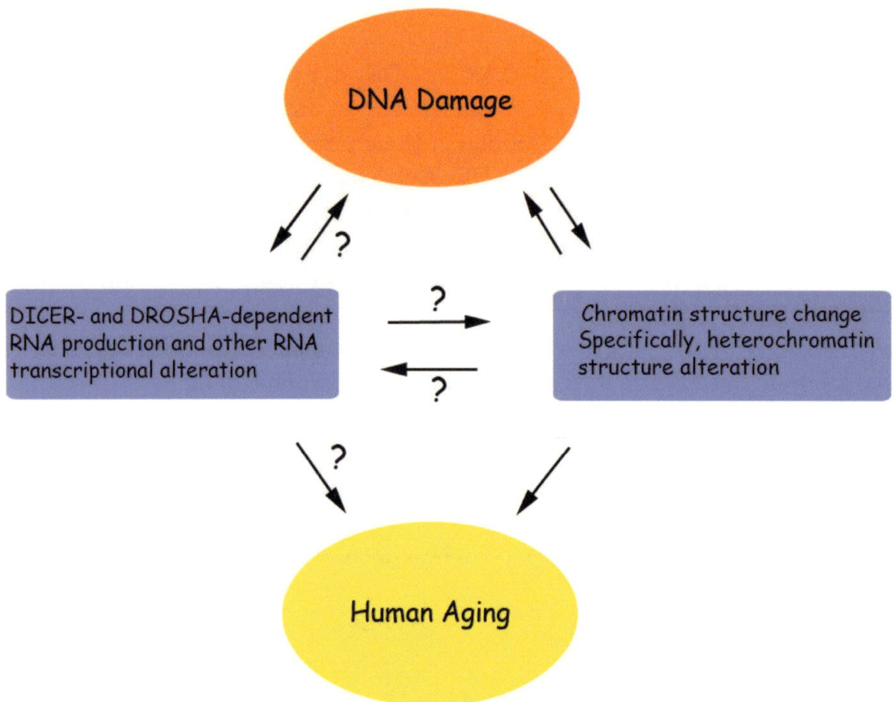

Figure 3. Interplay between DNA damage, chromatin remodeling and human aging. It is well recognized that DNA damage leads to chromatin remodeling. On the other hand, abnormal chromatin structures also contribute to DNA damage and correlate with human aging. Emerging evidence shed light on the DNA damage-induced global transcription regulation and also locus-specific production of small RNAs. It would be interesting to know through which mechanism the DNA damage-induced RNA regulates DNA damage response, and whether it affects the chromatin, especially, heterochromatin structures, and hence modulate human aging.

Author details

Lili Gong, Edward Wang and Shiaw-Yih Lin

Department of Systems Biology, The University of Texas M. D. Anderson Cancer Center, Houston, Texas, USA

References

[1] Kornberg RD. Chromatin structure: a repeating unit of histones and DNA. Science. 1974 May 24;184(4139):868-71.

[2] Polo SE, Jackson SP. Dynamics of DNA damage response proteins at DNA breaks: a focus on protein modifications. Genes Dev. 2011 Mar 1;25(5):409-33.

[3] Lukas J, Lukas C, Bartek J. More than just a focus: The chromatin response to DNA damage and its role in genome integrity maintenance. Nat Cell Biol. 2011 Oct;13(10): 1161-9.

[4] Gellert M. V(D)J recombination: RAG proteins, repair factors, and regulation. Annu Rev Biochem. 2002;71:101-32.

[5] Jackson SP, Bartek J. The DNA-damage response in human biology and disease. Nature. 2009 Oct 22;461(7267):1071-8.

[6] Friedberg EC. Nucleotide excision repair of DNA: The very early history. DNA Repair. 2011 Jul 15;10(7):668-72.

[7] Symington LS, Gautier J. Double-strand break end resection and repair pathway choice. Annu Rev Genet. 2011;45:247-71.

[8] Lieber MR. The mechanism of double-strand DNA break repair by the nonhomologous DNA end-joining pathway. Annu Rev Biochem. 2010;79:181-211.

[9] Weterings E, Chen DJ. The endless tale of non-homologous end-joining. Cell Res. 2008 Jan;18(1):114-24.

[10] Jeggo PA. DNA breakage and repair. Adv Genet. 1998;38:185-218.

[11] Haber JE. Partners and pathwaysrepairing a double-strand break. Trends Genet. 2000 Jun;16(6):259-64.

[12] Baumann P, West SC. Role of the human RAD51 protein in homologous recombination and double-stranded-break repair. Trends Biochem Sci. 1998 Jul;23(7):247-51.

[13] Gasior SL, Wong AK, Kora Y, Shinohara A, Bishop DK. Rad52 associates with RPA and functions with rad55 and rad57 to assemble meiotic recombination complexes. Genes Dev. 1998 Jul 15;12(14):2208-21.

[14] Sugawara N, Wang X, Haber JE. In vivo roles of Rad52, Rad54, and Rad55 proteins in Rad51-mediated recombination. Mol Cell. 2003 Jul;12(1):209-19.

[15] Rass E, Grabarz A, Plo I, Gautier J, Bertrand P, Lopez BS. Role of Mre11 in chromosomal nonhomologous end joining in mammalian cells. Nat Struct Mol Biol. 2009 Aug; 16(8):819-24.

[16] Rogakou EP, Pilch DR, Orr AH, Ivanova VS, Bonner WM. DNA double-stranded breaks induce histone H2AX phosphorylation on serine 139. J Biol Chem. 1998 Mar 6;273(10):5858-68.

[17] O'Hagan HM, Mohammad HP, Baylin SB. Double strand breaks can initiate gene silencing and SIRT1-dependent onset of DNA methylation in an exogenous promoter CpG island. PLoS Genet. 2008;4(8):e1000155.

[18] Cuozzo C, Porcellini A, Angrisano T, Morano A, Lee B, Di Pardo A, et al. DNA damage, homology-directed repair, and DNA methylation. PLoS Genet. 2007 Jul; 3(7):e110.

[19] Harper JW, Elledge SJ. The DNA damage response: ten years after. Mol Cell. 2007 Dec 14;28(5):739-45.

[20] Xiao A, Li H, Shechter D, Ahn SH, Fabrizio LA, Erdjument-Bromage H, et al. WSTF regulates the H2A.X DNA damage response via a novel tyrosine kinase activity. Nature. 2009 Jan 1;457(7225):57-62.

[21] Cook PJ, Ju BG, Telese F, Wang X, Glass CK, Rosenfeld MG. Tyrosine dephosphorylation of H2AX modulates apoptosis and survival decisions. Nature. 2009 Apr 2;458(7238):591-6.

[22] Singh N, Basnet H, Wiltshire TD, Mohammad DH, Thompson JR, Heroux A, et al. Dual recognition of phosphoserine and phosphotyrosine in histone variant H2A.X by DNA damage response protein MCPH1. Proc Natl Acad Sci U S A. 2012 Sep 4;109(36):14381-6.

[23] Langelier MF, Planck JL, Roy S, Pascal JM. Structural basis for DNA damage-dependent poly(ADP-ribosyl)ation by human PARP-1. Science. 2012 May 11;336(6082): 728-32.

[24] Messner S, Altmeyer M, Zhao H, Pozivil A, Roschitzki B, Gehrig P, et al. PARP1 ADP-ribosylates lysine residues of the core histone tails. Nucleic Acids Res. 2010 Oct; 38(19):6350-62.

[25] Mortusewicz O, Ame JC, Schreiber V, Leonhardt H. Feedback-regulated poly(ADP-ribosyl)ation by PARP-1 is required for rapid response to DNA damage in living cells. Nucleic Acids Res. 2007;35(22):7665-75.

[26] Chou DM, Adamson B, Dephoure NE, Tan X, Nottke AC, Hurov KE, et al. A chromatin localization screen reveals poly (ADP ribose)-regulated recruitment of the repressive polycomb and NuRD complexes to sites of DNA damage. Proc Natl Acad Sci U S A. 2010 Oct 26;107(43):18475-80.

[27] Wilkinson KA, Henley JM. Mechanisms, regulation and consequences of protein SUMOylation. Biochem J. 2010 Jun 1;428(2):133-45.

[28] Galanty Y, Belotserkovskaya R, Coates J, Polo S, Miller KM, Jackson SP. Mammalian SUMO E3-ligases PIAS1 and PIAS4 promote responses to DNA double-strand breaks. Nature. 2009 Dec 17;462(7275):935-9.

[29] Morris JR, Boutell C, Keppler M, Densham R, Weekes D, Alamshah A, et al. The SUMO modification pathway is involved in the BRCA1 response to genotoxic stress. Nature. 2009 Dec 17;462(7275):886-90.

[30] Galanty Y, Belotserkovskaya R, Coates J, Jackson SP. RNF4, a SUMO-targeted ubiquitin E3 ligase, promotes DNA double-strand break repair. Genes Dev. 2012 Jun 1;26(11):1179-95.

[31] Yin Y, Seifert A, Chua JS, Maure JF, Golebiowski F, Hay RT. SUMO-targeted ubiquitin E3 ligase RNF4 is required for the response of human cells to DNA damage. Genes Dev. 2012 Jun 1;26(11):1196-208.

[32] Dou H, Huang C, Singh M, Carpenter PB, Yeh ET. Regulation of DNA repair through deSUMOylation and SUMOylation of replication protein A complex. Mol Cell. 2010 Aug 13;39(3):333-45.

[33] Cremona CA, Sarangi P, Yang Y, Hang LE, Rahman S, Zhao X. Extensive DNA damage-induced sumoylation contributes to replication and repair and acts in addition to the mec1 checkpoint. Mol Cell. 2012 Feb 10;45(3):422-32.

[34] Huisinga KL, Brower-Toland B, Elgin SC. The contradictory definitions of heterochromatin: transcription and silencing. Chromosoma. 2006 Apr;115(2):110-22.

[35] Cheutin T, McNairn AJ, Jenuwein T, Gilbert DM, Singh PB, Misteli T. Maintenance of stable heterochromatin domains by dynamic HP1 binding. Science. 2003 Jan 31;299(5607):721-5.

[36] Grewal SI, Jia S. Heterochromatin revisited. Nat Rev Genet. 2007 Jan;8(1):35-46.

[37] Peng JC, Karpen GH. Heterochromatic genome stability requires regulators of histone H3 K9 methylation. PLoS Genet. 2009 Mar;5(3):e1000435.

[38] Yamada T, Fischle W, Sugiyama T, Allis CD, Grewal SI. The nucleation and maintenance of heterochromatin by a histone deacetylase in fission yeast. Mol Cell. 2005 Oct 28;20(2):173-85.

[39] Motamedi MR, Verdel A, Colmenares SU, Gerber SA, Gygi SP, Moazed D. Two RNAi complexes, RITS and RDRC, physically interact and localize to noncoding centromeric RNAs. Cell. 2004 Dec 17;119(6):789-802.

[40] Sugiyama T, Cam H, Verdel A, Moazed D, Grewal SI. RNA-dependent RNA polymerase is an essential component of a self-enforcing loop coupling heterochromatin assembly to siRNA production. Proc Natl Acad Sci U S A. 2005 Jan 4;102(1):152-7.

[41] Cam HP, Sugiyama T, Chen ES, Chen X, FitzGerald PC, Grewal SI. Comprehensive analysis of heterochromatin- and RNAi-mediated epigenetic control of the fission yeast genome. Nat Genet. 2005 Aug;37(8):809-19.

[42] Muchardt C, Guilleme M, Seeler JS, Trouche D, Dejean A, Yaniv M. Coordinated methyl and RNA binding is required for heterochromatin localization of mammalian HP1alpha. EMBO Rep. 2002 Oct;3(10):975-81.

[43] Keller C, Adaixo R, Stunnenberg R, Woolcock KJ, Hiller S, Buhler M. HP1(Swi6) mediates the recognition and destruction of heterochromatic RNA transcripts. Mol Cell. 2012 Jul 27;47(2):215-27.

[44] Cowell IG, Sunter NJ, Singh PB, Austin CA, Durkacz BW, Tilby MJ. gammaH2AX foci form preferentially in euchromatin after ionising-radiation. PLoS One. 2007;2(10):e1057.

[45] Vasireddy RS, Karagiannis TC, El-Osta A. gamma-radiation-induced gammaH2AX formation occurs preferentially in actively transcribing euchromatic loci. Cell Mol Life Sci. 2010 Jan;67(2):291-4.

[46] Cann KL, Dellaire G. Heterochromatin and the DNA damage response: the need to relax. Biochem Cell Biol. 2011 Feb;89(1):45-60.

[47] Kruhlak MJ, Celeste A, Dellaire G, Fernandez-Capetillo O, Muller WG, McNally JG, et al. Changes in chromatin structure and mobility in living cells at sites of DNA double-strand breaks. J Cell Biol. 2006 Mar 13;172(6):823-34.

[48] Falk M, Lukasova E, Gabrielova B, Ondrej V, Kozubek S. Chromatin dynamics during DSB repair. Biochim Biophys Acta. 2007 Oct;1773(10):1534-45.

[49] Falk M, Lukasova E, Kozubek S. Chromatin structure influences the sensitivity of DNA to gamma-radiation. Biochim Biophys Acta. 2008 Dec;1783(12):2398-414.

[50] Chiolo I, Minoda A, Colmenares SU, Polyzos A, Costes SV, Karpen GH. Double-strand breaks in heterochromatin move outside of a dynamic HP1a domain to complete recombinational repair. Cell. 2011 Mar 4;144(5):732-44.

[51] Goodarzi AA, Noon AT, Deckbar D, Ziv Y, Shiloh Y, Lobrich M, et al. ATM signaling facilitates repair of DNA double-strand breaks associated with heterochromatin. Mol Cell. 2008 Jul 25;31(2):167-77.

[52] Noon AT, Shibata A, Rief N, Lobrich M, Stewart GS, Jeggo PA, et al. 53BP1-dependent robust localized KAP-1 phosphorylation is essential for heterochromatic DNA double-strand break repair. Nat Cell Biol. 2010 Feb;12(2):177-84.

[53] Lechner MS, Begg GE, Speicher DW, Rauscher FJ, 3rd. Molecular determinants for targeting heterochromatin protein 1-mediated gene silencing: direct chromoshadow domain-KAP-1 corepressor interaction is essential. Mol Cell Biol. 2000 Sep;20(17): 6449-65.

[54] Schultz DC, Friedman JR, Rauscher FJ, 3rd. Targeting histone deacetylase complexes via KRAB-zinc finger proteins: the PHD and bromodomains of KAP-1 form a cooperative unit that recruits a novel isoform of the Mi-2alpha subunit of NuRD. Genes Dev. 2001 Feb 15;15(4):428-43.

[55] Pearson CE, Nichol Edamura K, Cleary JD. Repeat instability: mechanisms of dynamic mutations. Nat Rev Genet. 2005 Oct;6(10):729-42.

[56] Torres-Rosell J, Sunjevaric I, De Piccoli G, Sacher M, Eckert-Boulet N, Reid R, et al. The Smc5-Smc6 complex and SUMO modification of Rad52 regulates recombinational repair at the ribosomal gene locus. Nat Cell Biol. 2007 Aug;9(8):923-31.

[57] Peterson CL. The ins and outs of heterochromatic DNA repair. Dev Cell. 2011 Mar 15;20(3):285-7.

[58] Kudlow BA, Kennedy BK, Monnat RJ, Jr. Werner and Hutchinson-Gilford progeria syndromes: mechanistic basis of human progeroid diseases. Nat Rev Mol Cell Biol. 2007 May;8(5):394-404.

[59] De Sandre-Giovannoli A, Bernard R, Cau P, Navarro C, Amiel J, Boccaccio I, et al. Lamin a truncation in Hutchinson-Gilford progeria. Science. 2003 Jun 27;300(5628): 2055.

[60] Eriksson M, Brown WT, Gordon LB, Glynn MW, Singer J, Scott L, et al. Recurrent de novo point mutations in lamin A cause Hutchinson-Gilford progeria syndrome. Nature. 2003 May 15;423(6937):293-8.

[61] Scaffidi P, Misteli T. Lamin A-dependent nuclear defects in human aging. Science. (Research Support, N.I.H., Intramural). 2006 May 19;312(5776):1059-63.

[62] Pegoraro G, Misteli T. The central role of chromatin maintenance in aging. Aging (Albany NY). 2009 Dec;1(12):1017-22.

[63] Swedlow J, Danuser G. Scale integration: the structure and dynamics of macromolecular assemblies, cells and tissues. Curr Opin Cell Biol. 2012 Feb;24(1):1-3.

[64] Goldman RD, Shumaker DK, Erdos MR, Eriksson M, Goldman AE, Gordon LB, et al. Accumulation of mutant lamin A causes progressive changes in nuclear architecture in Hutchinson-Gilford progeria syndrome. Proc Natl Acad Sci U S A. 2004 Jun 15;101(24):8963-8.

[65] Scaffidi P, Misteli T. Reversal of the cellular phenotype in the premature aging disease Hutchinson-Gilford progeria syndrome. Nat Med. 2005 Apr;11(4):440-5.

[66] Shumaker DK, Dechat T, Kohlmaier A, Adam SA, Bozovsky MR, Erdos MR, et al. Mutant nuclear lamin A leads to progressive alterations of epigenetic control in premature aging. Proc Natl Acad Sci U S A. 2006 Jun 6;103(23):8703-8.

[67] Larson K, Yan SJ, Tsurumi A, Liu J, Zhou J, Gaur K, et al. Heterochromatin formation promotes longevity and represses ribosomal RNA synthesis. PLoS Genet. 2012 Jan; 8(1):e1002473.

[68] Hamilton B, Dong Y, Shindo M, Liu W, Odell I, Ruvkun G, et al. A systematic RNAi screen for longevity genes in C. elegans. Genes Dev. 2005 Jul 1;19(13):1544-55.

[69] Han S, Brunet A. Histone methylation makes its mark on longevity. Trends Cell Biol. 2012 Jan;22(1):42-9.

[70] Eickbush DG, Ye J, Zhang X, Burke WD, Eickbush TH. Epigenetic regulation of retrotransposons within the nucleolus of Drosophila. Mol Cell Biol. 2008 Oct;28(20): 6452-61.

[71] Hansen M, Taubert S, Crawford D, Libina N, Lee SJ, Kenyon C. Lifespan extension by conditions that inhibit translation in Caenorhabditis elegans. Aging Cell. 2007 Feb;6(1):95-110.

[72] Pan KZ, Palter JE, Rogers AN, Olsen A, Chen D, Lithgow GJ, et al. Inhibition of mRNA translation extends lifespan in Caenorhabditis elegans. Aging Cell. 2007 Feb; 6(1):111-9.

[73] Sedelnikova OA, Horikawa I, Redon C, Nakamura A, Zimonjic DB, Popescu NC, et al. Delayed kinetics of DNA double-strand break processing in normal and pathological aging. Aging Cell. 2008 Jan;7(1):89-100.

[74] Sedelnikova OA, Horikawa I, Zimonjic DB, Popescu NC, Bonner WM, Barrett JC. Senescing human cells and ageing mice accumulate DNA lesions with unrepairable double-strand breaks. Nat Cell Biol. 2004 Feb;6(2):168-70.

[75] Pegoraro G, Kubben N, Wickert U, Gohler H, Hoffmann K, Misteli T. Ageing-related chromatin defects through loss of the NURD complex. Nat Cell Biol. 2009 Oct;11(10): 1261-7.

[76] Zhang Y, Ng HH, Erdjument-Bromage H, Tempst P, Bird A, Reinberg D. Analysis of the NuRD subunits reveals a histone deacetylase core complex and a connection with DNA methylation. Genes Dev. 1999 Aug 1;13(15):1924-35.

[77] Lombard DB, Chua KF, Mostoslavsky R, Franco S, Gostissa M, Alt FW. DNA repair, genome stability, and aging. Cell. 2005 Feb 25;120(4):497-512.

[78] Cao L, Li W, Kim S, Brodie SG, Deng CX. Senescence, aging, and malignant transformation mediated by p53 in mice lacking the Brca1 full-length isoform. Genes Dev. 2003 Jan 15;17(2):201-13.

[79] Beli P, Lukashchuk N, Wagner SA, Weinert BT, Olsen JV, Baskcomb L, et al. Proteomic investigations reveal a role for RNA processing factor THRAP3 in the DNA damage response. Mol Cell. 2012 Apr 27;46(2):212-25.

[80] Bahar R, Hartmann CH, Rodriguez KA, Denny AD, Busuttil RA, Dolle ME, et al. Increased cell-to-cell variation in gene expression in ageing mouse heart. Nature. 2006 Jun 22;441(7096):1011-4.

[81] Kim VN, Han J, Siomi MC. Biogenesis of small RNAs in animals. Nat Rev Mol Cell Biol. 2009 Feb;10(2):126-39.

[82] Francia S, Michelini F, Saxena A, Tang D, de Hoon M, Anelli V, et al. Site-specific DICER and DROSHA RNA products control the DNA-damage response. Nature. 2012 Aug 9;488(7410):231-5.

[83] Mudhasani R, Zhu Z, Hutvagner G, Eischen CM, Lyle S, Hall LL, et al. Loss of miRNA biogenesis induces p19Arf-p53 signaling and senescence in primary cells. J Cell Biol. 2008 Jun 30;181(7):1055-63.

Chapter 8

Chromatin Remodelling During Host-Bacterial Pathogen Interaction

Yong Zhong Xu, Cynthia Kanagaratham and Danuta Radzioch

Additional information is available at the end of the chapter

http://dx.doi.org/10.5772/55977

1. Introduction

Eukaryotic DNA is tightly packaged into nucleosome repeats, which form the basic unit of cellular chromatin. The nucleosome consists of an octamer core wrapped with a segment of 146 base pairs of double stranded DNA. Each octamer core is composed of two molecules of each core histone proteins H2A, H2B, H3 and H4 (Figure 1). A fifth histone protein, linker H1, binds to the nucleosomal core particle and assists in further compaction of the chromatin into higher-order structure(Lusser and Kadonaga, 2003;Roberts and Orkin, 2004). This compaction of genomic DNA into chromatin restricts access of a variety of DNA regulatory proteins to the DNA strand, which are involved in the processes of transcription, replication, DNA repair and recombination machinery. To overcome these barriers, eukaryotic cells possess a number of multi-protein complexes which can alter the chromatin structure and make DNA more accessible. These complexes can be divided into two groups, histone-modifying enzymes and ATP-dependent chromatin remodelling complexes. The histone-modifying enzymes post-translationally modify the N-terminal tails of histone proteins through acetylation, phosphorylation, ubiquitination, ADP-ribosylation and methylation. On the other hand, ATP-dependent chromatin remodelling complexes use the energy of ATP hydrolysis to disrupt the contact between DNA and histones, move nucleosomes along DNA, and remove or exchange nucleosomes(Kallin and Zhang, 2004;Lusser and Kadonaga, 2003;Roberts and Orkin, 2004). The importance of chromatin structure and its functional role in genome regulation and development is becoming increasingly evident, especially in diseases such as cancer.

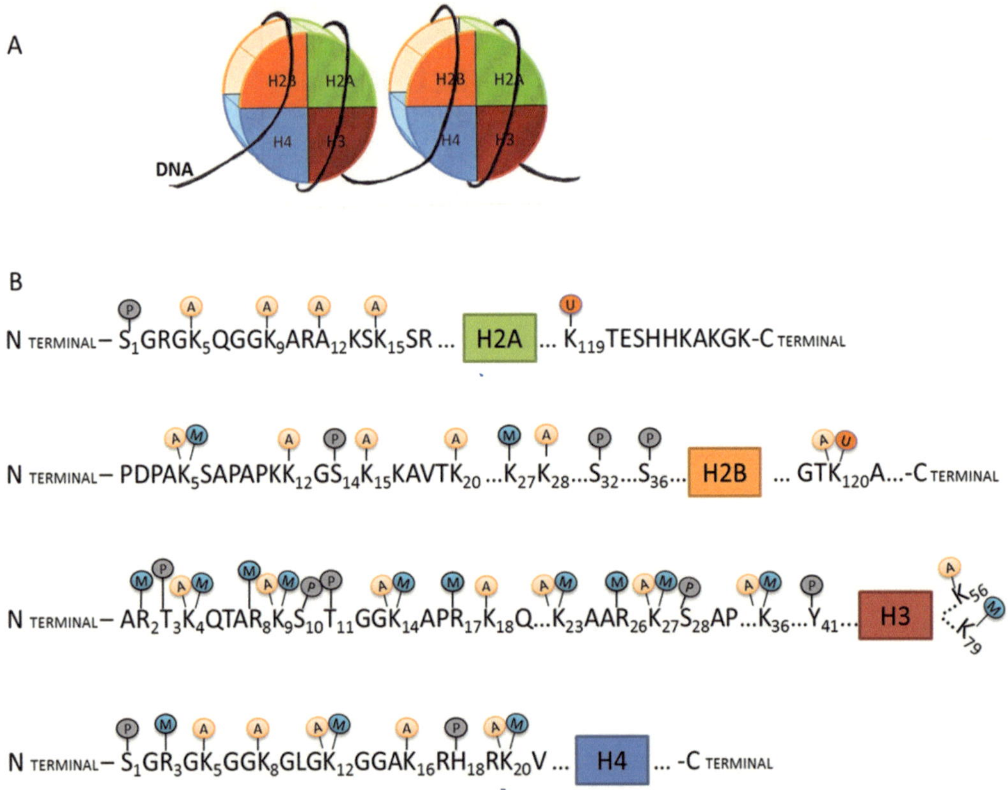

Figure 1. Schematic representation of a nucleosome (A) and major histone modifications (B). Modifications on histones are described in text. The major modifications shown include acetylation (A), methylation (M), phosphorylation (P) and ubiquitination (U). Histone modifications mainly occur on the N-terminal tails of histones but also on the C-terminal tails and globular domains, for example, ubiquitination of the C-terminal tails of H2A and H2B and acetylation and methylation of the globular domain of H3 at K56 and K79, respectively.

Intracellular pathogens, through a long-standing coexistence with host cells, have evolved mechanisms that provide pathogens with the amazing capacity to adapt and survive in the variable and often hostile environments of their hosts (Galan and Cossart, 2005). The concept of chromatin modification as a mechanism by which pathogens affect host immune responses to facilitate infection has emerged in recent years. For example, listeriolysin O (LLO), secreted by *Listeria monocytogenes*, induces a dramatic dephosphorylation of histone H3 at serine 10 and deacetylation of histone H4, and these modifications are associated with changes in host gene expression during early stages of infection (Hamon *et al.*, 2007). Arbibe and colleagues also indicate that *Shigella flexneri* effector OspF dephosphorylates ERK and p38 mitogen-activated protein kinase (MAPK) in the nucleus; this subsequently prevents histone H3 phosphorylation at Ser10 at the promoters of a specific subset of genes, which blocks the activation of nuclear factor –κB (NF-κB)- responsive genes leading to a compromised inflammation in the infected tissue(Arbibe *et al.*, 2007). These results suggest a strategy developed by microbial pathogens to manipulate the host cellular function through histone modification and subversion of host innate immune responses for their survival or to infect the host.

Histone acetylation/deacetylation is a key epigenetic regulator of chromatin structure and gene expression, in combination with other posttranslational modifications. These patterns of histone modification are maintained by histone modifying enzymes such as histone acetyl-transferases (HATs) and histone deacetylases (HDACs). While HATs acetylate histones, conferring an "open" chromatin structure that allows transcriptional activation, HDACs have the opposite effect resulting in transcriptional repression by closing chromatin structure. Global HDAC-mediated transcriptional changes can have a concomitant effect on cell function – an epigenetic mechanism often exploited by viruses to promote infection (Punga and Akusjarvi, 2000;Radkov *et al.*, 1999;Valls *et al.*, 2007). Recent reports also show that intracellular bacteria manipulate host cell epigenetics to facilitate infection (Arbibe *et al.*, 2007;Hamon *et al.*, 2007;Hamon and Cossart, 2008). Disruption of HDAC activity with inhibitors or by siRNA affects gene expression profilling in different cell types (Glaser *et al.*, 2003a;Glaser *et al.*, 2003b;Lee *et al.*, 2004;Zupkovitz *et al.*, 2006). The potential of HDAC inhibitors in treatment of infection has being studied.

In this chapter, the chromatin modifications in host cells induced by bacterial pathogens and their effects on host gene expression and infection will be reviewed. Furthermore, the potential role of HDAC inhibitors, as a therapeutic immunomodulator, in treatment of infections will also be discussed.

2. Chromatin structure in transcription regulation

The packaging of DNA into chromatin does not only simply facilitate the compaction of eukaryotic DNA genomes into the cell nucleus but also plays a profound and ubiquitous roles in almost all DNA-related cellular processes such as DNA replication, repair, recombination and transcription (Clapier and Cairns, 2009;Li *et al.*, 2007a). Chromatin structure is not a simple static unit. It possesses dynamic properties that are orchestrated by ATP-dependent chroma-tin-remodeling complexes and histone-modifying enzymes. In conjunction with other co-regulators, these chromatin remodelers modify histone-DNA interaction and regulate transcription at specific genomic loci.

2.1. Histone modifications and transcription

Histone sequences are highly conserved. A core histone protein typically consists of an unstructured N-terminal tail, a globular core including a central histone-fold domain, and a conformationally mobile C-terminal tail (Garcia *et al.*, 2007b;Mersfelder and Parthun, 2006). Both N-terminal tails and globular domains are subject to a variety of posttranslational modifications (Kouzarides T, Cell, 2007, 128:693-705) (Figure 1). At least fourteen different types of posttranslational (or covalent) modifications involving more than 60 different residues on histones have been reported to date including acetylation, methylation, phosphorylation, ubiquitination, poly-ADP ribosylation, sumoylation, butyrylation, formylation, deimination, citrullination, isomerisation, O-GlcNAcylation, crotonylation and hydroxylation (Martin and Zhang, 2007;Ruthenburg *et al.*, 2007;Sakabe *et al.*, 2010;Tan *et al.*, 2011). The majority of known histone modifications are located within the N-terminal tails of core histones. These modifications play an important role in the control of chromatin dynamics and its availability for transcription (Kouzarides, 2007). It has been suggested that all these modifications are combinatorial and interdependent and therefore may constitute a ``histone code`` (Jenuwein and Allis, 2001;Strahl and Allis, 2000). According to this hypothesis, the "histone code" is read by effector proteins (readers) which recognize and bind to modifications via specific domains and result in distinct and consistent cellular processes, such as replication, transcription, DNA repair and chromosome condensation (Kouzarides, 2007;Shi and Whetstine, 2007). Specific histone modifications are essential for partitioning the genome into functional domains, such as transcriptionally silent heterochromatin and transcriptionally active euchromatin (Martin and Zhang, 2005).

There are two major mechanisms underlying the function of histone modifications (Kouzarides, 2007;Ruthenburg *et al.*, 2007). The first is the modulation of chromatin structure either by altering DNA-nucleosome interaction or by altering nucleosome-nucleosome interactions via changing the histone charges or by addition of physical entities. For example, histone acetylation, a modification associated with transcriptional activation, has been proposed to unfold chromatin structure via neutralization of the basic charges of lysines (Kouzarides, 2007). Indeed, *in vitro* studies using recombinant nucleosomal arrays have demonstrated that acetylation of H4K16 restricts the formation of a 30-nanometer fiber and the generation of higher-order structures (Shogren-Knaak *et al.*, 2006;Shogren-Knaak and Peterson, 2006). Secondly, histone modifications provide docking sites for the recruitment of specific binding proteins, which recognize and interact with modified histones via specialized domains such as bromo-, chromo- and PHD (plant homeodomain) domains, thereby influence chromatin dynamics and function (Wysocka *et al.*, 2005;Wysocka *et al.*, 2006b;Zeng and Zhou, 2002). A number of proteins have been identified that are recruited to specific modifications. For example, methylation of H3K4, H3K9 and H3K27 can be recognized by inhibitor of growth (ING) proteins, heterochromatin protein 1 (HP1) and polycomb proteins, respectively. It has been shown that histone modification binding proteins can tether, directly or indirectly, an enzyme to chromatin. The activity of this recruited enzyme can be regulated (Pena *et al.*, 2006;Shi *et al.*, 2006;Wysocka *et al.*, 2006b). BPTF, a component of the NURF chromatin remodelling complex, binds to H3K4me3 via a PHD domain and tethers the SNF2L ATPase to H0XC8 gene and activates the expression of the latter (Wysocka *et al.*, 2006b). JMJD2A and CHD1, two other H3K4me-binding proteins, possess enzymatic activities themselves and can directly deliver enzymatic activities to chromatin when recruited (Huang *et al.*, 2006;Pray-Grant *et al.*, 2005;Sims, III *et al.*, 2005).

The link between histone modifications and transcriptional regulation has been widely studied. It has been found that a specific modification can be associated with transcriptional activation or repression. Among the histone modifications, methylation and acetylation of H3 and H4 play a major role in the regulation of transcriptional activity (Berger, 2007;Jenuwein and Allis, 2001;Li *et al.*, 2007a;Shahbazian and Grunstein, 2007). Methylation, which occurs on either a lysine or an arginine residue, is catalyzed by three different classes of methyltransferases: SET domain-containing histone methyltransferases (HMTs), non-SET domain-containing lysine methyltransferases as well as protein arginine methyltransferase (PRMT). Methylation is implicated in both activation and repression of transcription depending on the methylation site and the type of methyltransferase involved (Shilatifard, 2006;Wysocka *et al.*, 2006a). For example, methylation of lysine 4, 36 or 79 of H3 correlates with activation of transcription whereas methylation of lysine 9, 27 of H3 or lysine 20 of H4 is usually linked to transcriptional repression (Pawlak and Deckert, 2007). Type I PRMT, such as CARM1 (cofactor associated arginine methyltransferase 1), PRMT1 and PRMT2, catalyze the formation of monomethyl- and asymmetric dimethyl-arginine derivatives and is involved in transcriptional activation. Type II PRMT, such as PRMT5, catalyzes the formation of monomethyl- and symmetric dimethyl-arginine derivatives and is involved in transcriptional repression. In addition, a lysine can be mono-, di- or trimethylated with different effect on gene transcription (Santos-Rosa *et al.*, 2002;Schneider *et al.*, 2005). Both lysine and arginine methylations can be reversed by histone demethylases, which had been discovered many years after the discovery of HMTs. LSD1 was the first histone demethylase discovered in 2004 and was shown to demethylate H3K4 and to repress transcription (Shi *et al.*, 2004). However, LSD1 was also shown to demethylate H3K9 and activate transcription when present in a complex with the androgen receptor (Metzger *et al.*, 2005). Following the discovery of LSD1, a number of other related enzymes were subsequently discovered. Among them, Jumonji domain–containing 6 protein (JMJD6) is the only direct arginine demethylase reported to date shown to demethylate H3 at arginine 2 and H4 at arginine 3 (Chang *et al.*, 2007). In addition, human peptidylarginine deiminase 4 protein (Pad4) can regulate histone arginine methylation by converting mono-methylated arginine into citrulline via demethylimination or deimination (Cuthbert *et al.*, 2004;Wang *et al.*, 2004). Histone methylation may affect the binding of other histone-modifying enzymes to the chromatin, which then mediates other posttranscriptional modifications, such as histone phosphorylation and DNA methylation (Mosammaparast and Shi, 2010;Pedersen and Helin, 2010).

Acetylation, another well-characterized modification, occurs on lysine residues mainly in the N-terminal tail of core histones. However, a lysine 56 within the globular domain of H3 (H3K56) has been found to be acetylated in yeast. Yeast protein SPT10, a putative histone acetyltransferase (HAT), was shown to mediate the H3K56 acetylation of histone genes at their promoter regions. H3K56 acetylation allows the recruitment of Snf5, an essential component of SWI/SNF chromatin remodeling complex and subsequently regulating transcription (Xu *et al.*, 2005). Compared with the SPT10, the Rtt109 acetyltransferase mediates H3K56 acetylation more globally (Driscoll *et al.*, 2007;Han *et al.*, 2007;Schneider *et al.*, 2006). The acetylation level correlates with transcriptional activation (Davie, 2003;Legube and Trouche, 2003). The level of acetylation is balanced by HATs and HDACs. Generally, increased levels of histone acetylation by HATs enhance chromatin decondensation and DNA accessibility for transcription factors to activate gene expression. In contrast to acetylation, deacetylation of histones catalyzed by HDACs leads to chromatin condensation and gene silencing (Berger, 2007;Li *et al.*, 2007a). The relationship between histone acetylation and gene expression has been well documented (Verdone *et al.*, 2006). HATs can also acetylate non-histone proteins, such as transcription factors and nuclear receptors to facilitate gene expression (Bannister and Miska, 2000;Masumi, 2011)

Other histone modifications, such as phosphorylation, ubiquitylation and sumoylation, have also been shown to be involved in transcriptional regulation. For example, H3S10 phosphorylation has been demonstrated to be involved in the activation of NF-κB-regulated genes as well as "immediate early" genes, such as c-fos and c-jun (Macdonald *et al.*, 2005). Ubiquitination of H2AK119 and H2BK120 are associated with transcriptional repression and activation, respectively (Wang *et al.*, 2006;Zhu *et al.*, 2005).

2.2. Chromatin remodelling complex and transcription

The second major class of chromatin-modifying factors are the protein complexes that use energy from ATP hydrolysis to alter nucleosomal structure and DNA accessibility and hence are generally referred to as chromatin remodeling complex (Flaus and Owen-Hughes, 2004;Saha *et al.*, 2006). Each ATP-dependent chromatin-remodeling complex characterized to date contains a highly conserved ATPase subunit that belongs to the SNF2 ATPase superfamily (Marfella CGA, Mutate Res, 2007). Based on the similarities of their ATPase subunits and the presence of other conserved domains, these complexes can be classified into at least four different families (Figure 2): the SWI/SNF (mating type switching /sucrose non-fermenting) family; the ISWI (imitation switch) family; the NuRD/Mi-2/CHD (chromodomain helicase DNA-binding) family and INO80 (inositol requiring 80) family (Farrants, 2008;Saha *et al.*, 2006). The ATPase subunits of the SWI/SNF family members, including yeast Snf2 and Sth1, *Drosophila melangaster* brahma (BRM) and mammalian BRM and BRG1 (brahma-related gene 1), contain an C-terminal bromodomains which recognize and binds to acetylated histone tails (Hassan *et al.*, 2002;Marfella and Imbalzano, 2007). The members of ISWI family, such as yeast homologues ISW1 and ISW2, and mammalian homologues SNF2H and SNF2L, each contains an ATPase subunit with homology to *Drosophila* ISWI protein and has nucleosome-stimulated ATPase activity. These enzymes are characterized by the presence of a SANT (SWI3-ADA2-NCoR-TFIIIB) domain, which functions as a histone-tail-binding module (Boyer *et al.*, 2004;de la Serna *et al.*, 2006). SANT domain has been found in a number of transcriptional regulatory proteins and is therefore thought to play a role in transcriptional regulation (Aasland *et al.*, 1996;Boyer *et al.*, 2002). The NuRD/Mi-2/CHD family members include a number of proteins that are highly conserved from yeast to humans and are characterized by the presence of two N-terminal chromodomains involved in the remodeling of chromatin structure and regulation of transcription (Brehm *et al.*, 2004;Eissenberg, 2001;Jones *et al.*, 2000). The INO80 family contains the INO80 remodeling complex (INO80.com) and the SWR1 remodeling complex (SWR1.com), which are distinguished by the split ATPase domains and the presence of two RuvB-like proteins, Rvb1 and Rvb2 (Bao and Shen, 2007).

ATP-dependent chromatin remodelers can reposition (slide, twist, or loop) nucleosomes along the DNA, evict histones from DNA or facilitate exchange of histone variants, and thus creating nucleosome-free regions for gene activation (Figure 3) (Wang *et al.*, 2007).

http://dx.doi.org/10.5772/55977

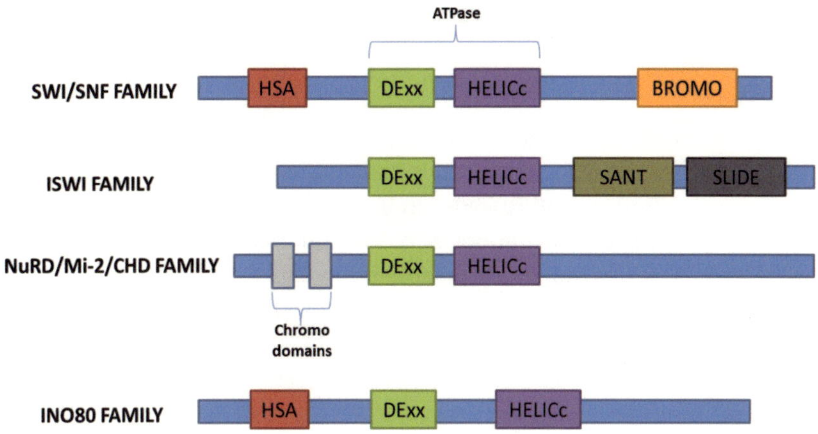

Figure 2. ATPase subunits of the four main families of ATP-dependent chromatin remodeling complexes. The ATPase subunit of each ATP-dependent chromatin-remodeling complex belongs to the SNF2 ATPase superfamily, whose ATPase domain comprises an N-terminal DExx and a C-terminal HELICc subdomain, separated by an insert region. The SWI/SNF family contains an HSA domain for actin binding, and a bromodomain which recognizes and binds to the acetylated histone tails. The ISWI family contains the SANT and SLIDE domains, important for histone binding. The CHD/NURD/Mi-2 family is characterized by the presence of two N-terminal chromodomains that is involved in the remodeling of chromatin structure and the transcriptional regulation of genes. The INO80 family, like the SWI/SNF family, also contains an HSA domain, however the insert region between the DExx and the HELICc subdomains is three times longer than that of other three families.

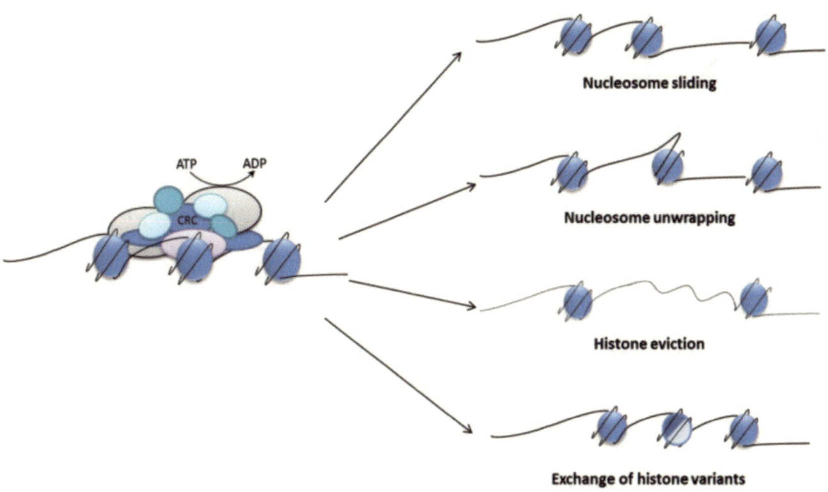

Figure 3. Mechanisms of ATP-dependent chromatin remodeling activity to alter the accessibility of nucleosomal DNA. Upon utilization of the energy from ATP hydrolysis, the nucleosomal structure is altered to make protected region of chromatin available to DNA binding protein complexes, such as transcription factors, which involves mobilization of nucleosome position(sliding), dissociation of DNA-histone contact (unwrapping), and eviction of histones (histone eviction). In some cases ATP dependent remodeling complexes can use the energy from ATP hydrolysis to introduce histone variants into the nucleosome (exchange of histone variants), such as H2A–H2B or H2A variants (H2Avar)–H2B dimers.

3. The role of chromatin remodelling in the regulation of inflammatory gene expression

The inflammatory response is a defense mechanism developed in higher organisms to protect themselves from infection with pathogens. It demands rapid and coordinated regulation of expression of multiple inflammatory genes in immune cells, including macrophages. It has increasingly become clear that alterations of chromatin architecture orchestrated by histone modifications and ATP-dependent chromatin remodeling complexes play a key role in controlling of inflammatory response genes (Medzhitov and Horng, 2009;Smale, 2010).

3.1. LPS-induced chromatin modification and target gene expression

LPS, a large molecule consisting of a lipid and a polysaccharide joined by a covalent bond, is the major component of the outer membrane of gram-negative bacteria and is one of the best-characterized agonist of host inflammatory response. LPS is recognized by Toll-like receptor 4 (TLR4) and activates the downstream signaling pathways, including the NF-κB signaling cascades, MAPK cascades and interferon regulatory factor (IRF) signaling cascades and induce the transcription of proinflammatory cytokine genes such as interleukin-6 (IL-6), IL-12 and tumor necrosis factor (TNF) (Akira and Takeda, 2004;Takeda *et al.*, 2003). The first evidence of the involvement of chromatin remodeling in LPS-induced gene expression dates back to 1999, when it was observed that nucleosome remodeling appears to contribute to the rapid induction of p40 subunit of IL-12 (IL-12p40). Upon activation by LPS, a positioned nucleosome, which spans the IL-12p40 gene promoter, is rapidly and selectively repositioned prior to initiation of transcription process (Weinmann *et al.*, 1999). Further studies demonstrated that the nucleosome remodeling by LPS requires TLR4 signaling but is independent of c-Rel, one of the NF-κB subunits required for transcription of integrated Il-12p40 promoter (Weinmann *et al.*, 2001). In the year 2000, Saccani and colleagues (Saccani *et al.*, 2002) revealed that upon LPS stimulation, H3 phosphorylation at serine 10 (H3S10) occurs selectively on the IL-12p40 promoter as well as promoters of a subset of other NF-κB-responsive proinflammatory genes such as IL-6, IL-8, and CC-chemokine ligand 2 (CCL2) but not TNF-α, MIP-1α and CCL3. This phosphorylation event was shown to be dependent on the activation of p38 MAPK signaling pathway by LPS, and specific inhibition of p38 activation blocks H3S10 phosphorylation, recruitment of NF-κB to the selective promoters and gene expression (Saccani *et al.*, 2002). Therefore, it is postulated that phosphorylation of H3S10 via the p38 MAPK signaling pathway promotes the loosening of chromatin at certain selective promoters, thereby permitting accessibility to NF-κB and allowing transcription to occur. There are some evidence that link H3S10 mark with transcriptional activation. Serine to alanine substitution at position 10 of H3 or deletion of Snf1, a histone H3 kinase which phosphorylates the serine 10, abrogates transcriptional activation of LPS- inducible genes (Lo *et al.*, 2001;Lo *et al.*, 2000).

LPS activates TLR-dependent signaling to produce inflammatory cytokines and chemokines, which contribute to the efficient control and clearance of invading pathogens. However, production of these inflammatory mediators is tightly regulated because excessive production results in amplified inflammatory response and fatal illness characteristic of severe septic shock. Therefore, the host has readily available mechanisms in place which allow to dampen the response to LPS or even confer unresponsiveness to successive stimuli with LPS, a phenomenon named LPS or endotoxin tolerance (Cavaillon and Adib-Conquy, 2006;Cavaillon *et al.*, 2003). The mechanisms underlying endotoxin tolerance are not completely understood, but are characterized by impaired TLR-mediated activation of both NF-κB- and MAPK-dependent genes (Adib-Conquy *et al.*, 2006;Adib-Conquy *et al.*, 2000). Endotoxin tolerance has been shown to be associated with chromatin remodeling in the promoter regions of several tolerizable genes (Chan *et al.*, 2005;El *et al.*, 2007). Chang and colleagues have demonstrated that chromatin remodeling and NF-κB p65 recruitment at the IL-1β gene promoter are altered in LPS-tolerant THP-1 cells, when compared to normal THP-1 cells (Chan *et al.*, 2005). Upon LPS treatment, increased phosphorylation of H3S10 and demethylation of H3K9 are observed in normal THP-1 cells, which represent an "open" chromatin state; however, these modifications are impaired in LPS-tolerant cells. Concomitantly, recruitment of NF- κB p65 but not NF-κB p50 to the IL-1 gene promoter is impaired in LPS-tolerant cells despite that the activation and nuclear accumulation of NF- κB is not changed. Similar histone modifications and NF- κB binding were also observed at the TNF-α promoter during endotoxin tolerance (El *et al.*, 2007). Interestingly, LPS tolerance negatively regulates expression of proinflammatory mediators without affecting antimicrobial effectors. Using microarrays and real-time PCR, Foster and colleagues (Foster *et al.*, 2007) identified two classes of genes based on their responsiveness to re-stimulation with LPS: so called tolerizable genes, which include proinflammatory mediators, and non-tolerizable genes, which include antimicrobial effectors. Induction of tolerance to LPS inhibits expression of the proinflammatory genes, while the other group of genes remain inducible. Both classes of gene promoters show H4 acetylation and H3K4 tri-methylation, which mark an "open" chromatin state, upon initial stimulation with LPS; however, this kind of "open" chromatin state and recruitment of Brg1 are lost in tolerizable genes upon LPS re-stimulation. In contrast, these epigenetic marks are maintained in the genes that remain inducible. Aung and colleagues reported that HDACs are transiently repressed then induced to express in murine bone marrow-derived macrophages when treated with LPS. HDACs are recruited to different gene promoters to regulate the expression of the latter.

3.2. Manipulation of host chromatin remodelling process by bacteria to facilitate infection

Interestingly, intracellular pathogens, such as *Listeria monocytogenes*, *Shigella flexneri*, and *Helicobacter pylori*, affecting the expression of host defense gene via modulation of chromatin structure has also been reported in recent years. *Listeria monocytogenes* is a gram positive bacterium that causes listeriosis. Two different mechanisms have been reported to be used by *L. monocytogenes* to modify histones during the course of infection. In endothelial cells, *L. monocytogenes* has been shown to selectively induce serine 10 phosphorylation and lysine 14 acetylation of H3 and lysine 8 acetylation of H4 at the IL-8 but not the Interferon-γ (IFN-γ) gene promoter through the activation of p38 and ERK MAPK pathway. A subsequent study showed that activation of p38 MAPK signaling pathway and NF-κB by *L. monocytogenes* depends on nucleotide-binding oligomerization domain-containing protein 1 (NOD1). NOD1 is critical for *L. monocytogenes* induced secretion of IL-8. Interestingly, only invasive bacteria which can enter into the host cell cytoplasm induce IL-8 production in endothelial cells (Opitz *et al.*, 2006). In another study, *L. monocytogenes* has been found to induce a dramatic H3 dephosphorylation at serine 10 (H3S10) as well as a deacetylation of H4 during early phase of infection (Hamon *et al.*, 2007). In contrast to the report described as above, entry of bacteria into the host cells is not required for these histone modifications. The LLO released by *L. monocytogenes* is a member of CDC (cholesterol-dependent cytolysin) toxin family, which is identified as a major effector sufficient for induction of H3S10 dephosphorylation and H4 deacetylation. LLO –induced H3S10 dephosphorylation specifically occurs in the case of genes whose expression is regulated by LLO, a number of which are involved in immunity. Interestingly, other members of the large family of CDC toxins, such as PFO and PLY secreted by *Clostridium perfringens* and *Streptococcus pneumonia*, respectively, dephosphorylate H3S10 through a mechanism analogous to that of LLO (Hamon *et al.*, 2007), suggesting that different bacteria may subvert immune response through a similar mechanism.

Shigella flexneri is a human intestinal pathogen, causing dysentery by invading the epithelium of the colon and is responsible, worldwide, for more than one million deaths per year. Arbibe and colleagues have shown that *S. flexneri* infection abrogates phosphorylation of H3S10 at the promoters of a specific subset of genes, such as IL-8 and CCL-20. The underlying mechanism is that the type III effector protein, OspF, secreted by *S. flexneri* enters into the nucleus and specifically dephosphorylates ERK and p38 MAPKs and then blocks MAPK-dependent phosphorylation of H3S10. This occurs in a gene-selective way, and renders selected gene promoter sites inaccessible to NF-κB, thereby reducing the expression of a subset of NF-κB-responsive genes, including IL8 (Arbibe *et al.*, 2007). This specificity might be a consequence of OspF's ability to inactivate MAPKs, thereby preventing them from entering into nucleus. Once activated, MAPKs translocate into nucleus and are recruited to the chromatin covering their target genes, where they regulate the phosphorylation of transcription factors, histones and chromatin-remodeling enzymes (Chow and Davis, 2006). It has been shown that OspF–induced down-regulation of inflammatory response is accomplished through the interaction of OspF with host retinoblastoma (Rb) protein, which has been linked to histone modification (Zurawski *et al.*, 2009). OspF also has the phosphothreonine lyase activity, a unique activity that has been found in a family of conserved effectors secreted by type III secretion system including OspF, SpvC from nontyphoid *Salmonella species*, and HopAI1 from the plant pathogen *Pseudomonas syringae* (Kramer *et al.*, 2007;Li *et al.*, 2007b;Zhang *et al.*, 2007). These effectors specifically inactivate their host MAPK pathway by carrying out a β elimination reaction to irreversibly remove the phosphate moiety from the phosphothreonine in phosphorylated MAPKs. Inhibition of MAPK signaling by OspF attenuates the recruitment of polymorphonuclear leukocytes to *Shigella* infection sites by suppressing the activation of a portion of NF-κB-responsive genes in mice (Arbibe *et al.*, 2007), thereby contributing to the survival and persistent infection of the pathogens.

Helicobacter pylori is a Gram-negative bacterium that colonizes the human gastric mucosa. The chronic infection generates a state of inflammation which may develop toward chronic gastritis, peptic ulcers and gastric malignancies (Peek, Jr. and Crabtree, 2006). The virulence factors of *Helicobacter pylori* have been suggested to play a crucial role in the development of inflammation and in affecting the host immune system (Gebert *et al.*, 2003;Lu *et al.*, 2005). For example, in

http://dx.doi.org/10.5772/55977

mouse macrophage, *H. pylori* peptidyl prolyl cis-, trans-isomerase (HP0175) has been shown to induce H3S10 phosphorylation at the IL-6 promoter resulting in increased IL-6 gene transcription and protein expression (Pathak *et al.*, 2006). HP0175-induced IL-6 gene transcription is dependent on the TLR4 –dependent activation of ERK and p38 MAPKs, which subsequently activate mitogen- and stress-activated protein kinase 1 (MSK1), a serine kinase responsible for H3S10 phosphorylation. This modification allows for recruitment of NF-κB to the IL-6 promoter and activation of gene transactivation. Interestingly, *H. pylori* infection has also been shown to dephosphorylate H3S10 and deacetylate H3K23 in a time- and dose- dependent manner in gastric epithelial cells (Ding *et al.*, 2010). Therefore, the effect of a specific histone modification in host cells appears to be cell type specific and gene promoter specific. Further studies demonstrate that *cag* pathogenicity island (PAI) is responsible for the dephosphorylation of H3S10 and this modification is independent of ERK and p38 signaling pathways as well as IFN signaling. In addition, H3S10 dephosphorylation is associated with changes in the host gene expression, which contributes to bacterial infection and pathogenesis (Ding *et al.*, 2010). Treatment of gastric epithelial cells with TSA, a general inhibitor of HDACs which non-specifically increases histone H3 and H4 acetylation at multiple sites results in altered gene transcription pattern in both *IL-8* and *c-fos* genes upon *H. pylori* infection. TSA reduces IL-8 but increases c-fos gene transcription in the presence of *H. pylori* infection (Ding *et al.*, 2010). *H. pylori* has also been shown to regulate the cell cycle controlled protein p21(WAF), which is associated with the release of HDAC-1from the promoter and histone H4 acetylation (Xia *et al.*, 2008).

4. Chromatin remodeling and IFN-γ-induced transcriptional response

IFN-γ is a cytokine secreted by activated T cells and natural killer cells. IFN-γ can induce expression of the major histocompatibility complex class II (MHC-II) on the cell surface (Boehm *et al.*, 1997), which presents antigens to $CD4^+$ T cells and plays a crucial role in normal immune response. IFN-γ activates gene expression mainly via the activation of JAK (Janus tyrosine kinase)/STATI (signal transducer and activator of transcription) signaling pathway, leading to the translocation of active STAT1 homodimers into the nucleus. The STAT1 homodimers then bind to the IFN-γ -activated sites (GAS) present in the promoters of IFN-γ -responsive genes thereby mediating the transcription of these genes, including class II transactivator (CIITA), which is necessary for both constitutive and inducible expression of MHC-II (Schroder *et al.*, 2004).

Chromatin remodeling, mediated by ATP-dependent chromatin remodeling complex and or histone-modifying enzymes, has also been shown to be involved in the activation of IFN-γ -responsive genes, such as CIITA and HLA-DR (Ni *et al.*, 2005;Pattenden *et al.*, 2002;Zika *et al.*, 2003). SWI/SNF complex often cooperates with histone-modifying enzymes to regulate transcription of genes, including those which are induced by IFN-γ (Chi, 2004;Wright and Ting, 2006). Studies have demonstrated that the SWI/SNF complex and CREB-binding protein (CBP), a transcriptional co-activator with histone acetyltransferase activity, are recruited to CIITA promoter in an IFN-γ-inducible fashion, leading to transcriptional activation of CIITA (Kretsovali *et al.*, 1998;Pattenden *et al.*, 2002). HLA-DR is a MHC–II surface molecule whose transcriptional activation is tightly associated with CIITA. However, forced expression of CIITA in BRG1- and BRM-deficient SW13 cells cannot activate expression of the MHC-II genes (Mudhasani and Fontes, 2002). BRG1 or BRM represent the catalytic subunit of mammalian SWI/SNF chromatin remodeling complex, suggesting that the SWI/SNF complex, which contains BRG1 might play additional roles in MHC-II expression. Further studies have indicated that BRG1 is recruited by CIITA to the MHC-II gene promoters and this recruitment is essential for activation of MHC-II gene expression (Mudhasani and Fontes, 2002). Interestingly, CIITA itself has intrinsic HAT activity, which can bind not onlyBRG1 but also HATs, such as CBP and/or p300 (Ting and Trowsdale, 2002). Furthermore, CIITA is associated with increased acetylation modifications of H3 and H4 at MHC-II promoter mediated directly through its intrinsic HAT activity or by the recruitment of HATs, such as CBP (Beresford and Boss, 2001;Kretsovali *et al.*, 1998). IFN-γ induced transactivation of CIITA and expression of MHC-II is inhibited by HDACs/mSin3A corepressor complex whereas enhanced by TSA, a general inhibitor of HDAC. Co-immunoprecipitation assay revealed that CIITA interacts strongly with HDAC1 and weakly with HDAC2 (Zika *et al.*, 2003). All these data suggest that CIITA may act as a modulator to coordinate functions of chromatin remodeling complex, HATs and HDACs.

In the context of host-pathogen interaction, intracellular pathogens have been shown to subvert the host immune response by affecting the macrophage responsiveness to IFN-γ but the underlying mechanism remains unclear. Intracellular pathogens may affect IFN-γ response via different ways. For example, *Leishamania donovani* inhibited IFN-γ response through down-regulation of IFN-γ receptor expression or interfering with the JAK/STAT1 signaling pathway (Nandan and Reiner, 1995;Ray *et al.*, 2000). By contrast, mycobacteria such as *Mycobacterium avium* and *Mycobacterium tuberculosis* impair IFN-γ response through inhibition of IFN-γ -responsive gene expression without interfering with the JAK/STAT1 signaling pathway (Kincaid EZ, J Immunol, 2003, 171:2042-2049). Interestingly, only a subset of IFN-γ responsive genes get affected, including CIITA, HLA-DR and CD64, while others remained unaffected (Pennini *et al.*, 2006;Wang *et al.*, 2005). Further studies showed that infection with *M. tuberculosis* affects the chromatin remodeling on CIITA gene since IFN-γ -induced histone acetylation and recruitment of BRG1 were both impaired (Pennini *et al.*, 2006). Additionally, LpqH, a mycobacterial cell wall protein, induces binding of the C/EBP transcriptional repressor to the CIITA promoter and inhibits IFN-γ -induced CIITA transcription (Pennini *et al.*, 2007). It has been shown that C/EBP can recruit HDAC-1-containing transcriptional repressor complex to the promoter of peroxisome proliferator-activated receptor beta thereby inhibiting its transcription (Di-Poi *et al.*, 2005). Therefore, *M. tuberculosis* might induce the recruitment of C/EBP resulting in transcriptional repression. The exact molecular mechanism by which *M. tuberculosis* inhibits IFN-γ -induced CIITA transcription remains to be elucidated. Similarly to CIITA, IFN-γ -induced histone acetylation gets impaired at the HLA-DR promoter and HLA-DR transcription becomes inhibited when the cells get infected with *M. tuberculosis*. Furthermore, inhibition of HDAC activities rescues histone acetylation, suggesting a role of HDACs in the transcriptional repression induced by *M. tuberculosis* (Wang *et al.*, 2005). Indeed, Mycobacterial infection increases the expression of mSin3A (a co-repressor associated HDACs), enabling competition with CBP for binding to the HLA-DR promoter.

A recent study has demonstrated that infection with *Toxoplasma gondii* renders murine macrophages globally unresponsive to IFN-γ stimulation without affecting the nuclear translocation of STAT1 triggered by IFN-γ in infected macrophages. However, the binding of STAT1 to the STAT1-responsive promoters is aberrant. A number of genes, which were induced by IFN-γ in uninfected macrophages, were not induced in the *T. gondii*-infected cells. Among them, there are several genes previously shown to be repressed by *T. gondii*, such as CIITA, MHC class II molecule H2-Eα, and interferon- regulatory factor 1(IRF-1) (Lang *et al.*, 2012). By analyzing the underlying mechanism, the authors revealed that assembly of chromatin remodeling complex and histone acetylation at the IFN-γ -responsive promoters are impaired upon infection with *T. gondii*. Treatment with HADC inhibitor restores the responsiveness of *T. gondii*-infected macrophages to IFN-γ, leading to an increase in the expression of IFN-γ-inducible genes, such as CIITA and H2-A/E.

5. The potential role of HDAC inhibitors in treatment of infection

HDAC inhibitors have been developed clinically for cancer therapy due to their abilities to induce cell-cycle arrest and apoptosis (Adcock, 2007). Studies have demonstrated that HDAC inhibitors can exert anti-inflammatory effects via the suppression of cytokine and nitric oxide production (Blanchard and Chipoy, 2005;Dinarello *et al.*, 2011), suggesting their therapeutic potential in inflammatory diseases including infectious diseases. For example, HDAC inhibitors have been examined for the treatment of HIV infection and the current results are exciting and encouraging (Wightman *et al.*, 2012). Couple of other studies have demonstrated that HDAC inhibitors, TSA and apicidin, can inhibit the growth of *Plasmodium falciparum*, the main parasite causing malaria in humans (Colletti *et al.*, 2001a;Colletti *et al.*, 2001b). Similarly, azelaic bishydroxamic acid and suberohydroxamic acid, two other HDAC inhibitors, also show anti-malarial activity against *P. falciparum* (Andrews *et al.*, 2000). The potential of HDAC inhibitors as anti-bacterial agents has also been investigated; however, the results are contradictory.

5.1. Inhibition of infection by targeting histone modifying enzymes in the pathogen

Candida albicans is an opportunistic pathogen that is normally found in the gut microflora of healthy individuals; however, *C. albicans* can cause severe and life-threatening diseases in immuosuppressed patients such as HIV infected, organ transplant and cancer chemotherapy patients (Tzung *et al.*, 2001). There is a very high rate of mortality from systemic candidiasis, ranging between 14 and 90% and averaging between 30 to 40%, depending on the disease group studied (Blot *et al.*, 2003). For patients with *Candida* infections, antifungal drug resistance is a major clinical problem. H3K56 acetylation is mediated by HAT Rtt109 and seems to be much more abundant in yeasts than in mammals (Garcia *et al.*, 2007a;Xie *et al.*, 2009), and close homologues of Rtt109 have not yet been detected in mammals (Bazan, 2008). Therefore, it is expected that Rtt109 might be a unique target for antifungal therapeutics. Indeed, Wurtele and colleagues demonstrated that modulation of the acetylation of H3K56 exhibits potential as an anti-fungal therapy (Wurtele *et al.*, 2010). Interestingly, similar results have been found in a study by Lopes da Rosa *et al* (Lopes da *et al.*, 2010). Wurtele and colleagues showed that deleting Rtt109, an acetyltransferase of H3K56, leads to increased sensitivity to some anti-fungal drugs. Both teams also demonstrated that Rtt109 mutants are considerably less virulent in a mouse model infected with *C.albicans.* Wurtele and colleagues further investigated how the growth of *C. albicans* is affected by chemical modification of H3 *in vitro* and *in vivo*. They have observed that the growth of *C. albicans* is greatly inhibited when HST3, the H3 deacetylase acting on lysine 56, is inhibited by nicotinamide (a form of Vitamin B3 and product of the NAD+-dependent deacetylation reaction). Furthermore, modulation of H3K56 acetylation reduces the virulence of wild-type *C. albicans* in mice when nicotinamide was given in the drinking water of mice to repress HST3 (Wurtele *et al.*, 2010). These results, together with the study by Lopes da Rosa and colleagues, provide basis for targeting H3 modifying enzymes to fight fungal infections. Although important catalytic residues in Rtt109 are much different from those in mammalian homologues, it is still a challenge to find suitable fungal-specific inhibitors of H3 modifying enzymes in the future.

5.2. Effects of HDAC inhibitors on host defense against bacterial infection

In a mouse model of septic shock induced by LPS, administration of of suberoylanilide hydroxamic acid (SAHA) (50mg/kg intraperitoneally), improves long-term survival rates of mice whether given before or post a lethal dose of LPS, which may be due to the down-regulation of MyD88-dependent pathway and decreased expression of proinflammatory mediators such as TNF-alpha, IL-1β, and IL-6 (Li *et al.*, 2010;Li *et al.*, 2009). Further studies demonstrated that treatment with SAHA increases anti-inflammatory IL-10 levels while decreasing proinflammatory IL-6 and MAP kinase production in the liver of septic shock mice (Finkelstein *et al.*, 2010). In contrast, it has also been shown that treatment with HDAC inhibitors lead to impaired host defense against bacterial infections. Studies have shown that HDAC inhibitors, TSA, SAHA, and VPA, can impair innate immune responses to TLR agonists by down-regulating the expression of genes involved in microbial sensing, such as C-type lectins and adhesion molecules, as well as genes involved in host defense, such as cytokines and chemokines, thereby increasing susceptibility to infection (Roger *et al.*, 2011). Interestingly, while LPS-induced IFN-β production is enhanced by HDAC inhibitors, the expression of a number of IFN-β /STAT1-dependent genes is strongly inhibited by TSA and VPA, suggesting that increased IFN-β production cannot overcome the potent inhibitory effects of HDAC inhibitors. Surprisingly, VPA was shown to increase the mortality of mice infected with *C. albicans* or *K. pneumonia*, but protect mice from toxic shock and severe sepsis in mouse models (Roger *et al.*, 2011). When murine macrophages were treated with TSA and VPA, their ability to kill *Escherichia coli* and *Staphyloccocus aureus* was attenuated, with impaired phagocytosis and production of reactive oxygen and nitrogen species (Mombelli *et al.*, 2011). Together, these

http://dx.doi.org/10.5772/55977

data reveal the complex effector mechanisms of HDAC inhibitors and suggest that more studies are required to fully understand this complex process.

6. Concluding remarks

The activation and suppression of innate immunity are central principles of host-pathogen interaction and need to be very well controlled. To establish persistent infection, intracellular pathogens must acquire efficient mechanisms to evade the host immune response. Interference with host posttranscriptional modifications by bacterial pathogens is a strategy widely used by the pathogens to promote survival and replication during the course of infection. MAPK, IFN-γ and transcription factor NF-κB signaling pathways are common targets for bacteria-induced posttranscriptional modifications (Ribet and Cossart, 2010). Interestingly, in the past few years, evidence has accumulated that targeting of histone modifications and chromatin remodeling, and subsequently subverting the host immune response, is a new and exciting field in the study of host-pathogen interaction. Phosphorylation of H3 and acetylation of H3 and/or H4 at lysine residues are frequently associated with transactivation. Conversely, dephosphorylation and methylation of histones are more often associated with gene suppression (Berger, 2002;Kouzarides, 2007;Verdone *et al.*, 2006). Several strains of bacteria, including *L. monocytogenes, C. perfringens, S. pneumonia* and *H. pylori,* induce the same dephosphorylation of H3S10, while *S. flexneri* blocks phosphorylation of H3S10; all of which lead to decreased phosphorylation of H3S10 and are associated with altered host immune response.

The molecular mechanisms by which bacterial infection induces histone modification and chromatin remodeling remain to be understood. For many pathogens, it is very difficult to hypothesize about the extent or the mechanics of epigenetic change they might induce. Currently available data largely provide snapshots of what is happening to the usual host genes studied in an infection model. More comprehensive global studies, such as ChIP-on–chip (chromatin immunoprecipitation coupled with expression microarray technology) for mapping global chromatin modifications, are now necessary and possible. This might provide fundamental clues to better understand the role and mechanism of chromatin regulation in the control of immune gene expression in inflammatory and infectious diseases.

Author details

Yong Zhong Xu, Cynthia Kanagaratham and Danuta Radzioch

*Address all correspondence to: danuta.radzioch@mcgill.ca

Department of Medicine, McGill University, Montreal, Canada

References

[1] Aasland, R, Stewart, A. F, & Gibson, T. (1996). The SANT domain: a putative DNA-binding domain in the SWI-SNF and ADA complexes, the transcriptional co-repressor N-CoR and TFIIIB. Trends Biochem. Sci. *8788*, 21

[2] Adcock, I. M. (2007). HDAC inhibitors as anti-inflammatory agents. Br. J. Pharmacol. *829831*, 150

[3] Adib-conquy, M, Adrie, C, Fitting, C, Gattolliat, O, Beyaert, R, & Cavaillon, J. M. (2006). Up-regulation of MyD88s and SIGIRR, molecules inhibiting Toll-like receptor signaling, in monocytes from septic patients. Crit Care Med. *23772385*, 34

[4] Adib-conquy, M, Adrie, C, Moine, P, Asehnoune, K, Fitting, C, Pinsky, M. R, Dhainaut, J. F, & Cavaillon, J. M. (2000). NF-kappaB expression in mononuclear cells of patients with sepsis resembles that observed in lipopolysaccharide tolerance. Am. J. Respir. Crit Care Med. *18771883*, 162

[5] Akira, S, & Takeda, K. (2004). Toll-like receptor signalling. Nat. Rev. Immunol. *499511*, 4

[6] Andrews, K. T, Walduck, A, Kelso, M. J, Fairlie, D. P, Saul, A, & Parsons, P. G. (2000). Anti-malarial effect of histone deacetylation inhibitors and mammalian tumour cyto-differentiating agents. Int. J. Parasitol. *761768*, 30

[7] Arbibe, L, Kim, D. W, Batsche, E, Pedron, T, Mateescu, B, Muchardt, C, Parsot, C, & Sansonetti, P. J. (2007). An injected bacterial effector targets chromatin access for transcription factor NF-kappaB to alter transcription of host genes involved in immune responses. Nat. Immunol. *4756*, 8

[8] Bannister, A. J, & Miska, E. A. (2000). Regulation of gene expression by transcription factor acetylation. Cell Mol. Life Sci. *11841192*, 57

[9] Bao, Y, & Shen, X. (2007). INO80 subfamily of chromatin remodeling complexes. Mutat. Res. *1829*, 618

[10] Bazan, J. F. (2008). An old HAT in human CBP and yeast Rtt109. Cell Cycle. *7*, 1884-1886., 300.

[11] Beresford, G. W, & Boss, J. M. (2001). CIITA coordinates multiple histone acetylation modifications at the HLA-DRA promoter. Nat. Immunol. *652657*, 2

[12] Berger, S. L. (2002). Histone modifications in transcriptional regulation. Curr. Opin. Genet. Dev. *142148*, 12

[13] Berger, S. L. (2007). The complex language of chromatin regulation during transcription. Nature. *407412*, 447

[14] Blanchard, F, & Chipoy, C. (2005). Histone deacetylase inhibitors: new drugs for the treatment of inflammatory diseases? Drug Discov. Today. *197204*, 10

[15] Blot, S. I, Hoste, E. A, Vandewoude, K. H, & Colardyn, F. A. (2003). Estimates of attributable mortality of systemic candida infection in the ICU. J. Crit Care. *130131*, 18

[16] Boehm, U, Klamp, T, Groot, M, & Howard, J. C. (1997). Cellular responses to interferon-gamma. Annu. Rev. Immunol. *74995*, 15

[17] Boyer, L. A, Langer, M. R, Crowley, K. A, Tan, S, Denu, J. M, & Peterson, C. L. (2002). Essential role for the SANT domain in the functioning of multiple chromatin remodeling enzymes. Mol. Cell. *935942*, 10

[18] Boyer, L. A, Latek, R. R, & Peterson, C. L. (2004). The SANT domain: a unique histone-tail-binding module? Nat. Rev. Mol. Cell Biol. *158163*, 5

[19] Brehm, A, Tufteland, K. R, Aasland, R, & Becker, P. B. (2004). The many colours of chromodomains. Bioessays. *133140*, 26

[20] Cavaillon, J. M, & Adib-conquy, M. (2006). Bench-to-bedside review: endotoxin tolerance as a model of leukocyte reprogramming in sepsis. Crit Care. *10*, 233.

[21] Cavaillon, J. M, Adrie, C, Fitting, C, & Adib-conquy, M. (2003). Endotoxin tolerance: is there a clinical relevance? J. Endotoxin. Res. *101107*, 9

[22] Chan, C, Li, L, Mccall, C. E, & Yoza, B. K. (2005). Endotoxin tolerance disrupts chromatin remodeling and NF-kappaB transactivation at the IL-1beta promoter. J. Immunol. *461468*, 175

[23] Chang, B, Chen, Y, Zhao, Y, & Bruick, R. K. (2007). JMJD6 is a histone arginine demethylase. Science. *% 19;318444447*

[24] Chi, T. view of the immune system. Nat. Rev. Immunol. *965977*, 4

[25] Chow, C. W, & Davis, R. J. (2006). Proteins kinases: chromatin-associated enzymes? Cell. *887890*, 127

[26] Clapier, C. R, & Cairns, B. R. (2009). The biology of chromatin remodeling complexes. Annu. Rev. Biochem. *273304doi:annurev.biochem.77.062706.153223.*, 273-304., 78

[27] Colletti, S. L. (2001a). Broad spectrum antiprotozoal agents that inhibit histone deacetylase: structure-activity relationships of apicidin. Part 1. Bioorg. Med. Chem. Lett. *107111*, 11

[28] Colletti, S. L. (2001b). Broad spectrum antiprotozoal agents that inhibit histone deacetylase: structure-activity relationships of apicidin. Part 2. Bioorg. Med. Chem. Lett. *113117*, 11

[29] Cuthbert, G. L. (2004). Histone deimination antagonizes arginine methylation. Cell. *545553*, 118

[30] Davie, J. R. (2003). Inhibition of histone deacetylase activity by butyrate. J. Nutr. *133,* 2485S-2493S.

[31] De La Serna, I. L, Ohkawa, Y, & Imbalzano, A. N. (2006). Chromatin remodelling in mammalian differentiation: lessons from ATP-dependent remodellers. Nat. Rev. Genet. *461473,* 7

[32] Di-poi, N, Desvergne, B, Michalik, L, & Wahli, W. (2005). Transcriptional repression of peroxisome proliferator-activated receptor beta/delta in murine keratinocytes by CCAAT/enhancer-binding proteins. J. Biol. Chem. *3870038710,* 280

[33] Dinarello, C. A, Fossati, G, & Mascagni, P. (2011). Histone deacetylase inhibitors for treating a spectrum of diseases not related to cancer. Mol. Med. *333352,* 17

[34] Ding, S. Z. (2010). Helicobacter pylori-induced histone modification, associated gene expression in gastric epithelial cells, and its implication in pathogenesis. PLoS. One. *5,* e9875.

[35] Driscoll, R, Hudson, A, & Jackson, S. P. (2007). Yeast Rtt109 promotes genome stability by acetylating histone H3 on lysine 56. Science. *649652,* 315

[36] Eissenberg, J. C. (2001). Molecular biology of the chromo domain: an ancient chromatin module comes of age. Gene. *1929,* 275

[37] El,Yoza, G. M, Hu, B. K, Cousart, J. Y, & Mccall, S. L. C.E. ((2007). Epigenetic silencing of tumor necrosis factor alpha during endotoxin tolerance. J. Biol. Chem. *2685726864,* 282

[38] Farrants, A. K. (2008). Chromatin remodelling and actin organisation. FEBS Lett. *20412050,* 582

[39] Finkelstein, R. A, Li, Y, Liu, B, Shuja, F, Fukudome, E, Velmahos, G. C, Demoya, M, & Alam, H. B. (2010). Treatment with histone deacetylase inhibitor attenuates MAP kinase mediated liver injury in a lethal model of septic shock. J. Surg. Res. *146154,* 163

[40] Flaus, A, & Owen-hughes, T. (2004). Mechanisms for ATP-dependent chromatin remodelling: farewell to the tuna-can octamer? Curr. Opin. Genet. Dev. *165173,* 14

[41] Foster, S. L, Hargreaves, D. C, & Medzhitov, R. (2007). Gene-specific control of inflammation by TLR-induced chromatin modifications. Nature. *972978,* 447

[42] Galan, J. E, & Cossart, P. (2005). Host-pathogen interactions: a diversity of themes, a variety of molecular machines. Curr. Opin. Microbiol. *13,* 8

[43] Garcia, B. A. (2007a). Organismal differences in post-translational modifications in histones H3 and H4. J. Biol. Chem. *76417655,* 282

[44] Garcia, B. A, Shabanowitz, J, & Hunt, D. F. (2007b). Characterization of histones and their post-translational modifications by mass spectrometry. Curr. Opin. Chem. Biol. *6673*, 11

[45] Gebert, B, Fischer, W, Weiss, E, Hoffmann, R, & Haas, R. (2003). Helicobacter pylori vacuolating cytotoxin inhibits T lymphocyte activation. Science. *10991102*, 301

[46] Glaser, K. B, Li, J, Staver, M. J, Wei, R. Q, Albert, D. H, & Davidsen, S. K. (2003a). Role of class I and class II histone deacetylases in carcinoma cells using siRNA. Biochem. Biophys. Res. Commun. *529536*, 310

[47] Glaser, K. B, Staver, M. J, Waring, J. F, Stender, J, Ulrich, R. G, & Davidsen, S. K. (2003b). Gene expression profiling of multiple histone deacetylase (HDAC) inhibitors: defining a common gene set produced by HDAC inhibition in T24 and MDA carcinoma cell lines. Mol. Cancer Ther. *151163*, 2

[48] Hamon, M. A, Batsche, E, Regnault, B, Tham, T. N, Seveau, S, Muchardt, C, & Cossart, P. (2007). Histone modifications induced by a family of bacterial toxins. Proc. Natl. Acad. Sci. U. S. A. *1346713472*, 104

[49] Hamon, M. A, & Cossart, P. (2008). Histone modifications and chromatin remodeling during bacterial infections. Cell Host. Microbe. *100109*, 4

[50] Han, J, Zhou, H, Horazdovsky, B, Zhang, K, Xu, R. M, & Zhang, Z. (2007). Rtt109 acetylates histone H3 lysine 56 and functions in DNA replication. Science. *653655*, 315

[51] Hassan, A. H, Prochasson, P, Neely, K. E, Galasinski, S. C, Chandy, M, Carrozza, M. J, & Workman, J. L. (2002). Function and selectivity of bromodomains in anchoring chromatin-modifying complexes to promoter nucleosomes. Cell. *369379*, 111

[52] Huang, Y, Fang, J, Bedford, M. T, Zhang, Y, & Xu, R. M. (2006). Recognition of histone H3 lysine-4 methylation by the double tudor domain of JMJD2A. Science. *748751*, 312

[53] Jenuwein, T, & Allis, C. D. (2001a). Translating the histone code. Science. *10741080*, 293

[54] Jones, D. O, Cowell, I. G, & Singh, P. B. (2000). Mammalian chromodomain proteins: their role in genome organisation and expression. Bioessays. *124137*, 22

[55] Kallin, E, & Zhang, Y. (2004). Chromatin Remodelling. In: Encyclopedia of Biological Chemistry., 456-463.

[56] Kouzarides, T. (2007). Chromatin modifications and their function. Cell. *693705*, 128

[57] Kramer, R. W, Slagowski, N. L, Eze, N. A, Giddings, K. S, Morrison, M. F, Siggers, K. A, Starnbach, M. N, & Lesser, C. F. (2007). Yeast functional genomic screens lead to identification of a role for a bacterial effector in innate immunity regulation. PLoS. Pathog. *3*, e21.

[58] Kretsovali, A, Agalioti, T, Spilianakis, C, Tzortzakaki, E, Merika, M, & Papamatheakis, J. (1998). Involvement of CREB binding protein in expression of major histocompatibility complex class II genes via interaction with the class II transactivator. Mol. Cell Biol. *67776783,* 18

[59] Lang, C, Hildebrandt, A, Brand, F, Opitz, L, Dihazi, H, & Luder, C. G. (2012). Impaired chromatin remodelling at STATregulated promoters leads to global unresponsiveness of Toxoplasma gondii-Infected macrophages to IFN-gamma. PLoS. Pathog. *8,* e1002483., 1.

[60] Lee, H. S, Park, M. H, Yang, S. J, Jung, H. Y, Byun, S. S, Lee, D. S, Yoo, H. S, Yeom, Y. I, & Seo, S. B. (2004). Gene expression analysis in human gastric cancer cell line treated with trichostatin A and S-adenosyl-L-homocysteine using cDNA microarray. Biol. Pharm. Bull. *14971503,* 27

[61] Legube, G, & Trouche, D. (2003). Regulating histone acetyltransferases and deacetylases. EMBO Rep. *944947,* 4

[62] Li, B, Carey, M, & Workman, J. L. (2007a). The role of chromatin during transcription. Cell. *707719,* 128

[63] Li, H, Xu, H, Zhou, Y, Zhang, J, Long, C, Li, S, Chen, S, Zhou, J. M, & Shao, F. (2007b). The phosphothreonine lyase activity of a bacterial type III effector family. Science. *10001003,* 315

[64] Li, Y. (2010). Surviving lethal septic shock without fluid resuscitation in a rodent model. Surgery. *246254,* 148

[65] Li, Y. (2009). Protective effect of suberoylanilide hydroxamic acid against LPS-induced septic shock in rodents. Shock. *517523,* 32

[66] Lo, W. S, Duggan, L, Emre, N. C, Belotserkovskya, R, Lane, W. S, Shiekhattar, R, & Berger, S. L. (2001). Snf1--a histone kinase that works in concert with the histone acetyltransferase Gcn5 to regulate transcription. Science. *11421146,* 293

[67] Lo, W. S, Trievel, R. C, Rojas, J. R, Duggan, L, Hsu, J. Y, Allis, C. D, Marmorstein, R, & Berger, S. L. (2000). Phosphorylation of serine 10 in histone H3 is functionally linked in vitro and in vivo to Gcn5-mediated acetylation at lysine 14. Mol. Cell. *917926,* 5

[68] Lopes daR.J., Boyartchuk,V.L., Zhu,L.J., and Kaufman,P.D. ((2010). Histone acetyltransferase Rtt109 is required for Candida albicans pathogenesis. Proc. Natl. Acad. Sci. U. S. A. *15941599,* 107

[69] Lu, H, Yamaoka, Y, & Graham, D. Y. (2005). Helicobacter pylori virulence factors: facts and fantasies. Curr. Opin. Gastroenterol. *653659,* 21

[70] Lusser, A, & Kadonaga, J. T. (2003). Chromatin remodeling by ATP-dependent molecular machines. Bioessays. *11921200,* 25

[71] Macdonald, N. (2005). Molecular basis for the recognition of phosphorylated and phosphoacetylated histone h3 by 14-3-3. Mol. Cell. *199211*, 20

[72] Marfella, C. G, & Imbalzano, A. N. (2007). The Chd family of chromatin remodelers. Mutat. Res. *3040*, 618

[73] Martin, C, & Zhang, Y. (2005). The diverse functions of histone lysine methylation. Nat. Rev. Mol. Cell Biol. *838849*, 6

[74] Martin, C, & Zhang, Y. (2007). Mechanisms of epigenetic inheritance. Curr. Opin. Cell Biol. *266272*, 19

[75] Masumi, A. (2011). Histone acetyltransferases as regulators of nonhistone proteins: the role of interferon regulatory factor acetylation on gene transcription. J. Biomed. Biotechnol. *2011:640610. doi:Epub;% 2010 Dec 29.*, 640610.

[76] Medzhitov, R, & Horng, T. (2009). Transcriptional control of the inflammatory response. Nat. Rev. Immunol. *692703*, 9

[77] Mersfelder, E. L, & Parthun, M. R. (2006). The tale beyond the tail: histone core domain modifications and the regulation of chromatin structure. Nucleic Acids Res. % *19;3426532662*

[78] Metzger, E, Wissmann, M, Yin, N, Muller, J. M, Schneider, R, Peters, A. H, Gunther, T, Buettner, R, & Schule, R. (2005). LSD1 demethylates repressive histone marks to promote androgen-receptor-dependent transcription. Nature. *436439*, 437

[79] Mombelli, M, Lugrin, J, Rubino, I, Chanson, A. L, Giddey, M, Calandra, T, & Roger, T. (2011). Histone deacetylase inhibitors impair antibacterial defenses of macrophages. J. Infect. Dis. *13671374*, 204

[80] Mosammaparast, N, & Shi, Y. (2010). Reversal of histone methylation: biochemical and molecular mechanisms of histone demethylases. Annu. Rev. Biochem. *15579doi:annurev.biochem.78.070907.103946.*, 155-179., 79

[81] Mudhasani, R, & Fontes, J. D. (2002). The class II transactivator requires brahma-related gene 1 to activate transcription of major histocompatibility complex class II genes. Mol. Cell Biol. *50195026*, 22

[82] Nandan, D, & Reiner, N. E. (1995). Attenuation of gamma interferon-induced tyrosine phosphorylation in mononuclear phagocytes infected with Leishmania donovani: selective inhibition of signaling through Janus kinases and Stat1. Infect. Immun. *44954500*, 63

[83] Ni, Z, Karaskov, E, Yu, T, Callaghan, S. M, Park, S, Xu, D. S, Pattenden, Z, & Bremner, S. G. R. ((2005). Apical role for BRG1 in cytokine-induced promoter assembly. Proc. Natl. Acad. Sci. U. S. A. *1461114616*, 102

[84] Opitz, B, Puschel, A, Beermann, W, Hocke, A. C, Forster, S, Schmeck, B, Chakraborty, L. , V, Suttorp, T, & Hippenstiel, N. S. ((2006). Listeria monocytogenes activated

MAPK and induced IL-8 secretion in a nucleotide-binding oligomerization domain 1-dependent manner in endothelial cells. J. Immunol. *176*, 484-490., 38.

[85] Pathak, S. K, Basu, S, Bhattacharyya, A, Pathak, S, Banerjee, A, Basu, J, & Kundu, M. B activation and mitogen- and stress-activated protein kinase 1-triggered phosphorylation events are central to Helicobacter pylori peptidyl prolyl cis-, trans-isomerase (HP0175)-mediated induction of IL-6 release from macrophages. J. Immunol. *79507958*, 177

[86] Pattenden, S. G, Klose, R, Karaskov, E, & Bremner, R. (2002). Interferon-gamma-induced chromatin remodeling at the CIITA locus is BRG1 dependent. EMBO J. *19781986*, 21

[87] Pawlak, S, & Deckert, J. (2007). Histone modifications under environmental stress. BIOLOGICAL LETT. *6573*, 44

[88] Pedersen, M. T, & Helin, K. (2010). Histone demethylases in development and disease. Trends Cell Biol. *662671*, 20

[89] Peek, R. M. Jr. and Crabtree,J.E. ((2006). Helicobacter infection and gastric neoplasia. J. Pathol. *233248*, 208

[90] Pena, P. V, Davrazou, F, Shi, X, Walter, K. L, Verkhusha, V. V, Gozani, O, Zhao, R, & Kutateladze, T. G. (2006). Molecular mechanism of histone H3K4me3 recognition by plant homeodomain of ING2. Nature. *100103*, 442

[91] Pennini, M. E, Liu, Y, Yang, J, Croniger, C. M, Boom, W. H, & Harding, C. V. (2007). CCAAT/enhancer-binding protein beta and delta binding to CIITA promoters is associated with the inhibition of CIITA expression in response to Mycobacterium tuberculosis 19-kDa lipoprotein. J. Immunol. *69106918*, 179

[92] Pennini, M. E, Pai, R. K, Schultz, D. C, Boom, W. H, & Harding, C. V. (2006). Mycobacterium tuberculosis 19-kDa lipoprotein inhibits IFN-gamma-induced chromatin remodeling of MHC2TA by TLR2 and MAPK signaling. J. Immunol. *43234330*, 176

[93] Pray-grant, M. G, Daniel, J. A, Schieltz, D, & Yates, J. R. III, and Grant,P.A. ((2005). Chd1 chromodomain links histone H3 methylation with SAGA- and SLIK-dependent acetylation. Nature. *434438*, 433

[94] Punga, T, & Akusjarvi, G. (2000). The adenovirus-2 E1B-55K protein interacts with a mSin3A/histone deacetylase 1 complex. FEBS Lett. *248252*, 476

[95] Radkov, S. A, Touitou, R, Brehm, A, Rowe, M, West, M, Kouzarides, T, & Allday, M. J. (1999). Epstein-Barr virus nuclear antigen 3C interacts with histone deacetylase to repress transcription. J. Virol. *56885697*, 73

[96] Ray, M, Gam, A. A, Boykins, R. A, & Kenney, R. T. (2000). Inhibition of interferon-gamma signaling by Leishmania donovani. J. Infect. Dis. *11211128*, 181

[97] Ribet, D, & Cossart, P. (2010). Post-translational modifications in host cells during bacterial infection. FEBS Lett. *27482758*, 584

[98] Roberts, C. W, & Orkin, S. H. (2004). The SWI/SNF complex--chromatin and cancer. Nat. Rev. Cancer. *133142*, 4

[99] Roger, T. (2011). Histone deacetylase inhibitors impair innate immune responses to Toll-like receptor agonists and to infection. Blood. *12051217*, 117

[100] Ruthenburg, A. J, Li, H, Patel, D. J, & Allis, C. D. (2007). Multivalent engagement of chromatin modifications by linked binding modules. Nat. Rev. Mol. Cell Biol. *983994*, 8

[101] Saccani, S, Pantano, S, & Natoli, G. (2002). marking of inflammatory genes for increased NF-kappa B recruitment. Nat. Immunol. *3*, 69-75., 38.

[102] Saha, A, Wittmeyer, J, & Cairns, B. R. (2006). Chromatin remodelling: the industrial revolution of DNA around histones. Nat. Rev. Mol. Cell Biol. *437447*, 7

[103] Sakabe, K, Wang, Z, & Hart, G. W. (2010). Beta-N-acetylglucosamine (O-GlcNAc) is part of the histone code. Proc. Natl. Acad. Sci. U. S. A. *1991519920*, 107

[104] Santos-rosa, H, Schneider, R, Bannister, A. J, Sherriff, J, Bernstein, B. E, Emre, N. C, Schreiber, S. L, Mellor, J, & Kouzarides, T. (2002). Active genes are tri-methylated at K4 of histone H3. Nature. *407411*, 419

[105] Schneider, J, Bajwa, P, Johnson, F. C, Bhaumik, S. R, & Shilatifard, A. (2006). Rtt109 is required for proper H3K56 acetylation: a chromatin mark associated with the elongating RNA polymerase II. J. Biol. Chem. *3727037274*, 281

[106] Schneider, J, Wood, A, Lee, J. S, Schuster, R, Dueker, J, Maguire, C, Swanson, S. K, Florens, L, Washburn, M. P, & Shilatifard, A. (2005). Molecular regulation of histone H3 trimethylation by COMPASS and the regulation of gene expression. Mol. Cell. *849856*, 19

[107] Schroder, K, Hertzog, P. J, Ravasi, T, & Hume, D. A. (2004). Interferon-gamma: an overview of signals, mechanisms and functions. J. Leukoc. Biol. *163189*, 75

[108] Shahbazian, M. D, & Grunstein, M. (2007). Functions of site-specific histone acetylation and deacetylation. Annu. Rev. Biochem. *75100*, 76

[109] Shi, X. (2006). ING2 PHD domain links histone H3 lysine 4 methylation to active gene repression. Nature. *9699*, 442

[110] Shi, Y, Lan, F, Matson, C, Mulligan, P, Whetstine, J. R, Cole, P. A, Casero, R. A, & Shi, Y. (2004). Histone demethylation mediated by the nuclear amine oxidase homolog LSD1. Cell. *941953*, 119

[111] Shi, Y, & Whetstine, J. R. (2007). Dynamic regulation of histone lysine methylation by demethylases. Mol. Cell. *114*, 25

[112] Shilatifard, A. (2006). Chromatin modifications by methylation and ubiquitination: implications in the regulation of gene expression. Annu. Rev. Biochem. *24369*, 75

[113] Shogren-knaak, M, Ishii, H, Sun, J. M, Pazin, M. J, Davie, J. R, & Peterson, C. L. K16 acetylation controls chromatin structure and protein interactions. Science. *844847*, 311

[114] Shogren-knaak, M, & Peterson, C. L. (2006). Switching on chromatin: mechanistic role of histone H4-K16 acetylation. Cell Cycle. *13611365*, 5

[115] Sims, R. J. III, Chen,C.F., Santos-Rosa,H., Kouzarides,T., Patel,S.S., and Reinberg,D. ((2005). Human but not yeast CHD1 binds directly and selectively to histone H3 methylated at lysine 4 via its tandem chromodomains. J. Biol. Chem. *4178941792*, 280

[116] Smale, S. T. (2010). Selective transcription in response to an inflammatory stimulus. Cell. *% 19;140833844*

[117] Strahl, B. D, & Allis, C. D. (2000). The language of covalent histone modifications. Nature. *4145*, 403

[118] Takeda, K, Kaisho, T, & Akira, S. (2003). Toll-like receptors. Annu. Rev. Immunol. *33576Epub;% 2001 Dec;% 19.*, 335-376., 21

[119] Tan, M. (2011). Identification of 67 histone marks and histone lysine crotonylation as a new type of histone modification. Cell. *10161028*, 146

[120] Ting, J. P, & Trowsdale, J. (2002). Genetic control of MHC class II expression. Cell. *109 Suppl:S2133*S21-S33.

[121] Tzung, K. W. (2001). Genomic evidence for a complete sexual cycle in Candida albicans. Proc. Natl. Acad. Sci. U. S. A. *32493253*, 98

[122] Valls, E, Blanco-garcia, N, Aquizu, N, Piedra, D, Estaras, C, & Martinez-balbas, l. C. , X. M.A. ((2007). Involvement of chromatin and histone deacetylation in SV40 T antigen transcription regulation. Nucleic Acids Res. *19581968*, 35

[123] Verdone, L, Agricola, E, Caserta, M, & Di, M. E. (2006a). Histone acetylation in gene regulation. Brief. Funct. Genomic. Proteomic. *209221*, 5

[124] Wang, G. G, Allis, C. D, & Chi, P. (2007). Chromatin remodeling and cancer, Part II: ATP-dependent chromatin remodeling. Trends Mol. Med. *373380*, 13

[125] Wang, H, Zhai, L, Xu, J, Joo, H. Y, Jackson, S, Erdjument-bromage, H, Tempst, P, Xiong, Y, & Zhang, Y. and H4 ubiquitylation by the CUL4-DDB-ROC1 ubiquitin ligase facilitates cellular response to DNA damage. Mol. Cell. *383394*, 22

[126] Wang, Y, Curry, H. M, Zwilling, B. S, & Lafuse, W. P. (2005). Mycobacteria inhibition of IFN-gamma induced HLA-DR gene expression by up-regulating histone deacetylation at the promoter region in human THP-1 monocytic cells. J. Immunol. *56875694*, 174

[127] Wang, Y. (2004). Human PAD4 regulates histone arginine methylation levels via demethylimination. Science. *279283*, 306

[128] Weinmann, A. S, Mitchell, D. M, Sanjabi, S, Bradley, M. N, Hoffmann, A, Liou, H. C, & Smale, S. T. (2001). Nucleosome remodeling at the IL-12 promoter is a TLR-dependent, Rel-independent event. Nat. Immunol. *2*, 51-57., 40.

[129] Weinmann, A. S, Plevy, S. E, & Smale, S. T. (1999). Rapid and selective remodeling of a positioned nucleosome during the induction of IL-12 transcription. Immunity. *11*, 665-675., 40.

[130] Wightman, F, Ellenberg, P, Churchill, M, & Lewin, S. R. (2012). HDAC inhibitors in HIV. Immunol. Cell Biol. *4754*, 90

[131] Wright, K. L, & Ting, J. P. (2006). Epigenetic regulation of MHC-II and CIITA genes. Trends Immunol. *405412*, 27

[132] Wurtele, H, Tsao, S, Lepine, G, Mullick, A, Tremblay, J, Drogaris, P, Lee, E. H, Thibault, P, Verreault, A, & Raymond, M. (2010). Modulation of histone H3 lysine 56 acetylation as an antifungal therapeutic strategy. Nat. Med. *774780*, 16

[133] Wysocka, J, Allis, C. D, & Coonrod, S. (2006a). Histone arginine methylation and its dynamic regulation. Front Biosci. *34455*, 11

[134] Wysocka, J, Swigut, T, Milne, T. A, Dou, Y, Zhang, X, Burlingame, A. L, Roeder, R. G, Brivanlou, A. H, & Allis, C. D. (2005). WDR5 associates with histone H3 methylated at K4 and is essential for H3 K4 methylation and vertebrate development. Cell. *859872*, 121

[135] Wysocka, J. (2006b). A PHD finger of NURF couples histone H3 lysine 4 trimethylation with chromatin remodelling. Nature. *8690*, 442

[136] Xia, G, Schneider-stock, R, Diestel, A, Habold, C, Krueger, S, Roessner, A, Naumann, M, & Lendeckel, U. (2008). Helicobacter pylori regulates WAF1) by histone H4 acetylation. Biochem. Biophys. Res. Commun. *369*, 526-531., 21.

[137] Xie, W. (2009). Histone h3 lysine 56 acetylation is linked to the core transcriptional network in human embryonic stem cells. Mol. Cell. *417427*, 33

[138] Xu, F, Zhang, K, & Grunstein, M. (2005). Acetylation in histone H3 globular domain regulates gene expression in yeast. Cell. *375385*, 121

[139] Zeng, L, & Zhou, M. M. (2002). Bromodomain: an acetyl-lysine binding domain. FEBS Lett. % *20;513124128*

[140] Zhang, J. (2007). A Pseudomonas syringae effector inactivates MAPKs to suppress PAMP-induced immunity in plants. Cell Host. Microbe. *175185*, 1

[141] Zhu, B, Zheng, Y, Pham, A. D, Mandal, S. S, Erdjument-bromage, H, Tempst, P, & Reinberg, D. (2005). Monoubiquitination of human histone H2B: the factors involved and their roles in HOX gene regulation. Mol. Cell. *601611*, 20

[142] Zika, E, Greer, S. F, Zhu, X. S, & Ting, J. P. (2003). Histone deacetylase 1/mSin3A disrupts gamma interferon-induced CIITA function and major histocompatibility complex class II enhanceosome formation. Mol. Cell Biol. *30913102*, 23

[143] Zupkovitz, G. (2006). Negative and positive regulation of gene expression by mouse histone deacetylase 1. Mol. Cell Biol. *79137928*, 26

[144] Zurawski, D. V, Mumy, K. L, Faherty, C. S, Mccormick, B. A, & Maurelli, A. T. (2009). Shigella flexneri type III secretion system effectors OspB and OspF target the nucleus to downregulate the host inflammatory response via interactions with retinoblastoma protein. Mol. Microbiol. *350368*, 71

Chapter 9

Rett Syndrome

Daniela Zahorakova

Additional information is available at the end of the chapter

http://dx.doi.org/10.5772/55020

1. Introduction

Defects in epigenetic mechanisms can give rise to several neurological and behavioral phenotypes. Rett syndrome (MIM 312750) is a pervasive neurodevelopmental disorder that is primarily caused by mutations in a gene encoding methyl-CpG-binding protein 2. The functions of the protein are related to DNA methylation, a key epigenetic mechanism that plays a critical role in gene silencing through chromatin remodeling. Rett syndrome was the first human disorder in which a link between epigenetic modification and neuronal dysfunction was discovered. In this chapter, the clinical features and the molecular pathology of Rett syndrome will be discussed.

1.1. History

Rett syndrome was first recognized by the Viennese pediatrician Andreas Rett. In 1965, he observed two girls sitting on their mothers' laps in his waiting room. Both girls were profoundly intellectually disabled and were continually wringing their hands in the same unusual manner. Dr. Rett recollected seeing such behavior in previous patients and searched for their files with his secretary. They found several girls with a similar developmental history and clinical features. He realized that these symptoms constituted something other than cerebral palsy, which was the usual designation at the time. In 1966, Dr. Rett published the first description of the disorder that now bears his name [1]. His paper, however, remained unnoticed by the medical community until the 1980s, when Swedish child neurologist Bengt Hagberg with colleagues published the same clinical findings and named the disorder Rett syndrome [2]. Later, diagnostic criteria were proposed [3], and Rett syndrome became recognized worldwide by pediatricians, neurologists, geneticists, and neuroscientists. Despite great effort, the genetic cause of the disorder was not determined until more than 30 years after the first clinical account. In 1999, mutations within the methyl-CpG-binding protein 2 gene (*MECP2*) were identified in patients with Rett syndrome [4], which became a turning point in

Rett syndrome research. This discovery allowed the molecular confirmation of clinical cases and contributed to amendments of the diagnostic criteria [5]. Most importantly, this finding started an extensive investigation into the molecular mechanisms that underlie the pathology of Rett syndrome.

1.2. Occurence

The estimated prevalence of Rett syndrome is 1:10,000 females by the age of 12 years old [6] with no specific ethnic or geographical preference. Rett syndrome is one of the leading genetic causes of profound mental retardation in females, second only to Down syndrome [7]. Male cases are very rare, and their phenotypic manifestations are different from those observed in girls with Rett syndrome.

2. Clinical aspects of Rett syndrome

2.1. Symptoms and stages

Rett syndrome, in its classic form, begins to manifest in early childhood and is characterized by neurodevelopmental regression that severely affects motor, cognitive, and communications skills.

Prenatal and perinatal periods are usually normal. Affected girls appear to develop normally during the first 6 to 18 months of life and seem to achieve appropriate developmental milestones. Nevertheless, retrospective analyses of home videos often show that, even during this period, affected female infants display some suboptimal development. This underdevelopment may include subtle motor and behavioral abnormalities, as well as hypotonia and feeding problems. General mobility and eye-hand coordination may be inadequate, and an excess of repetitive hand patting can be observed even during the first year of life. However, the overall developmental pattern is not obviously disturbed. The child is usually quiet and placid, and the parents often describe the child as "very good" [1, 8-11]. The characteristic clinical features appear successively over several stages, forming a distinctive disease progression pattern (Figure 1).

Stage I: Early onset stagnation (age of onset: 6-18 months). Psychomotor development begins to slow, but the general developmental pattern is not significantly abnormal. The deceleration of head growth (which eventually leads to microcephaly), growth retardation, and weight loss occur in most patients. The child is delayed or ceases in the acquisition of skills. Although babbling and new words may appear, language skills usually remain poor. A girl with Rett syndrome may become irritable and restless, and she may begin to display some autistic features, such as emotional withdrawal and indifference to the surrounding environment [11, 13, 14]

Stage II: Developmental regression (age of onset: 1-4 years). This stage may occur over a period of days to weeks and is characterized by a rapid reduction or loss of acquired skills, especially purposeful hand use, speech, and interpersonal contact [15]. In some patients, the

http://dx.doi.org/10.5772/55020

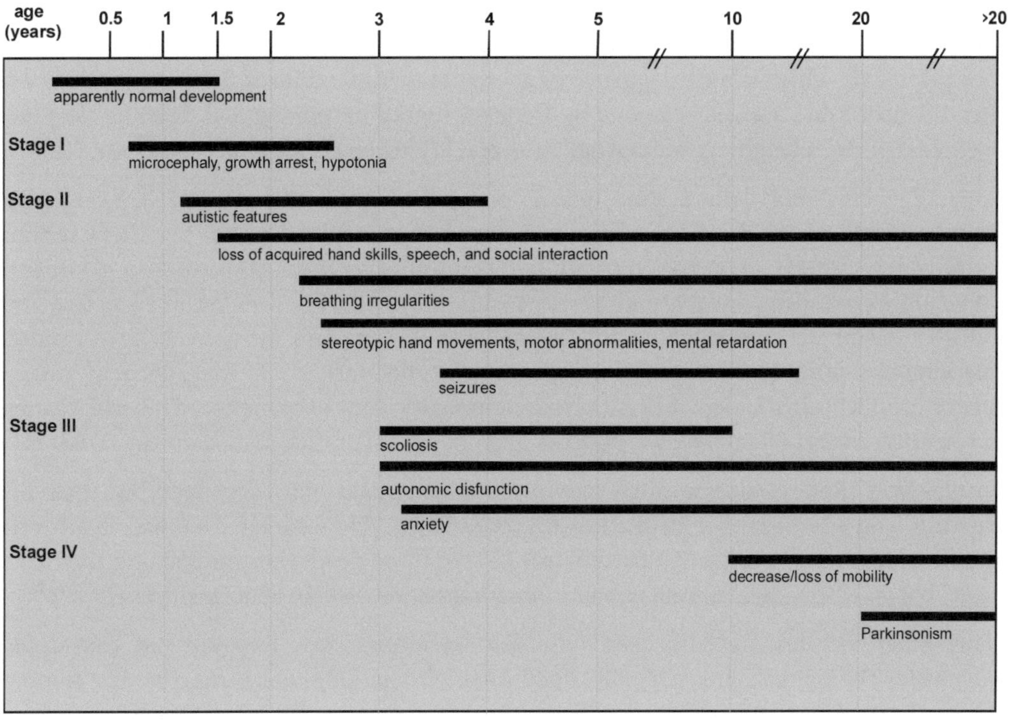

Figure 1. Onset and progression of Rett syndrome [12]

decline of motor and communicative performances is more gradual. Interest in people and objects is diminished, but eye contact may be preserved [11]. Voluntary hand use, such as grasping and reaching out for toys, is replaced with repetitive stereotypic hand movements, the hallmark of Rett syndrome. Patterns consisting of wringing, hand washing, mouthing, clapping, rubbing, squeezing, and other hand automatisms occur during waking hours [1, 16, 17]. Febrile seizures are often present, and epileptic paroxysms occur in most patients [18, 19]. The severity of seizures can vary, ranging from relatively mild or easily controlled by medication to severe drug-resistant episodes [20]. Irregular breathing patterns, such as episodes of hyperventilation, breath holding, and aerophagia, usually develop toward the end of the regression period. Panting, spitting, and hypersalivation are also frequent symptoms [8, 21].

Stage III: Pseudostationary period (age of onset: 4-7 years, after stage II). This stage can last for years or decades and is characterized by a relative stabilization of the disorder course. Patients may recover some skills, which were lost during the regression stage. Patients can become more joyful and sociable, and they may use eye pointing as a typical way to communicate and to express their needs. Some patients may even learn new words and use simple phrases in a meaningful way. Nevertheless, they continue to suffer from gross cognitive impairments [14]. Despite improved eye contact and non-verbal communication ability, the loss of motor functions further progresses in this stage. Stereotypic hand movements become prominent, as do breathing irregularities. Many patients develop scoliosis, which is often rapidly progressive and eventually requires surgical treatment. Cold feet and lower limbs, with or without color and atrophic changes, are also common. These conditions occur due to poor perfusion, which is a consequence of altered autonomic control. Sleeping patterns are often disturbed and are characterized by frequent nighttime waking and daytime sleeping. Unexplained night laughing, sudden agitation and crying spells may also be present [11].

Stage IV: Late motor deterioration (age of onset: 5-15 years, after stage III). Non-verbal communication and social skills continue to improve gradually. Despite persistent serious cognitive impairment, older patients with Rett syndrome are usually, in contrast to patients with childhood autism, sociable and pleasant with others [22]. Seizures become less frequent and less severe, and stereotypic hand movements become less intense. However, motor deterioration continues with age. Most patients, who previously could walk, become nonambulatory and wheelchair-dependent. Decreased mobility leads to pronounced muscle wasting and rigidity, and, at older ages, the patients often develop Parkinsonian features [11, 23, 24].

Females with Rett syndrome often survive into adulthood and older age, but their life expectancy is less than that of the healthy population. The estimated annual death rate from Rett syndrome is 1.2%. Approximately 25% of these deaths are sudden and they may occur due to autonomic nervous system disturbances or cardiac abnormalities [25-27].

Many other features are associated with Rett syndrome, but they are not considered diagnostic. The patients are generally small for their age [28], which may be due to poor self-feeding abilities and problems with chewing and swallowing. They often suffer from gastroesophageal reflux and bloating. Decreased intestinal motility often results in severe constipation. Electroencephalogram results tend to be abnormal but without any clear diagnostic pattern. A prolonged QT_c interval is observed in many patients and presents a risk for cardiac arrhythmia [26].

2.2. Rett syndrome variants

At least five atypical variants have been delineated in addition to classic Rett syndrome. These variants do not have all of the diagnostic features, and they are either milder or more severe than the classic form.

The most common atypical variant of Rett syndrome is "forme fruste". This mild variant is characterized by a protracted clinical course with partially preserved communication skills and gross motor functions. Other neurological abnormalities that are typical for Rett syndrome are more subtle and can be easily overlooked in this variant [30]. The mild forms of Rett syndrome also include the late regression variant, which manifests in patients of preschool or early school age [30], and the preserved speech variant (also called the Zappella variant) in which patients have preserved language skills and normal head sizes [31].

Severe variants include the early-onset seizure variant (the Hanefeld variant) with the onset of seizures before the age of 6 months [32] and the congenital variant, which is rare and lacks the early period of normal psychomotor development [33]. The Hanefeld variant is often caused by mutations in the *CDKL5* gene [34], and most cases of the congenital variant are related to mutations in the *FOXG1* gene [35]. These genetic abnormalities raise the question of

http://dx.doi.org/10.5772/55020

Consider Rett syndrome diagnosis when postnatal deceleration of head growth is observed
Required for classic Rett syndrome 1. A period of regression followed by recovery or stabilization 2. All main and all exclusive criteria 3. Supportive criteria are not required, although often present in classic Rett syndrome
Required for atypical or variant Rett syndrome 1. A period of regression followed by recovery or stabilization 2. At least 2 of 4 main criteria 3. 5 out 11 supportive criteria
Main criteria 1. Partial or complete loss of acquired purposeful hand skills 2. Partial of complete loss of acquired spoken language 3. Gait abnormalities: impaired ability (dyspraxia) or absence of ability (apraxia) 4. Stereotypic hand movements such as hand wringing/squeezing, clapping/tapping, mouthing and washing/ rubbing automatisms **Exclusion criteria for classic Rett syndrome** 1. Brain injury secondary to trauma (perinatally or postnatally), neurometabolic disease or severe infection that cause neurological problems 2. Grossly abnormal psychomotor development in the first 6 months of life **Supportive criteria for atypical or variant Rett syndrome** 1. Breathing disturbances when awake (hyperventilation, breath-holding, forced expulsion of air or saliva, air swallowing) 2. Bruxism when awake (grinding or clenching of the teeth) 3. Impaired sleep pattern 4. Abnormal muscle tone 5. Peripheral vasomotor disturbances 6. Scoliosis/kyphosis 7. Growth retardation 8. Small cold hands and feet 9. Inappropriate laughing/screaming spells 10. Diminished sensitivity to pain 11. Intense eye communication and eye-pointing behavior

Table 1. Diagnostic criteria for Rett syndrome [29]

whether these variants are separate clinical entities, different from *MECP2*-related Rett syndrome [11].

2.3. Diagnostic criteria

Despite a known genetic cause, Rett syndrome remains a clinical diagnosis. Its diagnosis is based on several well-defined criteria (Table 1), which were revised several times over the past few decades, most recently in 2010 [29].

3. The genetics of Rett syndrome

3.1. Mapping of the causative gene

The mode of inheritance of Rett syndrome was difficult to identify because more than 99% of the cases are sporadic, and the patients rarely reproduce. Therefore, the traditional genome-wide linkage analysis was not an applicable method for mapping the disease locus. The lack of males manifesting the classic Rett syndrome phenotype together with the occurrence of families with affected half-sisters suggested an X-linked dominant inheritance with lethality in hemizygous males [2, 36]. Focused exclusion mapping of the X chromosome in available familial cases was used to narrow down the candidate region, and the subsequent analysis of candidate genes in the patients finally revealed disease-causing mutations in the *MECP2* gene [4].

3.2. *MECP2* gene

The *MECP2* gene (MIM 300005) is located on Xq28 and undergoes X chromosome inactivation (XCI) in females [37, 38]. The gene spans approximately 76 kb and consists of four exons, which encode methyl-CpG-binding protein 2 (MeCP2). Alternative splicing of exon 2 and several polyadenylation signals in a conserved and unusually long 3′ untranslated region (3′UTR) give rise to eight different transcripts regulated in a tissue-specific and developmental stage-specific manner [39-42]. For example, the shortest transcript (1.8 kb) is predominant in adult muscles, heart, blood, and liver. The longest transcript (10.2 kb) occurs at the highest levels in the brain [41, 42]. The unique expression patterns of each transcript suggest a specific biological significance, such as a role in mRNA stability, nuclear export, folding, and sub-cellular localization, thus affecting the levels of the resulting protein [39]. The longest transcript also has one of the longest 3′ UTR tails in the human genome (8.5 kb), with several blocks of highly conserved residues between the human and mouse genomes. These findings argue in favor of a potential regulatory role of the 3′ UTR of the *MECP2* gene [43].

3.3. *MECP2* mutations

Mutations in the *MECP2* gene are identified in 90-95% of classic Rett syndrome patients [4, 44]. Because only the coding region and the adjacent non-coding parts of the gene are routinely analyzed, it is highly probable that mutations in more remote regulatory elements are responsible for the rest of the cases. The frequency of *MECP2* mutations in patients with atypical Rett syndrome variants varies considerably between studies. However, the frequency is generally lower (only 20-70% of patients have *MECP2* mutations) than in the classic form [44-46], suggesting that mutations of regulatory elements or other genes are involved more often in atypical Rett syndrome than in the classic Rett syndrome. The identification of *CDKL5* mutations in the Hanefeld variant and *FOXG1* mutations in the congenital variant strongly support the latter idea.

According to the Human Gene Mutation Database [47], more than 550 mutations have been identified in the *MECP2* gene in patients with Rett syndrome. The spectrum of mutations is heterogeneous, including missense and nonsense mutations, deletions, insertions, duplications, splice-site mutations, and large deletions of several exons or the entire *MECP2* gene. More than 99% of the mutations occur *de novo* and mostly originate on the paternal X chromosome, which explains the high occurrence of Rett syndrome in the female gender [4, 48, 49]. Familial cases of Rett syndrome (mostly affected sisters or maternal half-sisters) are very rare. *MECP2* mutations in these patients are inherited from an asymptomatic or very mildly affected mother, who carries a somatic mutation, but does not manifest the full pathogenic phenotype due to favorable XCI pattern [50, 51]. Another explanation for transmission of a *MECP2* mutation to the next generation is a germline mosaicism for a mutation. It is suggested when the *MECP2* mutation identified in several affected children is not present in somatic cells of their parents [51, 52].

The majority of point mutations in the *MECP2* gene are C>T transitions, presumably resulting from the spontaneous deamination of methylated cytosines [53]. The mutations are scattered throughout the coding sequence and splice sites, with the exception of exon 2. The eight most common mutations, which are also C>T transitions, account for approximately 70% of the Rett syndrome cases. Approximately 10% of cases are due to deletions, which are mostly clustered in the terminal segment of the coding region [12].

3.4. *MECP2* mutations in males and other disorders

Mutations in the *MECP2* gene have long been considered lethal in hemizygous males, and Rett syndrome has been assumed to be exclusively a female disorder. More recently, *MECP2* mutations were not only identified in males but also in females with phenotypes different from Rett syndrome. *MECP2*-related disorders thus represent a broad spectrum of phenotypes in both genders.

The estimated frequency of *MECP2* mutations in boys with mental retardation is 1.3-1.7% [54]. Typical Rett syndrome features have been observed almost exclusively in boys with Klinefelter syndrome (47,XXY) [55] or somatic mosaicism for a *MECP2* mutation [56, 57]. Other phenotypes include severe congenital encephalopathy with death in the first years of life [58-60] and mild to severe intellectual disability with or without various neurological and psychiatric symptoms [54, 61]. The most common *MECP2* mutations detected in males are duplications of the whole *MECP2* gene (and usually genes in its vicinity). This finding indicates that, besides the lack, an overabundance of fully functional MeCP2 protein is also harmful to the CNS. *MECP2* duplication syndrome is usually very mild or does not manifest in females. In boys, this syndrome is characterized by infantile hypotonia, severe mental retardation, loss of speech, recurrent respiratory infections, seizures, and spasticity [62-64].

In females, *MECP2* mutations have been detected in patients with mild mental retardation, learning disabilities or autism [65, 66]. More severe cases include severe mental retardation with seizures and Angelman-like syndrome [67, 68].

3.5. MeCP2 protein

The MeCP2 protein is ubiquitously expressed, but it is particularly abundant in the brain [41, 69]. The protein levels are low during embryogenesis, but they progressively increase during postnatal neuronal maturation and synaptogenesis [70-75]. High expression of MeCP2 in mature neurons implies its involvement in postmitotic neuronal functions, such as the modulation of neuronal activity and plasticity [12].

MeCP2 occurs in two isoforms that arise from alternative splicing of exon 2, and they differ only by their N-termini (Figure 2). MeCP2 e1 (498 amino acids), generated by exons 1, 3, and 4, is the dominant MeCP2 isoform in the brain [76-78]. The MeCP2 e2 isoform (486 amino acids) is encoded by exons 2, 3, and 4. Both isoforms were initially assumed to be functionally equivalent, but recent observations imply that additional isoform-specific functions may exist. This idea is strongly supported by the fact that no mutations in exon 2 have been found in Rett syndrome patients, which contrasts with the finding of identified mutations in exon 1. Thus, defects in MeCP2 e2 may lead to non-Rett phenotypes or fatally affect embryo viability [79, 80].

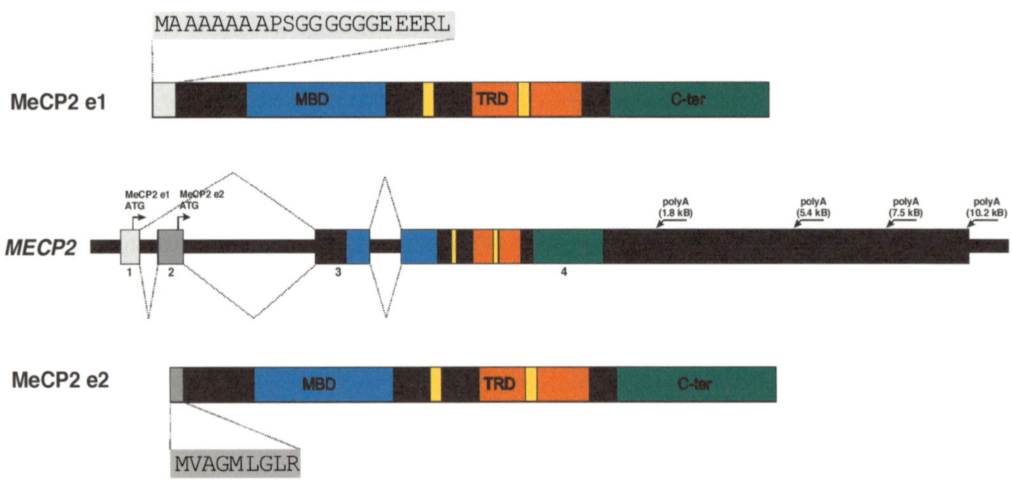

MBD: methyl-CpG-binding domain, TRD: transcriptional repression domain, C-ter: C-terminal domain, yellow boxes: nuclear localization signals.

Figure 2. *MECP2* gene structure and the isoforms MeCP2 e1 and MeCP2 e2 with different N-termini due to alternative splicing of exon 2 and different translation start sites.

Apart from different N-terminal regions, both isoforms share the same amino acid sequence, including at least three functional domains and two nuclear localization signals (Figure 2). The methyl-CpG-binding domain (MBD) (amino acids 78-162) mediates binding to symmetrically methylated CpG dinucleotides [81, 82], with a preference for CpGs with adjacent A/T-rich motifs [83]. The MBD also binds to unmethylated four-way DNA junctions, which suggests the role of MeCP2 in higher-order chromatin interactions [84]. The transcriptional repression domain (TRD) (amino acids 207-310) interacts with numerous proteins, such as co-repressor factors and histone deacetylases, HDAC1 and HDAC2. The nuclear localization signals (NLS) (amino acids 173-193 and 255-271) mediate transportation of the protein into the nucleus [85]. The C-terminal domain (amino acids 325-486) facilitates binding to DNA [86] and it most likely increases protein stability [87]. This domain also contains conserved poly-proline motifs that can bind to group II WW domain splicing factors [88].

3.6. MeCP2 function

The original model suggested that MeCP2 is a global transcriptional repressor [89], and it was based on *in vitro* experiments in which MeCP2 inhibited transcription from methylated promoters. Briefly, the protein binds to the promoters of target genes via its MBD, and the TRD then recruits the co-repressor Sin3A and HDACs [90, 91]. These interactions lead to the deacetylation of histones, resulting in chromatin condensation and the repression of downstream genes. In addition to Sin3A, other co-repressors, such as c-Ski and N-CoR, may interact with MeCP2 [92]. The compaction of chromatin can also be promoted through direct interaction with the C-terminal domain [93], which is an example of HDAC-independent MeCP2-mediated transcriptional repression. The TRD may also directly interact with transcription factor IIB; therefore, MeCP2 may silence transcription by interfering with the assembly of the transcriptional preinitiation complex [94]. Additional factors interacting with the TRD include Brahma, which is a catalytic component of the SWI/SNF-related chromatin-remodeling complex (at least in NIH 3T3 cells) [95], DNA methyltransferase 1 [96], and ATRX, a SWI2/SNF2 DNA helicase/ATPase [97].

Surprisingly, transcriptional profiling studies did not reveal major gene expression changes caused by the lack of functional MeCP2 protein [98, 99]. These observations, together with additional evidence, implied that MeCP2 regulates the transcription of tissue-specific genes in specific brain regions during certain developmental stages instead of acting as a global repressor [98, 100-102]. However, recent studies suggest that MeCP2 reduces genome-wide transcriptional noise, potentially by repressing spurious transcription of repetitive elements [103, 104]. Surprisingly, MeCP2 also interacts with the transcriptional activator CREB, and its genomic distribution is often associated with actively transcribed genes [105, 106]. MeCP2 apparently has dual roles in transcriptional regulation as a repressor and as an activator, and it performs different downstream responses depending on the context.

MeCP2 additionally acts as an architectural chromatin protein that is involved in chromatin remodeling and nucleosome clustering, which is consistent with the fact that the majority of MeCP2-binding sites are located outside of genes [105, 107]. MeCP2 can bind *in vitro* to chromatin fibers and compact them into higher order structures [93, 108, 109].

For further complexity, MeCP2 may also be involved in RNA splicing. Its interaction with the RNA-binding protein Y box-binding protein 1 (YB-1) has been observed, and MeCP2-deficient mice showed aberrant alternative splicing patterns [110].

MeCP2 functions are undeniably much more complex than initially anticipated (Figure 3), although the precise mechanisms of their regulation remain unknown.

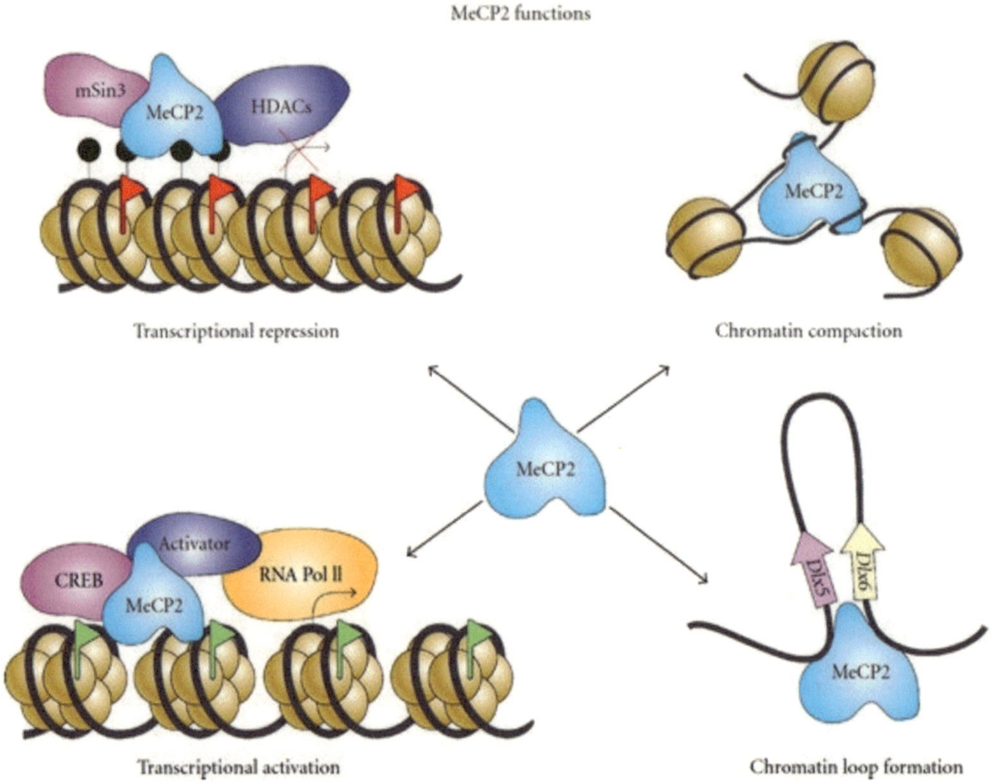

Figure 3. Representation of multiple MeCP2 roles [111].

3.7. MeCP2 target genes

A comprehensive knowledge of the target genes that are controlled by MeCP2 is essential for understanding the pathomechanisms of Rett syndrome and subsequently developing effective therapeutic strategies. Multiple studies have attempted to identify genes with altered expression in neuronal and nonneuronal tissues from Rett syndrome patients and mouse models, but these studies have often yielded conflicting results [102, 106, 112, 113]. Nevertheless, several candidate target genes have been proposed (Table 2). One of the most extensively studied target genes is the brain-derived neurotrophic factor gene (*Bdnf*), which has been shown to be up and down regulated in an activity-dependent manner through MeCP2 phosphorylation in mice [113-115]. Other targets, such as the imprinted genes *Dlx5* and *Dlx6*, also revealed a novel mode of gene repression mediated by MeCP2 through the formation of a silent chromatin loop (Figure 3) [116, 117].

http://dx.doi.org/10.5772/55020

Gene	Function	Reference
UBE3A	member of ubiquitin proteasome pathway, transcriptional co-activator	[118]
GABRB3	neurotransmission (GABA-A receptor)	[118]
PCDHB1	cell adhesion	[119]
PCDH7	cell adhesion	[119]
Bdnf	neuronal development and survival, neuronal plasticity, learning and memory (brain derived neurotropic factor)	[113, 114]
Dlx5	neuronal transcription factor (probably involved in control of GABAergic differentiation)	[116]
Sgk1	hormone signaling (regulation of renal functions and blood pressure)	[120]
Fkbp5	hormone signaling (regulation of glucocorticoid receptor sensitivity)	[120]
Uqcrc1	member of mitochondrial respiratory chain	[121]
ID1, ID2, ID3, ID4	transcription factors (involved in cell differentiation and neural development)	[122]
FXYD1	ion channel regulator	[123]
IGFBP3	hormone signaling (regulation of cell proliferation and apoptosis)	[124]
GDI1	regulation of GDP/GTP exchange	[112]
APLP1	enhancer of neuronal apoptosis	[112]
CLU	Extracellular molecular chaperone	[112]
Crh	neuropeptide (regulation of neuroendocrine stress response)	[125]

Table 2. Some of MeCP2 target genes.

3.8. The effect of *MECP2* mutations on MeCP2 function

Mutations in the *MECP2* gene are not likely to act in a dominant-negative mechanism because only one allele is active in each female cell due to XCI. The functional consequences of missense mutations on the function of the MeCP2 protein are sometimes especially difficult to predict. This difficulty is because testing the protein's various functions can be problematic because there are still many MeCP2 roles that are as yet unknown or not fully understood. Generally, mutations in the NLS prevent the transportation of the protein to the nucleus. Mutations located within the MBD reduce the affinity of the protein for methylated DNA [87, 126]. However, several mutant proteins with mutations in the MBD have been shown to bind to heterochromatin [127]. Proteins with an intact MBD but with a mutated TRD retain their ability to bind to methylated DNA, but they have impaired repressing activity [87]. Other mutations may affect the stability or the structure (secondary or tertiary) of the protein, and they may interfere with other functions of the protein.

3.9. Genotype-phenotype correlation

The severity of the clinical manifestations in Rett syndrome patients is widely variable and is relevant beyond the context of classic vs. atypical variants. Therefore, much effort has been devoted to uncovering the relationships between various *MECP2* mutations and the variability of clinical features. Such knowledge may provide information on the likely clinical profile of new cases with specific *MECP2* mutations and may be useful in designing specific preventive therapeutic interventions.

The general genotype-phenotype correlations were confirmed by numerous studies. As expected, patients with early truncating mutations (specifically p.R168X, p.R270X, p.R255X), large deletions of several exons, or the entire *MECP2* gene usually have the most severe clinical presentations. A milder phenotype is often associated with late truncating mutations that do not affect the MBD or the TRD, such as p.R294X. Interestingly, late truncating mutations together with the missense mutation p.R133C, which is located in the MBD, are frequently detected in patients with a preserved speech variant of Rett syndrome [128-133].

Despite some overall trends, considerable variability in clinical severity is often observed among patients with the same *MECP2* mutation [128, 130, 134]. Such variations may be caused by a different XCI pattern. Favorable skewing of XCI has been observed in some patients with milder phenotypes [135-137] and in asymptomatic carrier mothers [58, 135, 138]. However, XCI cannot be used as the single predictor because, according to several studies, it has limitations in explaining all of the differences of Rett syndrome severity [139-141]. Other modulation factors have been considered, such as *BDNF* [142, 143] and *APOE* [144].

3.10. Genetic counseling

A negative result from the *MECP2* analysis (usually including analysis of the entire coding region and copy number analysis of large deletions/duplications) does not rule out the diagnosis of Rett syndrome because regulatory and non-coding regions are not routinely analyzed. The recurrence risk in a family with a single Rett syndrome case and an otherwise negative family history is very low (less than 0.5%) because the majority of *MECP2* mutations arise *de novo*. Mothers of the patients, however, should be tested for *MECP2* mutations found in their daughters to rule out the possibility of being asymptomatic carriers. In such case, the recurrence risk is 50%. Prenatal diagnosis may be performed even in pregnancies of non-carrier mothers due to the likelihood of germline mosaicism.

4. Management of Rett syndrome

Currently, there is no effective cure for Rett syndrome. However, hopes for developing a targeted therapy have risen following the announcement of a study that rescued the pathological phenotype in a mouse model after postnatal reactivation of *Mecp2* [145, 146]. Treatment strategies are currently symptomatic and preventive. These strategies are aimed at ameliorating specific symptoms, such as seizures, mood disturbances, sleeping and feeding problems, as well as maintaining and improving motor and communication functions.

Rehabilitation programs and physical therapy help to control and improve balance and movement, maintain flexibility and strengthen muscles. These programs should be adapted to the patient's individual state and needs. Proper physical therapy is also important for preventing joint contractures and other deformities, such as scoliosis. Occupational therapy is recommended for improving purposeful hand use and to attenuate stereotypic hand movements. Particular care should be taken to preserve and maintain alternative communication (eye contact, eye pointing, facial expressions, signs, etc.) and thereby improving social interactions. Receiving necessary nutrients and maintaining an adequate weight may result in improved growth. To ensure appropriate caloric and nutritional intake, a high-fat, high-calorie diet or gastrostomy feeding may be required. Sufficient intake of fluid and high-fiber food is necessary to prevent constipation. The patients with cardiac conduction defects (such as prolonged QT_c intervals) should avoid certain medications, which may worsen the condition. These medications include several antipsychotics (thioridazine, tricyclic antidepressants), certain antiarrhythmics (quinidine, sotalol, amiodarone), and antibiotics (erythromycin) [147].

Early diagnosis and intervention, together with life-long management focused on each patient's specific needs, can significantly improve the health, quality of life, and longevity of patients with Rett syndrome.

5. Conclusion

Much progress has been made in the identification of the multiple roles of the MeCP2 protein in the brain since its discovery. Nevertheless, many mysteries still remain in understanding the precise mechanisms of how *MECP2* mutations affect protein function and subsequently contribute to the pathogenesis of Rett syndrome. A significant phenotypic overlap between Rett syndrome and several neurodevelopmental disorders implies that a common pathogenic process may induce or at least contribute to these conditions. The identification of pathogenic *MECP2* mutations in a portion of patients without the classic Rett syndrome phenotype strengthens this theory. Understanding the molecular pathology underlying Rett syndrome will therefore shed more light on the role of epigenetic modifications in neuronal development and function, and it may provide insight into the pathogenesis of other neurodevelopmental disorders.

Acknowledgements

I would like to thank prof. Pavel Martasek, MD, Ph.D. for helpful discussions and critical reading of the manuscript. The author was supported by grants NT 13120-4/2012, MZCR RVO-VFN64165/2012, P24/LF1/3, and UNCE 204011/2012.

Author details

Daniela Zahorakova*

Address all correspondence to: Daniela.Zahorakova@lf1.cuni.cz

Department of Pediatrics and Adolescent Medicine, First Faculty of Medicine Charles University and General Teaching Hospital, Prague, Czech Republic

References

[1] Rett A. [On a unusual brain atrophy syndrome in hyperammonemia in childhood]. Wiener Medizinische Wochenschrift 1966;116(37): 723-6.

[2] Hagberg B, Aicardi J, Dias K, Ramos O. A progressive syndrome of autism, dementia, ataxia, and loss of purposeful hand use in girls: Rett's syndrome: report of 35 cases. Annals of Neurology 1983;14(4): 471-9.

[3] Hagberg B, Goutieres F, Hanefeld F, Rett A, Wilson J. Rett syndrome: criteria for inclusion and exclusion. Brain and Development 1985;7(3): 372-3.

[4] Amir RE, Van den Veyver IB, Wan M, Tran CQ, Francke U, Zoghbi HY. Rett syndrome is caused by mutations in X-linked MECP2, encoding methyl-CpG-binding protein 2. Nature Genetics 1999;23(2): 185-8.

[5] Hagberg B, Hanefeld F, Percy A, Skjeldal O. An update on clinically applicable diagnostic criteria in Rett syndrome. Comments to Rett Syndrome Clinical Criteria Consensus Panel Satellite to European Paediatric Neurology Society Meeting, Baden Baden, Germany, 11 September 2001. European Journal of Paediatric Neurology 2002;6(5): 293-7.

[6] Laurvick CL, de Klerk N, Bower C, Christodoulou J, Ravine D, Ellaway C, et al. Rett syndrome in Australia: a review of the epidemiology. Journal of Pediatrics 2006;148(3): 347-52.

[7] Ellaway C, Christodoulou J. Rett syndrome: clinical update and review of recent genetic advances. Journal of Paediatrics and Child Health 1999;35(5): 419-26.

[8] Kerr AM. Early clinical signs in the Rett disorder. Neuropediatrics 1995;26(2): 67-71.

[9] Burford B, Kerr AM, Macleod HA. Nurse recognition of early deviation in development in home videos of infants with Rett disorder. Journal of Intellectual Disability Research 2003;47(Pt 8): 588-96.

[10] Einspieler C, Kerr AM, Prechtl HF. Abnormal general movements in girls with Rett disorder: the first four months of life. Brain and Development 2005;27 Suppl 1: S8-S13.

[11] Smeets EE, Pelc K, Dan B. Rett Syndrome. Molecular Syndromology 2011;2(3-5): 113-27.

[12] Chahrour M, Zoghbi HY. The story of Rett syndrome: from clinic to neurobiology. Neuron 2007;56(3): 422-37.

[13] Nomura Y, Segawa M. Natural history of Rett syndrome. Journal of Child Neurology 2005;20(9): 764-8.

[14] Shahbazian MD, Zoghbi HY. Rett syndrome and MeCP2: linking epigenetics and neuronal function. American Journal of Human Genetics 2002;71(6): 1259-72.

[15] Nomura Y. Early behavior characteristics and sleep disturbance in Rett syndrome. Brain and Development 2005;27 Suppl 1: S35-S42.

[16] Nomura Y, Segawa M. Motor symptoms of the Rett syndrome: abnormal muscle tone, posture, locomotion and stereotyped movement. Brain and Development 1992;14 Suppl: S21-8.

[17] Hagberg B. Rett syndrome: clinical peculiarities and biological mysteries. Acta Paediatrica 1995;84(9): 971-6.

[18] Glaze DG, Frost JD, Jr., Zoghbi HY, Percy AK. Rett's syndrome. Correlation of electroencephalographic characteristics with clinical staging. Archives of Neurology 1987;44(10): 1053-6.

[19] Steffenburg U, Hagberg G, Hagberg B. Epilepsy in a representative series of Rett syndrome. Acta Paediatrica 2001;90(1): 34-9.

[20] Jian L, Nagarajan L, de Klerk N, Ravine D, Bower C, Anderson A, et al. Predictors of seizure onset in Rett syndrome. Journal of Pediatrics 2006;149(4): 542-7.

[21] Witt Engerstrom I. Age-related occurrence of signs and symptoms in the Rett syndrome. Brain and Development 1992;14 Suppl: S11-20.

[22] Mount RH, Hastings RP, Reilly S, Cass H, Charman T. Behavioural and emotional features in Rett syndrome. Disability and Rehabilitation 2001;23(3-4): 129-38.

[23] Hagberg B, Witt-Engerstrom I. Rett syndrome: a suggested staging system for describing impairment profile with increasing age towards adolescence. American Journal of Medical Genetics Suppl 1986;1: 47-59.

[24] Roze E, Cochen V, Sangla S, Bienvenu T, Roubergue A, Leu-Semenescu S, et al. Rett syndrome: an overlooked diagnosis in women with stereotypic hand movements, psychomotor retardation, Parkinsonism, and dystonia? Movement Disorders 2007;22(3): 387-9.

[25] Kerr AM, Armstrong DD, Prescott RJ, Doyle D, Kearney DL. Rett syndrome: analysis of deaths in the British survey. European Child & Adolescent Psychiatry 1997;6 Suppl 1: 71-4.

[26] Guideri F, Acampa M, Hayek G, Zappella M, Di Perri T. Reduced heart rate variability in patients affected with Rett syndrome. A possible explanation for sudden death. Neuropediatrics 1999;30(3): 146-8.

[27] Kerr AM, Julu PO. Recent insights into hyperventilation from the study of Rett syndrome. Archives of Disease in Childhood 1999;80(4): 384-7.

[28] Holm VA. Physical growth and development in patients with Rett syndrome. American Journal of Medical Genetics Suppl 1986;1: 119-26.

[29] Neul JL, Kaufmann WE, Glaze DG, Christodoulou J, Clarke AJ, Bahi-Buisson N, et al. Rett syndrome: revised diagnostic criteria and nomenclature. Annals of Neurology 2010;68(6): 944-50.

[30] Hagberg B. Clinical manifestations and stages of Rett syndrome. Mental Retardation and Developmental Disabilities Research Reviews 2002;8(2): 61-5.

[31] Zappella M. The Rett girls with preserved speech. Brain and Development 1992;14(2): 98-101.

[32] Hanefeld F. The clinical pattern of the Rett syndrome. Brain and Development 1985;7(3): 320-5.

[33] Hagberg BA, Skjeldal OH. Rett variants: a suggested model for inclusion criteria. Pediatric Neurology 1994;11(1): 5-11.

[34] Tao J, Van Esch H, Hagedorn-Greiwe M, Hoffmann K, Moser B, Raynaud M, et al. Mutations in the X-linked cyclin-dependent kinase-like 5 (CDKL5/STK9) gene are associated with severe neurodevelopmental retardation. American Journal of Human Genetics 2004;75(6): 1149-54.

[35] Ariani F, Hayek G, Rondinella D, Artuso R, Mencarelli MA, Spanhol-Rosseto A, et al. FOXG1 is responsible for the congenital variant of Rett syndrome. American Journal of Human Genetics 2008;83(1): 89-93.

[36] Killian W. On the genetics of Rett syndrome: analysis of family and pedigree data. American Journal of Medical Genetics Suppl 1986;1: 369-76.

[37] D'Esposito M, Quaderi NA, Ciccodicola A, Bruni P, Esposito T, D'Urso M, et al. Isolation, physical mapping, and northern analysis of the X-linked human gene encoding methyl CpG-binding protein, MECP2. Mammalian Genome 1996;7(7): 533-5.

[38] Sirianni N, Naidu S, Pereira J, Pillotto RF, Hoffman EP. Rett syndrome: confirmation of X-linked dominant inheritance, and localization of the gene to Xq28. American Journal of Human Genetics 1998;63(5): 1552-8.

[39] Coy JF, Sedlacek Z, Bachner D, Delius H, Poustka A. A complex pattern of evolutionary conservation and alternative polyadenylation within the long 3"-untranslated region of the methyl-CpG-binding protein 2 gene (MeCP2) suggests a regulatory role in gene expression. Human Molecular Genetics 1999;8(7): 1253-62.

[40] Reichwald K, Thiesen J, Wiehe T, Weitzel J, Poustka WA, Rosenthal A, et al. Comparative sequence analysis of the MECP2-locus in human and mouse reveals new transcribed regions. Mammalian Genome 2000;11(3): 182-90.

[41] Shahbazian MD, Antalffy B, Armstrong DL, Zoghbi HY. Insight into Rett syndrome: MeCP2 levels display tissue- and cell-specific differences and correlate with neuronal maturation. Human Molecular Genetics 2002;11(2): 115-24.

[42] Pelka GJ, Watson CM, Christodoulou J, Tam PP. Distinct expression profiles of Mecp2 transcripts with different lengths of 3'UTR in the brain and visceral organs during mouse development. Genomics 2005;85(4): 441-52.

[43] Santos M, Yan J, Temudo T, Oliveira G, Vieira JP, Fen J, et al. Analysis of highly conserved regions of the 3'UTR of MECP2 gene in patients with clinical diagnosis of Rett syndrome and other disorders associated with mental retardation. Disease Markers 2008;24(6): 319-24.

[44] Percy AK. Rett syndrome: recent research progress. Journal of Child Neurology 2008;23(5): 543-9.

[45] Psoni S, Sofocleous C, Traeger-Synodinos J, Kitsiou-Tzeli S, Kanavakis E, Fryssira-Kanioura H. MECP2 mutations and clinical correlations in Greek children with Rett syndrome and associated neurodevelopmental disorders. Brain and Development 2012;34(6): 487-95.

[46] Raizis AM, Saleem M, MacKay R, George PM. Spectrum of MECP2 mutations in New Zealand Rett syndrome patients. The New Zealand Medical Journal 2009;122(1296): 21-8.

[47] Stenson PD, Ball EV, Mort M, Phillips AD, Shiel JA, Thomas NS, et al. Human Gene Mutation Database (HGMD): 2003 update. Human Mutation 2003;21(6): 577-81.

[48] Girard M, Couvert P, Carrie A, Tardieu M, Chelly J, Beldjord C, et al. Parental origin of de novo MECP2 mutations in Rett syndrome. European Journal of Human Genetics 2001;9(3): 231-6.

[49] Trappe R, Laccone F, Cobilanschi J, Meins M, Huppke P, Hanefeld F, et al. MECP2 mutations in sporadic cases of Rett syndrome are almost exclusively of paternal origin. American Journal of Human Genetics 2001;68(5): 1093-101.

[50] Knudsen GP, Neilson TC, Pedersen J, Kerr A, Schwartz M, Hulten M, et al. Increased skewing of X chromosome inactivation in Rett syndrome patients and their mothers. European Journal of Human Genetics 2006;14(11): 1189-94.

[51] Wan M, Lee SS, Zhang X, Houwink-Manville I, Song HR, Amir RE, et al. Rett syndrome and beyond: recurrent spontaneous and familial MECP2 mutations at CpG hotspots. American Journal of Human Genetics 1999;65(6): 1520-9.

[52] Mari F, Caselli R, Russo S, Cogliati F, Ariani F, Longo I, et al. Germline mosaicism in Rett syndrome identified by prenatal diagnosis. Clinical Genetics 2005;67(3): 258-60.

[53] Lee SS, Wan M, Francke U. Spectrum of MECP2 mutations in Rett syndrome. Brain and Development 2001;23 Suppl 1: S138-43.

[54] Villard L. MECP2 mutations in males. Journal of Medical Genetics 2007;44(7): 417-23.

[55] Schwartzman JS, Bernardino A, Nishimura A, Gomes RR, Zatz M. Rett syndrome in a boy with a 47,XXY karyotype confirmed by a rare mutation in the MECP2 gene. Neuropediatrics 2001;32(3): 162-4.

[56] Armstrong J, Pineda M, Aibar E, Gean E, Monros E. Classic Rett syndrome in a boy as a result of somatic mosaicism for a MECP2 mutation. Annals of Neurology 2001;50(5): 692.

[57] Pieras JI, Munoz-Cabello B, Borrego S, Marcos I, Sanchez J, Madruga M, et al. Somatic mosaicism for Y120X mutation in the MECP2 gene causes atypical Rett syndrome in a male. Brain and Development 2011;33(7): 608-11.

[58] Villard L, Kpebe A, Cardoso C, Chelly PJ, Tardieu PM, Fontes M. Two affected boys in a Rett syndrome family: clinical and molecular findings. Neurology 2000;55(8): 1188-93.

[59] Geerdink N, Rotteveel JJ, Lammens M, Sistermans EA, Heikens GT, Gabreels FJ, et al. MECP2 mutation in a boy with severe neonatal encephalopathy: clinical, neuropathological and molecular findings. Neuropediatrics 2002;33(1): 33-6.

[60] Lundvall M, Samuelsson L, Kyllerman M. Male Rett phenotypes in T158M and R294X MeCP2-mutations. Neuropediatrics 2006;37(5): 296-301.

[61] Moog U, Smeets EE, van Roozendaal KE, Schoenmakers S, Herbergs J, Schoonbrood-Lenssen AM, et al. Neurodevelopmental disorders in males related to the gene causing Rett syndrome in females (MECP2). European Journal of Paediatric Neurology 2003;7(1): 5-12.

[62] Van Esch H, Bauters M, Ignatius J, Jansen M, Raynaud M, Hollanders K, et al. Duplication of the MECP2 region is a frequent cause of severe mental retardation and progressive neurological symptoms in males. American Journal of Human Genetics 2005;77(3): 442-53.

[63] Van Esch H. MECP2 Duplication Syndrome. Molecular Syndromology 2012;2(3-5): 128-36.

[64] Ramocki MB, Tavyev YJ, Peters SU. The MECP2 duplication syndrome. American Journal of Medical Genetics Part A 2010;152A(5): 1079-88.

http://dx.doi.org/10.5772/55020

[65] Lam CW, Yeung WL, Ko CH, Poon PM, Tong SF, Chan KY, et al. Spectrum of mutations in the MECP2 gene in patients with infantile autism and Rett syndrome. Journal of Medical Genetics 2000;37(12): E41.

[66] Carney RM, Wolpert CM, Ravan SA, Shahbazian M, Ashley-Koch A, Cuccaro ML, et al. Identification of MeCP2 mutations in a series of females with autistic disorder. Pediatric Neurology 2003;28(3): 205-11.

[67] Watson P, Black G, Ramsden S, Barrow M, Super M, Kerr B, et al. Angelman syndrome phenotype associated with mutations in MECP2, a gene encoding a methyl CpG binding protein. Journal of Medical Genetics 2001;38(4): 224-8.

[68] Milani D, Pantaleoni C, D'Arrigo S, Selicorni A, Riva D. Another patient with MECP2 mutation without classic Rett syndrome phenotype. Pediatric Neurology 2005;32(5): 355-7.

[69] LaSalle JM, Goldstine J, Balmer D, Greco CM. Quantitative localization of heterogeneous methyl-CpG-binding protein 2 (MeCP2) expression phenotypes in normal and Rett syndrome brain by laser scanning cytometry. Human Molecular Genetics 2001;10(17): 1729-40.

[70] Cohen DR, Matarazzo V, Palmer AM, Tu Y, Jeon OH, Pevsner J, et al. Expression of MeCP2 in olfactory receptor neurons is developmentally regulated and occurs before synaptogenesis. Molecular and Cellular Neuroscience 2003;22(4): 417-29.

[71] Jung BP, Jugloff DG, Zhang G, Logan R, Brown S, Eubanks JH. The expression of methyl CpG binding factor MeCP2 correlates with cellular differentiation in the developing rat brain and in cultured cells. Journal of Neurobiology 2003;55(1): 86-96.

[72] Samaco RC, Nagarajan RP, Braunschweig D, LaSalle JM. Multiple pathways regulate MeCP2 expression in normal brain development and exhibit defects in autism-spectrum disorders. Human Molecular Genetics 2004;13(6): 629-39.

[73] Kishi N, Macklis JD. Dissecting MECP2 function in the central nervous system. Journal of Child Neurology 2005;20(9): 753-9.

[74] Smrt RD, Eaves-Egenes J, Barkho BZ, Santistevan NJ, Zhao C, Aimone JB, et al. Mecp2 deficiency leads to delayed maturation and altered gene expression in hippocampal neurons. Neurobiology of Disease 2007;27(1): 77-89.

[75] Swanberg SE, Nagarajan RP, Peddada S, Yasui DH, LaSalle JM. Reciprocal co-regulation of EGR2 and MECP2 is disrupted in Rett syndrome and autism. Human Molecular Genetics 2009;18(3): 525-34.

[76] Mnatzakanian GN, Lohi H, Munteanu I, Alfred SE, Yamada T, MacLeod PJ, et al. A previously unidentified MECP2 open reading frame defines a new protein isoform relevant to Rett syndrome. Nature Genetics 2004;36(4): 339-41.

[77] Dragich JM, Kim YH, Arnold AP, Schanen NC. Differential distribution of the MeCP2 splice variants in the postnatal mouse brain. The Journal of Comparative Neurology 2007;501(4): 526-42.

[78] Kriaucionis S, Bird A. The major form of MeCP2 has a novel N-terminus generated by alternative splicing. Nucleic Acids Research 2004;32(5): 1818-23.

[79] Itoh M, Tahimic CG, Ide S, Otsuki A, Sasaoka T, Noguchi S, et al. Methyl CpG-binding protein isoform MeCP2_e2 is dispensable for Rett syndrome phenotypes but essential for embryo viability and placenta development. The Journal of Biological Chemistry 2012;287(17): 13859-67.

[80] Dastidar SG, Bardai FH, Ma C, Price V, Rawat V, Verma P, et al. Isoform-specific toxicity of Mecp2 in postmitotic neurons: suppression of neurotoxicity by FoxG1. Journal of Neuroscience 2012;32(8): 2846-55.

[81] Lewis JD, Meehan RR, Henzel WJ, Maurer-Fogy I, Jeppesen P, Klein F, et al. Purification, sequence, and cellular localization of a novel chromosomal protein that binds to methylated DNA. Cell 1992;69(6): 905-14.

[82] Nan X, Meehan RR, Bird A. Dissection of the methyl-CpG binding domain from the chromosomal protein MeCP2. Nucleic Acids Research 1993;21(21): 4886-92.

[83] Klose RJ, Sarraf SA, Schmiedeberg L, McDermott SM, Stancheva I, Bird AP. DNA binding selectivity of MeCP2 due to a requirement for A/T sequences adjacent to methyl-CpG. Molecular Cell 2005;19(5): 667-78.

[84] Galvao TC, Thomas JO. Structure-specific binding of MeCP2 to four-way junction DNA through its methyl CpG-binding domain. Nucleic Acids Research 2005;33(20): 6603-9.

[85] Nan X, Tate P, Li E, Bird A. DNA methylation specifies chromosomal localization of MeCP2. Molecular and Cellular Biology 1996;16(1): 414-21.

[86] Chandler SP, Guschin D, Landsberger N, Wolffe AP. The methyl-CpG binding transcriptional repressor MeCP2 stably associates with nucleosomal DNA. Biochemistry 1999;38(22): 7008-18.

[87] Yusufzai TM, Wolffe AP. Functional consequences of Rett syndrome mutations on human MeCP2. Nucleic Acids Research 2000;28(21): 4172-9.

[88] Buschdorf JP, Stratling WH. A WW domain binding region in methyl-CpG-binding protein MeCP2: impact on Rett syndrome. Journal of Molecular Medicine 2004;82(2): 135-43.

[89] Nan X, Campoy FJ, Bird A. MeCP2 is a transcriptional repressor with abundant binding sites in genomic chromatin. Cell 1997;88(4): 471-81.

[90] Jones PL, Veenstra GJ, Wade PA, Vermaak D, Kass SU, Landsberger N, et al. Methylated DNA and MeCP2 recruit histone deacetylase to repress transcription. Nature Genetics 1998;19(2): 187-91.

[91] Nan X, Ng HH, Johnson CA, Laherty CD, Turner BM, Eisenman RN, et al. Transcriptional repression by the methyl-CpG-binding protein MeCP2 involves a histone deacetylase complex. Nature 1998;393(6683): 386-9.

[92] Kokura K, Kaul SC, Wadhwa R, Nomura T, Khan MM, Shinagawa T, et al. The Ski protein family is required for MeCP2-mediated transcriptional repression. The Journal of Biological Chemistry 2001;276(36): 34115-21.

[93] Nikitina T, Shi X, Ghosh RP, Horowitz-Scherer RA, Hansen JC, Woodcock CL. Multiple modes of interaction between the methylated DNA binding protein MeCP2 and chromatin. Molecular and Cellular Biology 2007;27(3): 864-77.

[94] Kaludov NK, Wolffe AP. MeCP2 driven transcriptional repression in vitro: selectivity for methylated DNA, action at a distance and contacts with the basal transcription machinery. Nucleic Acids Research 2000;28(9): 1921-8.

[95] Harikrishnan KN, Chow MZ, Baker EK, Pal S, Bassal S, Brasacchio D, et al. Brahma links the SWI/SNF chromatin-remodeling complex with MeCP2-dependent transcriptional silencing. Nature Genetics 2005;37(3): 254-64.

[96] Kimura H, Shiota K. Methyl-CpG-binding protein, MeCP2, is a target molecule for maintenance DNA methyltransferase, Dnmt1. The Journal of Biological Chemistry 2003;278(7): 4806-12.

[97] Nan X, Hou J, Maclean A, Nasir J, Lafuente MJ, Shu X, et al. Interaction between chromatin proteins MECP2 and ATRX is disrupted by mutations that cause inherited mental retardation. Proceedings of the National Academy of Sciences of the United States of America 2007;104(8): 2709-14.

[98] Tudor M, Akbarian S, Chen RZ, Jaenisch R. Transcriptional profiling of a mouse model for Rett syndrome reveals subtle transcriptional changes in the brain. Proceedings of the National Academy of Sciences of the United States of America 2002;99(24): 15536-41.

[99] Traynor J, Agarwal P, Lazzeroni L, Francke U. Gene expression patterns vary in clonal cell cultures from Rett syndrome females with eight different MECP2 mutations. BMC Medical Genetics 2002;3: 12.

[100] Colantuoni C, Jeon OH, Hyder K, Chenchik A, Khimani AH, Narayanan V, et al. Gene expression profiling in postmortem Rett Syndrome brain: differential gene expression and patient classification. Neurobiology of Disease 2001;8(5): 847-65.

[101] Ballestar E, Ropero S, Alaminos M, Armstrong J, Setien F, Agrelo R, et al. The impact of MECP2 mutations in the expression patterns of Rett syndrome patients. Human Genetics 2005;116(1-2): 91-104.

[102] Jordan C, Li HH, Kwan HC, Francke U. Cerebellar gene expression profiles of mouse models for Rett syndrome reveal novel MeCP2 targets. BMC Medical Genetics 2007;8: 36.

[103] Muotri AR, Marchetto MC, Coufal NG, Oefner R, Yeo G, Nakashima K, et al. L1 retrotransposition in neurons is modulated by MeCP2. Nature 2010;468(7322): 443-6.

[104] Skene PJ, Illingworth RS, Webb S, Kerr AR, James KD, Turner DJ, et al. Neuronal MeCP2 is expressed at near histone-octamer levels and globally alters the chromatin state. Molecular Cell 2010;37(4): 457-68.

[105] Yasui DH, Peddada S, Bieda MC, Vallero RO, Hogart A, Nagarajan RP, et al. Integrated epigenomic analyses of neuronal MeCP2 reveal a role for long-range interaction with active genes. Proceedings of the National Academy Sciences of the United States of America 2007;104(49): 19416-21.

[106] Chahrour M, Jung SY, Shaw C, Zhou X, Wong ST, Qin J, et al. MeCP2, a key contributor to neurological disease, activates and represses transcription. Science 2008;320(5880): 1224-9.

[107] Hite KC, Adams VH, Hansen JC. Recent advances in MeCP2 structure and function. Biochemistry and Cell Biology 2009;87(1): 219-27.

[108] Georgel PT, Horowitz-Scherer RA, Adkins N, Woodcock CL, Wade PA, Hansen JC. Chromatin compaction by human MeCP2. Assembly of novel secondary chromatin structures in the absence of DNA methylation. The Journal of Biological Chemistry 2003;278(34): 32181-8.

[109] Nikitina T, Ghosh RP, Horowitz-Scherer RA, Hansen JC, Grigoryev SA, Woodcock CL. MeCP2-chromatin interactions include the formation of chromatosome-like structures and are altered in mutations causing Rett syndrome. The Journal of Biological Chemistry 2007;282(38): 28237-45.

[110] Young JI, Hong EP, Castle JC, Crespo-Barreto J, Bowman AB, Rose MF, et al. Regulation of RNA splicing by the methylation-dependent transcriptional repressor methyl-CpG binding protein 2. Proceeding of the National Academy of Sciences of the United States of America 2005;102(49): 17551-8.

[111] Zachariah RM, Rastegar M. Linking epigenetics to human disease and Rett syndrome: the emerging novel and challenging concepts in MeCP2 research. Neural Plasticity 2012;2012: 415825.

[112] Gibson JH, Slobedman B, K NH, Williamson SL, Minchenko D, El-Osta A, et al. Downstream targets of methyl CpG binding protein 2 and their abnormal expression in the frontal cortex of the human Rett syndrome brain. BMC Neuroscience 2010;11: 53.

[113] Martinowich K, Hattori D, Wu H, Fouse S, He F, Hu Y, et al. DNA methylation-related chromatin remodeling in activity-dependent BDNF gene regulation. Science 2003;302(5646): 890-3.

[114] Chen WG, Chang Q, Lin Y, Meissner A, West AE, Griffith EC, et al. Derepression of BDNF transcription involves calcium-dependent phosphorylation of MeCP2. Science 2003;302(5646): 885-9.

[115] Zhou Z, Hong EJ, Cohen S, Zhao WN, Ho HY, Schmidt L, et al. Brain-specific phosphorylation of MeCP2 regulates activity-dependent Bdnf transcription, dendritic growth, and spine maturation. Neuron 2006;52(2): 255-69.

[116] Horike S, Cai S, Miyano M, Cheng JF, Kohwi-Shigematsu T. Loss of silent-chromatin looping and impaired imprinting of DLX5 in Rett syndrome. Nature Genetics 2005;37(1): 31-40.

[117] Miyano M, Horike S, Cai S, Oshimura M, Kohwi-Shigematsu T. DLX5 expression is monoallelic and Dlx5 is up-regulated in the Mecp2-null frontal cortex. Journal of Cellular and Molecular Medicine 2008;12(4): 1188-91.

[118] Samaco RC, Hogart A, LaSalle JM. Epigenetic overlap in autism-spectrum neurodevelopmental disorders: MECP2 deficiency causes reduced expression of UBE3A and GABRB3. Human Molecular Genetics 2005;14(4): 483-92.

[119] Miyake K, Hirasawa T, Soutome M, Itoh M, Goto Y, Endoh K, et al. The protocadherins, PCDHB1 and PCDH7, are regulated by MeCP2 in neuronal cells and brain tissues: implication for pathogenesis of Rett syndrome. BMC Neuroscience 2011;12: 81.

[120] Nuber UA, Kriaucionis S, Roloff TC, Guy J, Selfridge J, Steinhoff C, et al. Up-regulation of glucocorticoid-regulated genes in a mouse model of Rett syndrome. Human Molecular Genetics 2005;14(15): 2247-56.

[121] Huppke P, Gartner J. Molecular diagnosis of Rett syndrome. Journal of Child Neurology 2005;20(9): 732-6.

[122] Peddada S, Yasui DH, LaSalle JM. Inhibitors of differentiation (ID1, ID2, ID3 and ID4) genes are neuronal targets of MeCP2 that are elevated in Rett syndrome. Human Molecular Genetics 2006;15(12): 2003-14.

[123] Deng V, Matagne V, Banine F, Frerking M, Ohliger P, Budden S, et al. FXYD1 is an MeCP2 target gene overexpressed in the brains of Rett syndrome patients and Mecp2-null mice. Human Molecular Genetics 2007;16(6): 640-50.

[124] Itoh M, Ide S, Takashima S, Kudo S, Nomura Y, Segawa M, et al. Methyl CpG-binding protein 2 (a mutation of which causes Rett syndrome) directly regulates insulin-like growth factor binding protein 3 in mouse and human brains. Journal of Neuropathology & Experimental Neurology 2007;66(2): 117-23.

[125] McGill BE, Bundle SF, Yaylaoglu MB, Carson JP, Thaller C, Zoghbi HY. Enhanced anxiety and stress-induced corticosterone release are associated with increased Crh

expression in a mouse model of Rett syndrome. Proceedings of the National Academy of Sciences of the United States of America 2006;103(48): 18267-72.

[126] Ballestar E, Yusufzai TM, Wolffe AP. Effects of Rett syndrome mutations of the methyl-CpG binding domain of the transcriptional repressor MeCP2 on selectivity for association with methylated DNA. Biochemistry 2000;39(24): 7100-6.

[127] Kudo S, Nomura Y, Segawa M, Fujita N, Nakao M, Hammer S, et al. Functional characterisation of MeCP2 mutations found in male patients with X linked mental retardation. Journal of Medical Genetics 2002;39(2): 132-6.

[128] Bebbington A, Anderson A, Ravine D, Fyfe S, Pineda M, de Klerk N, et al. Investigating genotype-phenotype relationships in Rett syndrome using an international data set. Neurology 2008;70(11): 868-75.

[129] Neul JL, Fang P, Barrish J, Lane J, Caeg EB, Smith EO, et al. Specific mutations in methyl-CpG-binding protein 2 confer different severity in Rett syndrome. Neurology 2008;70(16): 1313-21.

[130] Halbach NS, Smeets EE, van den Braak N, van Roozendaal KE, Blok RM, Schrander-Stumpel CT, et al. Genotype-phenotype relationships as prognosticators in Rett syndrome should be handled with care in clinical practice. American Journal of Medical Genetics Part A 2012;158A(2): 340-50.

[131] Young D, Bebbington A, de Klerk N, Bower C, Nagarajan L, Leonard H. The relationship between MECP2 mutation type and health status and service use trajectories over time in a Rett syndrome population. Research in Autism Spectrum Disorders 2011;5(1): 442-9.

[132] Bebbington A, Percy A, Christodoulou J, Ravine D, Ho G, Jacoby P, et al. Updating the profile of C-terminal MECP2 deletions in Rett syndrome. Journal of Medical Genetics 2010;47(4): 242-8.

[133] Renieri A, Mari F, Mencarelli MA, Scala E, Ariani F, Longo I, et al. Diagnostic criteria for the Zappella variant of Rett syndrome (the preserved speech variant). Brain and Development 2009;31(3): 208-16.

[134] Scala E, Longo I, Ottimo F, Speciale C, Sampieri K, Katzaki E, et al. MECP2 deletions and genotype-phenotype correlation in Rett syndrome. American Journal of Medical Genetics Part A 2007;143A(23): 2775-84.

[135] Hardwick SA, Reuter K, Williamson SL, Vasudevan V, Donald J, Slater K, et al. Delineation of large deletions of the MECP2 gene in Rett syndrome patients, including a familial case with a male proband. European Journal of Human Genetics 2007;15(12): 1218-29.

[136] Amir RE, Van den Veyver IB, Schultz R, Malicki DM, Tran CQ, Dahle EJ, et al. Influence of mutation type and X chromosome inactivation on Rett syndrome phenotypes. Annals of Neurology 2000;47(5): 670-9.

[137] Huppke P, Maier EM, Warnke A, Brendel C, Laccone F, Gartner J. Very mild cases of Rett syndrome with skewed X inactivation. Journal of Medical Genetics 2006;43(10): 814-6.

[138] Villard L, Levy N, Xiang F, Kpebe A, Labelle V, Chevillard C, et al. Segregation of a totally skewed pattern of X chromosome inactivation in four familial cases of Rett syndrome without MECP2 mutation: implications for the disease. Journal of Medical Genetics 2001;38(7): 435-42.

[139] Takahashi S, Ohinata J, Makita Y, Suzuki N, Araki A, Sasaki A, et al. Skewed X chromosome inactivation failed to explain the normal phenotype of a carrier female with MECP2 mutation resulting in Rett syndrome. Clinical Genetics 2008;73(3): 257-61.

[140] Archer H, Evans J, Leonard H, Colvin L, Ravine D, Christodoulou J, et al. Correlation between clinical severity in patients with Rett syndrome with a p.R168X or p.T158M MECP2 mutation, and the direction and degree of skewing of X-chromosome inactivation. Journal of Medical Genetics 2007;44(2): 148-52.

[141] Xinhua B, Shengling J, Fuying S, Hong P, Meirong L, Wu XR. X chromosome inactivation in Rett Syndrome and its correlations with MECP2 mutations and phenotype. Journal of Child Neurology 2008;23(1): 22-5.

[142] Zeev BB, Bebbington A, Ho G, Leonard H, de Klerk N, Gak E, et al. The common BDNF polymorphism may be a modifier of disease severity in Rett syndrome. Neurology 2009;72(14): 1242-7.

[143] Nectoux J, Bahi-Buisson N, Guellec I, Coste J, De Roux N, Rosas H, et al. The p.Val66Met polymorphism in the BDNF gene protects against early seizures in Rett syndrome. Neurology 2008;70(22 Pt 2): 2145-51.

[144] Zahorakova D, Jachymova M, Kemlink D, Baxova A, Martasek P. APOE epsilon4: a potential modulation factor in Rett syndrome. Journal of Child Neurology 2010;25(5): 546-50.

[145] Guy J, Gan J, Selfridge J, Cobb S, Bird A. Reversal of neurological defects in a mouse model of Rett syndrome. Science 2007;315(5815): 1143-7.

[146] Giacometti E, Luikenhuis S, Beard C, Jaenisch R. Partial rescue of MeCP2 deficiency by postnatal activation of MeCP2. Proceedings of the National Academy of Sciences of the United States of America 2007;104(6): 1931-6.

[147] Ellaway CJ, Sholler G, Leonard H, Christodoulou J. Prolonged QT interval in Rett syndrome. Archives of Disease in Childhood 1999;80(5): 470-2.